AF696198

Contents

Preface

ALS, also known as Lou Gehrig's Disease, is the most common of the motor neuron diseases that cause muscle atrophy. ALS is a chronic, progressively debilitating disease characterized by progressive muscle atrophy starting in the limbs and spreading to the rest of the body, often accompanied by overactive reflexes. It usually manifests itself after the age of 40. The exact cause of ALS is unknown and there is no cure at this time. ALS may be fatal in one year or continue for 10 or more years. This new book includes leading edge research from around the world and covers the etiology, pathogenesis, symptoms, diagnosis, and treatment of amyotrophic lateral sclerosis (ALS).

As reported in chapter I, Amyotrophic lateral sclerosis (ALS), a fatal disorder primarily affecting motor neurons, is characterized by a combination of upper and lower motor neuron signs with progression. Approximately 10% of the ALS patients suffer from a familial form (FALS). Contrary to sporadic ALS (SALS), the onset of FALS is, on the average, 10 years earlier than that of SALS and the female:male ratio is 1:1. Otherwise, FALS phenotypes do not markedly differ from SALS. The etiology of FALS is quite heterogeneous. So far, mutations were detected in a gene on chromosome 21q21, encoding for superoxid-dismutase 1 (SOD1), in a gene on chromosome 2q32-34, encoding for alsin, and in a gene on chromosome 17q21-22 encoding for the tau-protein. SOD1 functions as anti-oxidant and alsin as a putative GTPase regulator. The function of the tau-protein is yet unknown. More than 100 SOD1 mutations and seven alsin mutations associated with a FALS phenotype have been reported. Phenotypes of the various SOD1 mutations differ with regard to disease onset, severity and prognosis. In addition to the SOD1, alsin and tau genes, genome-wide linkage-analysis detected 7 further loci associated with FALS. They were localized to chromosomes 18q21, 9q34, 15q5-q21, 9q21-22, 16q12, 20, and Xp11-q12 respectively. The pathogenesis of SOD1 mutations is actually explained by: the oligomerization hypothesis, according to which mutated SOD1 protein is misfolded and consecutively oligomerized into high-molecular-weight aggregates, manifesting as axonal inclusions. Aggregates impair axonal transport, protein degradation and apoptosis; The oxidative damage hypothesis according to which mutant SOD1 catalyses oxidative reactions, which damage substrates critical for the viability of motor neurons. The role of neurofilaments, glutamate, copper, mitochondria and apoptosis, autoimmunity, growth factors, infections, and environmental factors in the pathogenesis and expression of FALS is under debate. To diagnose FALS an extensive family history and thorough clinical and electrophysiological investigations of all family members are required. As for SALS only symptomatic and supportive therapy is available for FALS.

In chapter II, Amyotrophic Lateral Sclerosis (ALS) is a neurodegenerative disease causing progressive death of the motor neurons in both brain cortex and spinal cord. Twenty per cent of ALS familial cases (fALS) are caused by a mutation in the SOD1 gene. The SOD1 gene is located in the short arm of human chromosome 21 and consists of 5 exons encoding for 153 amino acids. More than 100 mutations have been identified that are spred in all parts of the SOD1 gene; the majority of them are missense mutations but there are both insertions and deletions. Two mutations, in 126 and 141 codons, define a signal stop that produces a shorter protein. Mutations have been found also in intronic parts of the gene in two ALS cases. All mutations behave as autosomal dominant traits except for the D90A and the L84F, that exist in both dominant and recessive forms. Attempts to correlate genotype with phenotype demonstrated that prediction of disease severity based on age of onset and disease duration on the basis of the single SOD1 mutation remains uncertain. Some mutations are associated with early onset (L38V, G37S), while others are associated with particularly short (A4V) or relatively long (D100G) disease duration. Mutations in SOD1 gene were also found in ALS patients with no family history. Subjects with SOD1 mutations (L84F, L144F and D76V) that did not develop the disease were reported. Epidemiological data underline that, in some cases, a mutation is present only in a single population: A4T mutation in the Japanese population , D76V in the hispanic one, the L144F mutation in several patients coming from Slavic regions (Yugoslavia, Croatia). Correlation between sex, regional disease onset, age of onset and SOD1 gene mutations have not been found. SOD1 mutations have been divided in three groups considering the three-dimensional structure of the wt protein. One group of mutations occurs within the dimer interface (A4V), while another group is positioned in loop regions at the end of beta strands (G93A). Mutant proteins falling into these two groups appear to have full SOD1 activity and biophysical properties similar to the wt SOD1 protein. The third group of mutations is located near the metal binding site, in particular the protein region that binds copper ion. These mutant proteins (H46R, H48Q) carry little amount of copper or zinc and have biophysical properties quite different from the wt SOD1 protein. In fALS carrying a SOD1 mutation the mutated protein is the cause for the development of ALS. In fALS various mutated SOD1 proteins show unaltered enzymatic activity, thus suggesting that the mutations in SOD1 gene may act causing a toxic "gain of function" in SOD1 rather than a loss of function. In fALS SOD1 accumulates within the cytoplasm of the motor neurons. Similarly in sporadic ALS, intracellular aggregates in motor neurons have been found, possibly containing SOD1. As ALS, several other neurodegenerative disorders, like Alzheimer's disease, Parkinson's disease and prion diseases, are characterized by the accumulation of specific proteins in the brain areas in which neuronal loss occurs. The majority of neurodegenerative disorders have both familial and sporadic presentation and the gene involved in the familial form encodes for the protein that accumulates in both familial and sporadic form. Moreover, the mutated proteins may function normally, but tend to accumulate in a conformation that hampers degradation (amyloid). While the specific features of each disorder is related to the affected neuronal population and to the protein involved, the common aspect relies in the mechanisms of cell death. In fact, many experimental data demonstrate that in neurodegenerative disorders a common apoptotic mechanism causes the neuronal death through the activation of different factors (such as cdk5, Apaf-1 and JNK) belonging to the same pathway. The authors think that the neuronal cell peculiar condition of being unable to replicate is of fundamental importance in understanding neurodegeneration. In the CNS the condition of permanent neuronal cells throughout the individual life span exists only by the strict interaction between neurons and glial cells. In ALS peripheral blood cells express mutated SOD1 and display alterations in mitochondrial metabolism and calcium homeostasis, but they show no degeneration. In their hypothesis neurodegenerative diseases are the expression of a general difficulty in degradation of misfolded proteins that are toxic to the cell. Whereas replicating tissues can resolve such problem by replacing itscellular components, nervous tissue can not. This is the reason why only neurons contain the aggregated protein. This could also explain why neurodegeneration and aging are so closely related.

As reported in chapter III, the current gap between hypothesized pathogenic mechanisms and efficacy of therapeutics in patients affected by amyotrophic lateral sclerosis (ALS) constitutes a major problem, whose solution represents a serious commitment for researchers. ALS pathogenesis can be viewed as the consequence of a complex neurodegenerative process involving neuron-glia interactions. Excitotoxicity, oxidative stress, mitochondrial dysfunction and apoptosis are all putative mechanisms which seem to operate in ALS and might be amenable of pharmacological intervention. Disturbances of glutamatergic transmission are a well-established feature of ALS, documented by increased glutamate levels in cerebrospinal fluid, reduced glutamate transport and downregulation of the excitatory amino acid transporter EAAT2 in the affected areas. Glutamate toxicity in motor neurons is thought to be principally mediated by the GluR2-defective, calcium-permeable AMPA receptors. Moreover, after the demonstration that mutations in the copper/zinc superoxide dismutase (SOD1) gene are associated with familial ALS, oxidative damage was shown in samples from ALS patients. The recent finding that a substantial amount of SOD1 is localized in the mitochondrial intermembrane space has provided a new rationale for the mitochondrial damage occurring in ALS, which is now regarded as an important step in the pathogenesis of the disease. Interestingly, the excitotoxic and oxidative stress theories of ALS are not mutually exclusive and several experimental evidences suggest the existence of a deep interplay between oxidative stress and excitotoxicity. Free radical-mediated damage could sensitize neurons to glutamate-mediated excitotoxic mechanisms and, conversely, the increase in intracellular calcium concentrations that accompanies excitotoxicity can increase free radical production. Assessing the role of excitotoxicity in each single patient may provide useful indications as far as prognosis and response to therapy. In fact, molecular and biochemical markers of glutamatergic transmission can be easily assessed in peripheral tissues, such as platelets and fibroblasts, which physiologically express the three major glutamate transporters. In conclusion, considering this crosstalk between excitotoxicity and oxidative stress, it is conceivable that combination therapies or drugs with multiple mechanisms of actions are likely to be the only way forward for ALS therapeutics.

In chapter IV, accumulating evidence indicates that alterations of the mithochondrial pool in motor neurons are implicated in the pathogenesis of Amyotrophic Lateral Sclerosis (ALS) and therefore mitochondrial damage has become an important area of the investigation in the causes of this pathology. Ultrastructural investigations have shown that morphological abnormalities of mitochondria in spinal motor neurons are a very early sign in the disease progression in murine models of familial ALS represented by transgenic mice carrying a mutated form of the gene coding for human Cu, Zn superoxide dismutase (SOD1). In particular, in a transgenic line of mice expressing human SOD1 with a glycine to alanine mutation in position 93 (Tg SOD1G93A mice) swollen mitochondria with dilated and disorganized cristae in spinal motor neurons as early as two weeks after birth, when the animals are completely asymptomatic have been detected. Similar mitochondrial abnormalities were detected also in motor neurons of the hypoglossal and trigeminal motor nuclei of young Tg SOD1G93A mice and do not seem to depend on the number of transgene copies expressed as they are present even in low expressor mice with a late onset of the pathology. The mechanisms that can lead to mitochondrial damage, which include excitotoxicity, oxidation of mitochondrial components and accumulation of protein aggregates are discussed in light of possible therapeutic interventions.

Chapter V focuses on, the majority of cases of amyotrophic lateral sclerosis (ALS) are sporadic (primary or idiopathic ALD), while about 5 to 10% are familial (familial ALS). In sporadic ALS, recent studies showed abnormalities of glutamate metabolism, which would be responsible for motor neuron degeneration via neuroexcitotoxic mechanisms. Part of the familial forms of ALS have been linked with mutations of Cu,Zn-superoxide dismutase (Cu,Zn-SOD), an enzyme which is involved in the defense against superoxide free radicals. It has been shown that these mutations lead to a gain of toxic function of the enzyme rather than a loss of activity. Expression of the mutant human Cu,Zn-SOD in transgenic mice causes motor neuron disease while expression of wild type human Cu,Zn-SOD does not. Various hypotheses on the toxicity of the mutant SOD have been proposed such as increased access of the substrate to the active site, leading to increased oxidation of the substrate; disruption of the active site of the enzyme, allowing access of peroxynitrite to copper and leading to increased nitration by peroxynitrite. Oxidative stress may also be related to impaired ability of mutant SOD to bind zinc. Moreover, glutamate excitotoxicity would be associated with increased oxidative stress, which could constitute a linkage between sporadic and familial forms of ALS. In relation with this mechanism, riluzole (2-amino-6-trifluoromethoxybenzothiazole) demonstrated a therapeutic activity in ALS patients. In chapter V, a study was conducted aiming to evaluate the blood oxidative stress status in a large population of 167 definite or probable ALS patients (without detected SOD mutation), with or without treatment with riluzole, in comparison with age- and sex-matched healthy control subjects. The data supported an imbalance of the oxidant/antioxidant systems in favor of an oxidative stress in ALS, in patients without treatment as well as in patients treated with riluzole, as compared with healthy age-matched controls. No correlation was found between the level of oxidative stress markers and the disease duration nor the riluzole treatment duration. Patients treated with riluzole exhibited an erythrocyte Cu,Zn-SOD activity intermediate between the elevated SOD activity of ALS patients without treatment and that of controls. This suggests a possible activity of the drug on the oxidative stress. Therapeutic trials using classical antioxidants alone, such as vitamin E, showed no effect on the survival and motor function in ALS. However, when using the ALS Health State scale, patients receiving riluzole plus alpha-tocopherol remained longer in a better condition and they showed changes in biochemical markers of oxidative stress. Additional studies are in course which could provide more information. These results suggest that oxidative processes may play a critical role in the pathogenic mechanisms of neurodegeneration in ALS and therapeutic interventions targeted against this mechanism appear promising.

In chapter VI, the excitability and potentials (intracellular and electrotonic) of human motor and sensory axons in amyotrophic lateral sclerosis (ALS) types (termed as ALS1, ALS2 and ALS3, respectively) can be reliably studied using double cable models of the fibres. The intracellular potentials can be then used as input to a line source model that allows the calculation of the corresponding spatial and temporal distributions of the extracellular potentials at various radial distances in the surrounding volume conductor. The potentials and indices of the axonal excitability delivered from single or pairs of threshold stimuli, such as strength-duration and charge-duration curves, strength-duration time constants, rheobasic currents and recovery cycles depend on the methods of fibre stimulation. Two cases of fibre stimulation are considered in the present investigations. The first case of point application of current intra-axonally at the center of the first node closely approximates the effects of point application of current extra-axonally at the node and realizes a point fibre polarization. The second case of simultaneous intracellular current application at the midpoints of all available internodal segments closely approximates the effects of external surface stimulation with a large electrode and realizes a periodic kind of uniform fibre polarization. Each of these investigations also depends on the electrophysiological cable characteristics of the axons. Together they can provide new information about the pathophysiology underlying abnormalities in the excitability and potentials of the human fibres in ALS. Simulated results indicate that the used models are rather promising tools in studying the prominent feature (fasciculation) of ALS which up till now has not been sufficiently well understood.

As reported in chapter VII, the characters of the degeneration of the white matter of the spinal cord of amyotrophic lateral sclerosis (ALS) were examined, and the origins of the degenerated fibers were discussed.

1. The degree of large myelinated fiber loss in the lateral corticospinal tract (l-CST) did not correlate with either the duration of their illness or their history of respirator use. Direct correlation of disease mechanism was absent between the anterior horn cells and the l-CST in classic ALS.

2. The patients who required respirator support showed more severe degeneration of the anterolateral funiculus (ALF) in the ALS than those who required none, and the degree of myelinated fiber loss in the l-CST did not correspond with either the illness duration or the history of respirator use. Thus the large myelinated fibers in the l-CST and ALF degenerate independently in classic ALS.

3. The large myelinated fibers in the ALF of the mid-cervical spinal cord of humans originate from the tegmentum of the brain stem and the lower cervical spinal cord, not from the cerebrum, or the thoracic or lumbar spinal cord. The origin of the large myelinated fibers in the ALF of the spinal cord in humans, is considered to be the long-descending neurons in the brain stem tegmentum and the propriospinal neurons in the spinal cord.

For maintenance and normal functionality, spinal motoneurons depend on a continuous retrograde neurotrophic supply of muscular factors, in particular neurotrophins. Therefore, disturbances in normal neurotrophin signaling are considered to contribute - either primary or secondary - to the pathogenesis of ALS. These disturbances may not only include abnormalities in the amount and pattern of muscular neurotrophin production but also alterations in the expression of the neurotrophin receptor repertory by the motoneurons and in particularly the appearance of the neurotrophin receptor $p75^{NTR}$, an alleged 'death receptor'.

In chapter VIII, post-mortem studies performed in the past years in our lab concerning the neurotrophin production in muscles of ALS patient and the expression of the $p75^{NTR}$ neurotrophin receptor by the spinal motoneurons was reported. Moreover, using a hSOD1 transgenic animal model that lacked the genetic information for the $p75^{NTR}$ receptor (hSOD1/$p75^{NTR-/-}$ mice) the significance of this receptor for the ALS pathogenesis process has been examined. The data suggests that the severe imbalances that were found in neurotrophin- and $p75^{NTR}$-levels are most likely not primary phenomena in the pathology of ALS. However, the gender related differences in clinical symptom gravity and disease endpoint that were observed in the hSOD1/$p75^{NTR-/-}$ mice indicate that this neurotrophin receptor is of importance for secondary pathogenic events contributing to ALS disease progress.

In chapter IX, a diagnosis of definite amyotrophic lateral sclerosis (ALS) requires the presence of motor neuron degeneration signs on at least three spinal levels or two spinal and bulbar levels. In the initial stage of the disease there is a group of patients in whom only limbs involvement is apparent. EMG studies of bulbar region muscles are of limited value. There is a need for development of new diagnostic tools facilitating the early detection of bulbar involvement in ALS patients. To evaluate the usefulness of acoustic speech analysis (ASA) and dysarthria profile tests (DPT) in the early detection of speech disturbances in ALS. The authors studied 56 sporadic, definite and probable ALS subjects. Te disease severity was scored on the Norris scale. The evidence of dysarthria was measured using two independent, quantitative and semiquantitative methods such as ASA, which is based on the sounds test and DPT including tests of the respiration, phonation, articulation, speech intelligibility, prosody, face movements, diadochokinesis and reflexes, respectively. Firstly, DPT and ASA were carried out in ALS subjects and 67 healthy age-matched controls. Secondly, limb and bulbar onset ALS subjects were compared separately in three consecutive examinations. The mean sound distances from the pattern of all the sounds measured by ASA were greater both in bulbar and limb onset ALS subjects as compared to the controls ($p<0.001$). The mean sound distances from the pattern for 4 out of 5 sounds measured were greater in the bulbar than in limb onset ALS patients: "W" ($p<0.001$), "I" ($p<0.05$), "O" ($p<0.05$), "B" ($p<0.05$). The mean score of DPT in the whole ALS group was significantly lower as compared to the controls ($p<0.001$). A comparison between bulbar and limb onset ALS subjects, as well as between the limb onset group and healthy controls revealed in each case the significant difference in the mean DPT score ($p<0.01$). The results obtained confirm the usefulness of ASA and DPT in the early detection of bulbar pathology in limb onset ALS patients.

In chapter X, There are currently only few techniques available to reliably assess the stages of swallowing dysfunction due to ALS, including mainly videofluoroscopy and different clinical scales which are based on symptomatology only. The occurrence of the oropharyngeal phases of swallowing in ALS patients has been well documented. The authors suggest that the oesophageal manometry (OM) can be useful in determining the degree of dysphagia even on the level of the oesophageal body. To evaluate the use of oesophageal manometry as the diagnostic procedure in amyotrophic lateral sclerosis' (ALS) patients with dysphagia. The study was carried out in 20 bulbar onset ALS patients with dysphagia, fulfilling WFN criteria (aged from 36 to 74 yr.) and 20 sex- and age matched healthy volunteers. The standard transnasal oesophageal manometry was performed in all subjects using a flexible catheter with the solid state transducers (Synectics, Sweden). The proximal part of oesophageal body was evaluated by locating the proximal transducer 3 cm below the distal border of the upper oesophageal sphincter (UOS). Five ml of water (wet swallows) and saliva (dry swallows) were given at 30-sec intervals. The comparison of mean oesophageal contractile amplitude, mean oesophageal contractile duration and mean oesophageal contractile velocity during the wet swallows between ALS and control subjects were: 99± 58 vs. 60±22mmHg ($p=0.009$), 3.91±1.4 vs. 2.7±0.7 sec ($p=0.001$), 4.6±1.8 vs. 2.8±0.4 cm/sec ($p<0.001$), respectively and during the dry swallows were: 96 ±59 vs. 44±25 mm Hg ($p<0.001$), 4.8±1.9 vs. 2.5±1.7 sec($p<0.001$), 5.4±2.0 vs. 3.9±0.5 cm/sec ($p=0.002$), respectively. The differences of the results of these parameters during wet vs. dry swallows in the studied groups were statistically significant only for the amplitude and the velocity in controls ($p<0.001$) but not in ALS subjects. The most remarkable result of the study is the evidence that all ALS patients with dysphagia showed significant abnormalities in all parameters measured by oesophageal manometry as compared to controls. Our study showed the presence of oesophageal dysmotility in all ALS patients with dysphagia, which had not been systematically studied before.

As reported in chapter XI, the coordination between grip and load force profiles in patients with ALS performing vertical point-to-point arm movements with a hand-held instrumented object has been analyzed. This task necessitates a complex temporal coupling of motor activity in the proximal arm and shoulder muscles responsible for transporting the object and in the fingers used to grasp it. In healthy subjects, the precise regulation of grasping forces is reflected in (a) modulation of the grip force profile in parallel with the movement-induced fluctuations in load and (b) scaling of grip force in such a way that grip force is only a small amount greater than load at all phases of the movement. The grip force control of ALS patients exhibits two major pathologies: (a) they apply inefficiently high grip forces against a hand-held object and (b) there is a desynchronisation of the temporo-spatial coupling between grip and load force profiles. Current rehabilitation concepts commonly focus on the measurement of maximum grip force to objectively evaluate the progress in rehabilitation. Based on the authors' theory that an overflow in grip force contributes significantly to the disability in patients with ALS, it seems fruitful to define the reduction of unnecessarily high finger forces as the preferential goal in hand motor rehabilitation. A potential treatment scheme these patients should include the measurement of grip force during natural unencumbered arm movements with a hand-held load. The finding of uneconomically high grip force should motivate an individual training program to decrease the amount of force overshoot, facilitating fine finger movements and prevent early fatigue of affected hand muscles.

In chapter XII, The satellites of a motor unit potentials (MUP), i.e. late components distinct from the main component but time - locked to it, is a phenomenon found in electromyography. Satellite potentials are observed in EMG investigations in almost all neuromuscular disorders and occasionally in healthy muscles. In amyotrophic lateral sclerosis (ALS) satellite potentials are observed less frequently and have different features than in the case of other neurogenic processes. The aim of this study was to analyse the parameters of satellite potentials and to model a possible pathomechanism underlying generation of satellites in ALS. Motor unit potentials with satellites were characterized by the mean number of satellites per one motor unit potential, mean amplitude and duration of the main MUP component, mean amplitude and duration of the satellites. These parameters were compared between satellites recorded in the controls, ALS and spinal muscle atrophy (SMA, typ III). The prevalence index of satellites in SMA was significantly higher than that in ALS. In both, ALS and SMA, the prevalence index was significantly higher than that in the controls. The mean amplitudes and the mean duration of MUPs with satellites were significantly higher in SMA than in ALS, whereas there was no significant difference in the duration of the main components. The mean number of satellites per one MUP, and the duration of satellites have larger values in SMA than those in ALS. A simulation study indicates that in ALS a satellite is more often a potential of a single fiber whereas in SMA - groups of muscle fibers of small diameters are the sources of satellites. The range of delay of satellites caused by slower neuromuscular transmission and conductivity in terminal axon sprouts have been estimated. The reduced number of satellites and muscle fibers contributing to a single satellite in ALS probably depend on a failure of the compensation process.

In chapter XIII, it has long been known that central nervous lesions of amyotrophic lateral sclerosis (ALS) may extend beyond the spinal cord and the brain stem to involve the cerebral hemisphere. However, roles of degenerative changes of cerebral hemisphere have been controversial. Although it is a case that ALS has both upper and lower motor neuron signs and upper motor neuron signs may be resulted from degeneration in the motor related cerebral, whether degenerative changes in cerebral hemisphere develop higher cognitive dysfunction is not clear. Recent advent of neuroimaging techniques enables us to investigate these cerebral involvements in vivo and to study correlation between results of neuroimage and cognitive dysfunction. Among them magnetic resonance spectroscopy (MRS) present us a useful information about on-going changes of metabolites in the brain of ALS. Metabolites in the brain of patients with ALS by using MRS have been investigated. In the authors' reports, it is described that the NA (*N*-acetylaspartate and *N*-acetylaspartylglutamate)/ Cr (creatine and phosphocreatine), ratio was reduced in the motor area and the frontal lobe in patients with ALS. And the NA/Cr ratio in the brain had significant correlations with clinical signs including cognitive functions. In addition to those studies, several attempts have been conducting this field of investigation. From reviewing those same studies and literally evidences, the authors believe that the reduced NA/Cr ratio was a marker of cortical neuronal loss and dysfunction in ALS. Here, MRS investigations to detect abnormalities in the CNS of ALS are introduced by the authors, mainly according with themselves, and the usefulness of MRS to detect and to evaluate pathologic process in the brain of ALS is discussed.

As reported in chapter XIV, molecular genetic and biochemical study of 73 patients with sporadic motor neuron disease (MND) with definite diagnosis according to the Revised El Escorial Criteria (1998) was conducted. According to the Norris classification (1993), 57 patients (78%) had amyotrophic lateral sclerosis (ALS) form of the disease, and among them 35 had cervical onset (47.9%), 5 had truncal onset (6.8%), 13 had lumbar onset (17.8%) and

4 had diffuse onset (5.5%) of the disease. The remaining 16 patients (22%) had progressive bulbar palsy (PBP). All patients were assessed by the Norris ALS Score (1974) each six months until death. Patients with slow, moderate and rapid progression lost <4.5, 5-10 and >10 degrees each 6 months respectively ($r = -0.96$, $p < 0.0001$) and comprised 40 (54.8%), 21 (28.7%) and 12 (16.5%), respectively. The search for mutations in CuZn-superoxide dismutase gene showed that 3 individuals (4.1%) were the carriers of mutations. One female aged 67 was homozygous for the D90A mutation, whereas another female aged 55 was heterozygous for this mutation. The last female aged 71 was heterozygous for the G12R mutation. All patients had lumbar onset of ALS. The D90A homozygous patient had very slow progression lasting 24 years, and the heterozygous one deteriorated rapidly. That corresponded to the original findings by P.M. Andersen, who first described D90A associated ALS cases. However, identical haplotypes within polymorphic markers on both 21st chromosomes of the D90A homozygous and well as of D90A heterozygous ALS patient (D21S263-1, D21S223(SOD-1)-3, D21S63-10, D21S262-4, D21S261-2) were found. No cases of ALS in association with D90A heterozygosity and this so-called Scandinavian haplotype have been reported before. This was the first case when D90A heterozygosity was detected in an individual with ALS who has the "protective" Scandinavian haplotype shown to be typical only for the autosomal-recessive D90A carriers. The D90A heterozygous patient was thought to develop the disease due to ALS-causative factor other than D90A mutation with pathogenically strong action against the putative "protective" properties of the haplotype. The patient with G12R mutation had more rapid progression and elder age of onset than the Italian cohort of G12R ALS patients, although the same clinical phenotype. The study of alanine-9-valine (A9V) manganese-superoxide dismutase gene signal sequence polymorphism showed that there were no differences between frequencies of A9V alleles in patients and 50 neurologically normal controls from Moscow. The study of S/L-polymorphism of heavy neurofilament subunit gene (NEFH) showed that the homozygosity for short (S) allele had higher frequency in the MND group than in 45 neurologically normal controls (33.9% vs 6.7%, $\chi^2 = 10.37$, $p < 0.005$). Patients with different variants of S/L-polymorphism showed no difference in age or site of onset. A statistically significant correlation was established between the loss of total clinical score and the NEFH genotypes (Spearman correlation, $R = 0.335$, $p < 0.03$). The lowest values of loss of total clinical score were observed in patients with the LL genotype (mean ± SD, 18.8 ± 12.4), and the highest ones in patients with the SS genotype (mean ± SD, 31.1 ± 16.3). The dissimilarity in mean values of loss of total clinical score in the patients with LL and SS genotypes was statistically significant (Newman–Keuls test $q = 3.671$, $p < 0.05$). The activities of CuZn-superoxide dismutase in erythrocytes measured by Beauchamp and Fridovich (1971) of MND patients did not differ from those in control group, but was higher in S allele carriers vs LL genotype carriers (^730 vs ^677 U/g Hb; px2 < 0.05). Also, the content of thiobarbituric acid substances (TBARS) in cerebrospinal fluid measured by Ohkawa and Heikkila (1979) was higher in the SS genotype carriers vs controls (^0.425 vs ^0.307 nmol/ml, $p < 0.05$). These findings suggested that the SS genotype of the NEFH gene in the Russian population is a predisposition factor for both sporadic MND and oxidative stress possibly mediated by abnormal pro-oxidative interaction between short NEFH and CuZn-SOD.

In: Amyotrophic Lateral Sclerosis: New Research
Editor: Christine A. Murray, pp. 1-47
ISBN 1-59454-179-5

Chapter I

Familial Amyotrophic Lateral Sclerosis

Josef Finsterer [*]
Neurological Department, Krankenanstalt Rudolfstiftung,
Vienna, Austria

ABSTRACT

Amyotrophic lateral sclerosis (ALS), a fatal disorder primarily affecting motor neurons, is characterized by a combination of upper and lower motor neuron signs with progression. Approximately 10% of the ALS patients suffer from a familial form (FALS). Contrary to sporadic ALS (SALS), the onset of FALS is, on the average, 10 years earlier than that of SALS and the female:male ratio is 1:1. Otherwise, FALS phenotypes do not markedly differ from SALS. The etiology of FALS is quite heterogeneous. So far, mutations were detected in a gene on chromosome 21q21, encoding for superoxid-dismutase 1 (SOD1), in a gene on chromosome 2q32-34, encoding for alsin, and in a gene on chromosome 17q21-22 encoding for the tau-protein. SOD1 functions as anti-oxidant and alsin as a putative GTPase regulator. The function of the tau-protein is yet unknown. More than 100 SOD1 mutations and seven alsin mutations associated with a FALS phenotype have been reported. Phenotypes of the various SOD1 mutations differ with regard to disease onset, severity and prognosis. In addition to the SOD1, alsin and tau genes, genome-wide linkage-analysis detected 7 further loci associated with FALS. They were localized to chromosomes 18q21, 9q34, 15q5-q21, 9q21-22, 16q12, 20, and Xp11-q12 respectively. The pathogenesis of SOD1 mutations is actually explained by: the oligomerization hypothesis, according to which mutated SOD1 protein is misfolded and consecutively oligomerized into high-molecular-weight aggregates, manifesting as axonal inclusions. Aggregates impair axonal transport, protein degradation and apoptosis; the oxidative damage hypothesis according to which mutant SOD1 catalyses oxidative reactions, which damage substrates critical for the viability of motor neurons. The role of neurofilaments, glutamate, copper, mitochondria

[*] Correspondence concerning this article should be addressed to Dr. J. Finsterer, Schindlergasse 9/10, 1180 Vienna, Austria, Europe; Tel. and Fax. +43-1-4781711; E-mail: duarte@aonmail.at.

and apoptosis, autoimmunity, growth factors, infections, and environmental factors in the pathogenesis and expression of FALS is under debate. To diagnose FALS an extensive family history and thorough clinical and electrophysiological investigations of all family members are required. As for SALS only symptomatic and supportive therapy is available for FALS.

Keywords: hereditary disease, mutations, motor neuron, genetics, amyotrophic lateral sclerosis.

Abbreviations

AGE	advanced glycation end products
ALS	amyotrophic lateral sclerosis
AMPA	α-amino-3-hydroxy-5-methyl-n-isoxazol-proprionacid
APEX	apurinic/apurimidinic exonuclease
Bcl-2	B-cell lymphoma 2 (apoptosis related molecule)
BDNF	brain derived neurotrophic factor
BMAA	β-methyl-amino-L-alanine (cycad))
BOAA	beta-N-oxalyl amino-L-alanine
CCS	chaperone for SOD1
Cdk5	cyclo-dependent kinase 5
CNS	central nervous system
CTGF	connective tissue growth factor
DNA	desoxy-ribonucleic acid
EAAT 1and 2	excitatory amino-acid carrier 1 and 2 (glutamate transporters)
FALS	familial amyotrophic lateral sclerosis
Fas	death receptor-mediated signaling pathway
GLAST	rat glial glutamate and aspartate transporter
GLT1	rat glial glutamate transporter 1
GTP	guanine trinucleotide
HNE	4-hydroxynonenal
H_2O_2	hydrogen-peroxide
ICE	interleukin-1β-converting enzyme
JNK/SAPK	c-Jun N-terminal kinase/ stress activated protein kinase
KSP	Lysine-serine-proline repeat
LSP	lysine-serin-proline
MORN	membrane occupation and recognition motif
MRI	magnetic resonance imaging
MtDNA	mitochondrial DNA
NMDA	N-methyl-D-aspartate (ionotropic glutamate receptor)
NF	neurofilament
NFH	neurofilament heavy chain
NFL	neurofilament light chain

NFM	neurofilament medium chain
NO	nitrogen-oxide
NOS	nitric oxide synthetase
ODAP	β-N-oxalyl-L-α,β-diamino-proprionate
O_2^-	superoxide anion
OH^-	hydroxyl radical
$ONOO^-$	peroxynitrite
Par-4	prostate apoptosis response-4
PNS	peripheral nervous system
Rab5	small GTPase that controls endocytosis and early endosome dynamics
RLD	regulation of chromosome condensation (RCC1)-like domain
RNA	ribonucleic acid
ROS	reactive oxygen species
SALS	sporadic amyotrophic lateral sclerosis
SOD1	superoxide dismutase 1
TMS	transcranial magnetic stimulation
VPS9	vacuolar protein sorting 9

Introduction

Amyotrophic lateral sclerosis (ALS), also known as motor neuron disease, Lou Gehring's disease or Charcot's disease, is a disorder of the adult, characterized by degeneration predominantly of the upper and lower motor neuron, but also by degeneration of sensory, extrapyramidal and autonomic fibers and tracts [1,2,3]. Epidemiologically, ALS can be classified into sporadic, familial and endemic forms. Clinically, ALS manifests as initially asymmetric, rapidly progressive weakness, wasting of the limb and bulbar muscles and lastly death due to muscular respiratory insufficiency, mostly 3-5 years after onset of the clinical manifestations. In approximately 10% of the cases the family history is positive for the disease (familial ALS (FALS)), whereas the other 90% occur sporadically (SALS) [3,4]. Clinical and pathological characteristics of FALS and SALS are almost identical. FALS is genetically heterogeneous (FALS1-10), caused by mutations in genes encoding for the superoxid-dismutase-1 (SOD1), alsin, or the tau-protein, but there are indications that the genetic heterogeneity is even broader, suspecting various other genes to cause FALS [2,5,6]. SOD1 mutations result in the aggregation of mutant SOD1 protein and in the oxidation of essential cell proteins. The pathogenic role of factors likes neurofilaments (NFs), which are classified as heavy (NFH), medium (NFM), and light (NFL) NFs, glutamate, copper, mitochondrial damage and apoptosis, autoimmune-mechanisms, growth factors, infections and environmental factors is under debate. Aim of this review is to summarize recent findings, which further elucidate the pathogenic background of FALS.

Historical Remarks

The concept that ALS can be inherited dates to the earliest description of the disease. Among the 11 ALS patients reported by Aran in 1850, one obviously had FALS [7]. None of the ALS patients reported by Duchenne in 1860 or Charcot in 1869 had FALS. Among 13 adult ALS patients, Osler et al. in 1880 observed progressive muscular atrophy in 2 generations (Farr family) [7]. Vulpian in 1886 noted an ALS variant with predominant affection of the upper limbs, suggesting FALS [8]. In 1951 Brown and Whetherbee reported additional cases from the Farr family. In 1955 Mulder et al. reported six new FALS pedigrees [7]. In 1982 it has been shown that FALS can be inherited as a Mendelian dominant or recessive trait. In 1991 the first ALS gene (FALS1) was mapped to chromosome 21q22.1 [9]. In 1993 the SOD1 gene was identified to cause FALS1 [10]. In 2001 the alsin gene was identified to cause FALS2 [11,12,13].

Terminology

If there is predominant involvement of the upper motor neuron, the disorder is called primary lateral sclerosis. In case of predominant affection of the lower motor neuron, the disease is termed progressive muscular atrophy. In case of predominant affection of the bulbar muscles, the clinical picture is called progressive bulbar paralysis. For predominant affection of the limb muscles the term spinal ALS is used [3,5]. For severe weakness and wasting of the upper limbs without significant functional involvement of other regions the term "flail arm syndrome" was coined [14]. The "flail arm syndrome" is considered an ALS variant, showing striking male preponderance and a trend to prolonged survival [8].

Frequency

The incidence of ALS is 1-3/100000/year and increases with age. The prevalence of ALS is reported to amount 4-6/100000 and increases with age [5,6,15,16]. The prevalence of FALS with dementia is reported to be 2.8/100000 [17]. Local clusters have been reported among the Chamorros from the Mariana islands Guam, Saipan and Rota (7.5/100000/year) [18], the Kii peninsula in Japan (Hohara village) [19], the Miyakonojo basin in Japan (11.4/100000/year) [20], Oki island (Japan) [21], among the Auyu and Jakai of southern West Papua New Guinea (now Irian Jaya), in an isolated tribe at Anguru on Groote Eylandt in the Gulf of Carpentaria (North Australia), among the Amish community, in Guadeloupe, central Italy [22] and southern France [23]. Taking into account that on the average 10% of the ALS cases are FALS cases, the incidence of FALS is assumed to be 0.1-0.3/100000/year and the prevalence 0.4-0.6/100000. Altogether, the frequency of FALS between ALS cases ranges from 0.8 to 13.5% [brown=7]. Factors leading to misinterpretation of FALS as SALS are: low penetrance; retrospective design; inadequate recording of the family history; loss of contact between different branches of a family; reluctance to acknowledge ALS; early death of those who transmit the disease but do not develop it; misdiagnosis of ALS; and illegitimacy [7].

Gender Distribution

Before the age of 65 years the female:male ratio in SALS has been reported between 1:1.1, 1:1.2, 1:1.4, 1:1.7, 1:1.9 and 1:2.5 (mean: 1:1.7) in different population studies [7]. The sex ratio of FALS decreases after the age of 65 years until it approaches unity. The mean sex ratio in FALS is estimated to be 1:1 [5]. Overall, the female:male ratio is lower in SALS patients as compared to that of FALS.

Clinical Presentation

A) Symptoms

The disease course can be divided into a pre-paretic and a paretic phase. In the early, pre-paretic phase patients complain of a burning or aching pain in the lower back (lumbalgia, coxalgia), hips or knees (gonalgia), a sensation of unsteadiness, the feeling of restlessness, and clumsiness, stiffness, and occasionally cramps in the lower limb muscles [7]. Initial symptoms of the paretic phase frequently comprise unilateral weakness, hoarseness, dysarthria, dysphagia, head drop [24], chewing weakness, muscle cramps, or myocloni. In the later stages of the disease patients additionally complain about hypersomnia, dyspnea, frequent urinary urgency, and memory decline [25]. Intra-familial variation in site of onset is common in FALS pedigrees [7]. Within the same family, cases of progressive muscular atrophy, progressive bulbar paralysis, and primary lateral sclerosis can be found [7]. Urgency of micturition or difficulty in initiating urination has been found in more than two thirds of the FALS cases [7].

B) Signs

In relation to disease duration, and the amount of muscle impairment, clinical neurologic examination may reveal distal, initially frequently asymmetric weakness and wasting, fasciculations of the tongue, trunk and limb muscles, reduced, absent, normal or exaggerated deep tendon reflexes, upper motor neuron signs, reduced gag reflex, and exaggerated masseter reflex. In the late stages of the disease, eye movement abnormalities like limitation in horizontal and vertical gaze may develop [26]. Particularly patients maintained for years with assisted ventilation, often develop ophthalmoplegia. Supra-nuclear ophthalmoplegia, however, may also occur early in the evolution of the disease [27]. Contrary to SALS, upper motor neuron signs are rare or absent [2]. In 3-5% of the cases fronto-temporal dementia can be detected [28,29,30]. If patients undergo thorough neuropsychological investigation, frontal deficits can be found in up to 50% of the cases [4]. Language defects may be more common than hitherto appreciated and occasionally patients present with rapidly progressive aphasia. Extrapyramidal features, including tremor and rigidity, impaired postural reflexes and propulsion are sometimes present in FALS without dementia [8]. Nevertheless, differentiation between SALS and FALS patients on a clinical basis is difficult.

C) Laboratory Investigations

Creatine kinase may be elevated in the serum of FALS patients. In single patients also elevated GM1 and elevated GD2 antibody titers have been found [31]. In 22% of the FALS patients antibodies against the Fas-receptor are elevated [32]. However, activation of the peripheral immune system as reflected by anti-Fas antibodies is not specific for ALS [32]. Only in certain patients autoimmune mechanisms may participate in the development of ALS as related to anti-Fas antibodies [33]. In the cerebro-spinal fluid glutamate can be elevated. The vital capacity or sniff nasal capacity (more sensitive than the vital capacity) may be reduced, depending on the stage of the disease.

D) Electrophysiology

Electrophysiologic studies play an important role in the diagnostic evaluation of patients with suspected ALS [34]. Nerve conduction studies may reveal slowed nerve conduction and reduced amplitude of the compound muscle action potential, without indication of a conduction block [34]. Electromyography may reveal signs of acute or chronic denervation (fibrillations, positive sharp waves, fasciculations, complex repetitive discharges) and re-innervation, including giant motor unit action potentials [35,36]. Denervation and re-innervation may start already before evident clinical manifestations, particularly of bulbar muscles [37,38]. On transcranial magnetic stimulation (TMS) the central motor conduction time may be prolonged with normal amplitudes, mostly in patients carrying the D90A mutation or in the final stages of the disease [39]. TMS may reveal cortical hyperexcitability [40] and occult upper motor neuron affection [8]. TMS may also reveal reduction of the silent period and the absence of intra-cortical inhibition [8]. TMS can be also used to map area and volume of the motor cortex, which both get reduced over time [8]. Reduction of the motor cortex area or volume on TMS may be due to cortical or spinal hypoexcitability or due to loss of excitable neurons. Map parameters appear to be more sensitive for neuronal loss than other TMS parameters, like threshold, central motor conduction time, or potential amplitude [8]. Using peri-stimulus time histograms, it is possible to estimate the size of a unitary excitatory postsynaptic potential, which is typically desynchronized in ALS [35].

E) Imaging

Cerebral magnetic resonance imaging (MRI) occasionally shows wasting or hyperintensity of the pyramidal tract [41]. Diffusion tensor imaging shows significant increase in mean diffusivity and a reduction of fractional anisotropy in the corticospinal tract [41]. Single voxel proton magnetic resonance spectroscopy may show decreased V-acetylaspartate:creatine/phophocreatine ratio and elevated choline:phosphocreatine and inositol:phosphocreatine ratios in the motor cortex [42]. 18F-DOPA PET shows subclinical nigrostriatal dopaminergic dysfunction in some FALS patients [43]. Independent of the stage of the disease, the 133-Xenon washout-technique and tilting table investigations may demonstrate involvement of the central sympathetic system [44].

F) Neuropathology

At autopsy atrophy of the lateral and anterior funiculi can be found [20]. The number of anterior horn cells is decreased and there is prominent gliosis [20]. Living anterior horn cells may show degeneration with spheroid inclusions, ubiquinated inclusions, and SOD1 immuno-reactive inclusions [26,45]. Furthermore, there may be Bunina-bodies (eosinophilic intracellular aggregates of dense, granular, proteinaceous material, which is immunoreactive for cystatin C) [4] in the spinal cord and brain stem, or hyaline inclusions (suggestive but not pathognomonic of ALS) in the rostral interstitial nucleus of the medial longitudinal fasciculus and interstitial nucleus of Cajal's nuclei [26]. Neuropathological evaluation in FALS4 patients revealed degeneration of the dentate nucleus, nucleus gracilis, inferior olivary nucleus, and the dorsal roots [46]. Other autopsy studies have revealed aggregates and abnormal assembly of NFs in the perykarion and axon of motor neurons in both SALS and FALS patients with posterior column and spino-cerebellar tract involvement [7]. In patients with extrapyramidal features there may be degeneration of the substantia nigra, associated with skein-like and Lewy body-like inclusions in the pigmental neurons [8]. A double immunoflourescence study revealed that dorfin, a peri-nucleraly located E3 ubiquitin ligase, which participates in the formation of ubiquitylated inclusions, shows a distribution pattern parallel to that of ubiquitin [45]. In FALS patients with SOD1 mutations Lewy-body-like inclusions in anterior horn cells showed co-aggregation with c-Met, the receptor for the hepatocyte growth factor, suggesting partial disruption of this system, and thereby contributing to lower motor neuron degeneration [47]. Studies of the endosome-lysosome system, involved in proteolysis, showed decreased cathepsin B immunoreactivity preferentially in the lateral parts of the anterior gray horn [48]. In the Guam ALS syndrome and the atypical Parkinson syndrome with ALS from Guadaloupe accumulations of abnormally phosphorylated tau protein can be found [49].

G) Disease Course

The pre-paretic phase lasts from months to years. The paretic phase is characterized by slowly ascending weakness, which usually starts in the lower limbs. At onset of the paretic phase a few patients demonstrate ataxia [7]. When leg weakness is slight, the Achilles reflexes are weak or absent whereas the patella reflexes are brisk [7]. A pattern of brisk deep tendon reflexes is seen as the disease spreads to the upper limbs or the bulbar muscles [7].

Extensor plantar responses are noted in most patients but may disappear with disease progression, even before wasting is pronounced [7]. Disease duration shows a bimodal distribution. One group of patients survives <2 years and a second group >5 years [5]. The site of onset is variable, but bulbar onset is rare [5]. Survival time is, on the average, 2.4 years. Survival time does not correlate with age at onset or sex. The most extended survival is found in those patients in whom the disease starts in the upper limbs and progresses via the lower limbs to the bulbar muscles [5,7,]. Pure bulbar onset is rare [7]. In the majority of the cases there is no clinical difference between FALS and SALS. Only the average age at onset of 45.7 years in FALS patients is lower than that of 56 years in SALS patients [7]. Intra-familial variation in age at onset of the order of 15-25 years is a frequent finding in FALS families, but also a few families with small variation have been reported [7]. In 90% of the FALS patients the initial symptoms occur before age 70 years [28].

Table 1. Revised El Escorial criteria (Airlie House criteria) for the diagnosis of ALS [55]

Diagnosis of ALS requires:	Detection
Lesion of the 2. motor neuron in at least two limbs	Clinical findings, electrophysiology
Upper motor neuron lesion in at least 3 regions*	Clinical findings, magnetic stimulation
Progression of these abnormalities (at least progression on history)	Clinical findings
Exclude:	
Sensory disturbances	Clinical findings, electrophysiology
Clinically manifesting, progressive CNS or PNS disorder	Clinical findings, electrophysiology, imaging
Multifocal motor neuropathy	Clinical findings, electrophysiology
Kennedy disease	Clinical findings, genetics
Sensorimotor polyneuropathy	Clinical findings, electrophysiology
Lesion of the spinal cord (e.g. cervical spondylotic myelopathy)	Clinical findings, electrophysiology, imaging
Hyperthyroidism	Thyroidea function tests
Plexopathy	Clinical findings, electrophysiology
Hereditary spastic paraplegia	Clinical findings, electrophysiology, genetics
Hyperparathyroidism	Ca, P, parathormon, calcitonin, imaging
Monoclonal gammopathy associated with lymphoma or myeloma (benign gammopathy)	Immunoglobulines, bone marrow aspiration, blood cell count
Lead intoxication	Blood cell count, lead in the serum, electrophysiology
Aluminum intoxication	Serum aluminum
Radiation therapy of the cerebrum or myelon	History, imaging
Hexosaminidase A and B deficiency	Funduscopy, hexosaminidase A and B
Pick's disease	Clinical findings, neuropsychology
Mitochondriopathy	Clinical findings, CPK, lactacidosis, muscle biopsy, genetics

BB: whole blood cell count, KM: bone marrow, CK: creatine-kinase, the four body regions assessed are head, upper limbs, trunc, lower limbs.

H) Diagnosis

The correct diagnosis of ALS remains a complex clinical problem, despite increasing availability of improved diagnostic facilities, the development of scientific criteria for diagnosing ALS (El Escorial criteria), and the increasing awareness of neurologists for disorders mimicking ALS [50]. Except for desoxyribonucleic acid (DNA) analysis there is still no reliable diagnostic marker for FALS [8]. In addition to the El Escorial criteria, the revised El Escorial criteria (Airlie House criteria) [51,52,53], or sometimes the Lambert-criteria are applied [36]. According to the revised El Escorial criteria, clinical or electrophysiological signs of an upper and lower motor neuron lesion, which also have to show progression, are required for the diagnosis of ALS, in the absence of another disease that could explain the neurological abnormalities [5]. Upper motor neuron signs need to be present in at least 3 of the 4 body regions head, shoulder girdle/arm, trunk, lower limb girdle/leg. Lower motor neuron involvement needs to be present in at least two limbs (table 1). FALS is diagnosed if the El Escorial criteria or the Airlie House criteria are met and if there is a familial background (table 1) [54].

I) Differential Diagnoses

For diagnosing FALS a number of differential diagnoses has to be excluded (table 1) [54]. It has been estimated that up to 10% of the patients initially diagnosed as ALS are ultimately re-diagnosed as having a disease other than ALS [50]. Differential diagnoses which have to be excluded are: multi-focal motor neuropathy, which has been shown to be the most frequent condition misdiagnosed as ALS, Kennedy disease, sensorimotor polyneuropathy, hereditary spastic paraplegia, plexopathy, poliomyelitis, cervical and lumbar myelopathy (tandem stenoses), hyperthyroidism, hyper-parathyroidism, lead intoxication, a state after radiation therapy of the cerebrum or of the myelon, monoclonal gammopathy associated with lymphoma or myeloma, hexosaminidase A deficiency, multiple sclerosis, Pick's disease and mitochondriopathy (table 1) [54,55,56]. Factors leading to the suspicion of any of the differential diagnoses fall into three broad categories: evolution of atypical symptoms, failure of symptom progression, and the results of specific investigations [50].

Genetics

FALS is genetically heterogeneous (FALS1-10) (table 2). Eight of these FALS types are autosomal dominantly (FALS1, FALS3, FALS4, FALS6-10) and 2 types autosomal recessively transmitted (FALS2, FALS5). In FALS1 single SOD1 mutations may also be inherited via a recessive trait. In three of the FALS types (FALS 1, 2, 10) causative mutations have been identified. In the other 7 FALS types linkage-analyses disclosed loci of yet unidentified genes. Linkage describes the association of a certain phenotype with a certain haplotype (typical marker sequence for a distinct DNA-section). Generally, linkage analyses in FALS patients are difficult, because of the late disease onset, the age-dependent penetrance and the relatively short survival time. Due to these reasons, only a limited number of pedigree members is usually available for linkage analysis [5,6].

FALS1

FALS1 is an autosomal dominant and rarely autosomal recessive disorder with adult onset, which was first described in 23 families by Siddique et al. in 1991 [9]. Linkage analyses located the responsible gene within a 10cM long region on chromosome 21q22.1. Following these findings, the causative SOD1 gene was identified within this region in 1993 [10]. Mutations in this gene are associated with an ALS phenotype and are absent in healthy subjects [5].

Table 2. Genetic heterogeneity of FALS [4,6]

FALS type	Transmission	Locus	Gene	Onset	Reference
FALS1	AD, AR#	21q21	SOD1	Adulthood	[88]
FALS2	AR	2q32-34	Alsin	Juvenile	[13,90]
FALS3	AD	18q21	uk	Adulthood	[96]
FALS4	AD	9q34	uk	Juvenile	[97,99,100]
FALS5	AR	15q15-q21	uk	Juvenile	[89]
FALS6*	AD	9q21-q22	uk	uk	[98]
FALS 7	AD	16q12	uk	uk	[95,99,100]
FALS 8	AD	20	uk	uk	[99,100]
FALS 9	AD	Xp11-q12	uk	Juvenile	[99,100]
FALS10*	AD	17q21-22	Tau	Juvenile	[102]

Uk: unknown, SOD1: superoxid-dismutase 1, *: frontotemporal dementia, occasionally associated with ALS, is predominating, #: only the D90A and D96N mutations are inherited as a recessive trait.

A) SOD1 Gene/Gene Product

The SOD1 gene extends over a length of 11 kb and consists of five exons and 4 introns [57]. The gene sequence is highly conserved among species, including lemon, mouse, Drosophila, maize and yeast [58]. The SOD1 gene encodes for a 153-amino-acid, 16kDa protein, which functions as a homodimer and is highly expressed in nervous tissue, liver and erythrocytes [5]. Each subunit contains one atom of both copper and zinc. Two of these polypeptide chains join for a homodimer and are tightly packed and held together by strong hydrophobic interchain disulfide bonds [7]. Each polypeptide chain forms a flattened cylinder build up of eight strands of antiparallel β-structures, arranged in two interlocking Greek key motifs, forming the β-barrel or β-sandwich [5,59,60]. From both the top and bottom of the β-barrel, two large non-helical loops extend (β-barrel plug) [5]. One contains residues required for the electrostatic guidance of O_2^-. The second contributes to the dimer interface. The active site is located on one end of the β-barrel, with an opening facing out and away from the β-barrel and the other subunit. Superoxide anion is guided to the active site of the enzyme through a positively charged tunnel. Zinc is required for a stable pH and the rapid dissociation of H_2O_2 (hydrogen-peroxide). The SOD1 dimer is extremely stable. Three human types of SOD are differentiated: a CuZn SOD, which is located mainly in the cytosol (SOD1), a mitochondrial Mn SOD (SOD2), located within the intermembranous space, and an extra cellular CuZn SOD (SOD3) [61]. Recently it has been shown that SOD1 is not only a cytosolic enzyme, but also localizes to the inner membrane if mitochondria, thereby minimizing oxidative stress in and around the organelle [62]. SOD1 is an ubiquitously and abundantly occurring enzyme, comprising approximately 1% of all cytosolic proteins [57]. In the cerebrum the SOD1 constitutes 0.5-2% of the total soluble proteins [7,8].

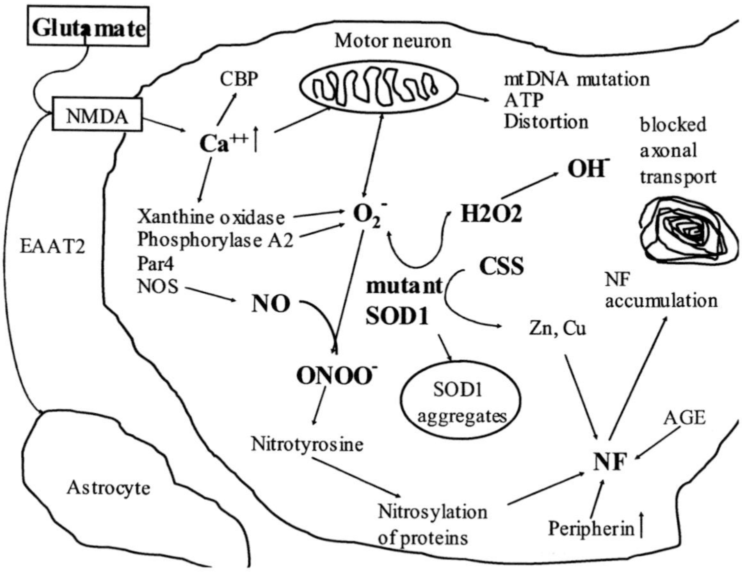

Figure 1. Pathways of motor neuron degeneration in ALS. After release from the pre-synaptic terminal, glutamate activates post-synaptic ionotropic and metabotropic glutamate receptors (e.g. NMDA). Glutamate is cleared from the synaptic cleft by glutamate transporters (e.g. EAAT2). Activation of glutamate receptors causes calcium influx. Calcium increases, also because of impaired calcium binding proteins (CBP, e.g. calbindin, parvalbumin). Increased calcium disturbs the mitochondrial metabolism. Calcium activates enzymes, which produce O_2^- and NO. O_2^- is also produced by mitochondria, due to the high energy requirement of motor neurons. NO reacts with O_2^- to generate $ONOO^-$. ONOO- nitrolyses proteins by use of copper (e.g. NFs). NO also inhibits the mitochondrial electron flow, resulting in further generation of O_2^- and ONOO-. A source of copper may be mutant SOD1which cannot accept copper from the copper chaperone for SOD1 (CCS). Mutant SOD1 also aggregates to immuno-reactive inclusions. Targets of nitrozylation are also NF subunits, resulting in NF accumulation and disruption of the NF network and blocking of the axonal transport, enhanced by increase of peripherin and advanced glycation end products (AGE).

B) Physiologic SOD1 Function

Together with the glutathion-peroxidase and the catalase, SOD1 compensates for the production of free radicals, also termed reactive oxygen species (ROS), like the superoxide-anion (O_2^-), hydroxyl-radical (OH^-), hydrogen-peroxide (H_2O_2), and peroxynitrite ($OONO^-$) (figure 1). SOD1, functioning as an anti-oxidans, catalyzes the dismutation of O_2^- to H_2O_2, dioxygen and water via the reduction of copper [7,63]. Superoxide is an aggressive molecule, which impairs cell function by affection of the cell membrane, proteins and DNA [5,57,64]. In addition to dismutase activity, SOD1 can function as a copper-dependent peroxidase, catalyzing oxidative reactions of substrates by hydrogen peroxide (H_2O_2) [5]. In the presence of nitrogen-oxide (NO) and O_2^- SOD1 forms peroxynitrite ($ONOO^-$). Peroxynitrite reacts to form hydroxyl radicals and nitronium ions, which nitrate tyrosin residues [65,66]. O_2^- reacts with NO three times faster than with wild-type SOD1. The glutathion-peroxidase and catalase convert hydrogen-peroxide into water and oxygen.

C) SOD1 Mutations

Rosen et al. described the first 11 SOD1 missense mutations in 1993 in 13 FALS families [10]. In 2000 the number of SOD1 mutations had reached 63 [67]. Meanwhile more than 100 SOD1 mutations in 64 codons have been described (table 3) [5,68,69,70,71]. The mutations are distributed over all 5 exons of the gene, with a maximum in exon 4 and 5. Why the least number of mutations occurs in exon 3 is unknown [7]. More than ten mutations result in shortened polypeptides [7]. They lie between codon 118 and 133. Most of the mutations affect the backbone of the protein or regions involved in the dimerization of the two subunits. Only 4 mutations reside in the active center of the enzyme. Additionally, there are a number of SOD1 variants (polymorphisms) (table 3). The most prevalent SOD1 mutation in North America is the A4V mutation (50% of all SOD1 mutations) [67,72], followed by the I113T mutation (11.7% of all SOD1-mutations) [6]. SOD1 mutations are responsible, on the average, for 20% (range: 14,3-23,4%) of the FALS cases [7]. SOD1 mutations may be also detected in SALS patients [21,26,57,64,67,73,74,75,76,77].

Table 3. SOD1 and alsin mutations currently known [71]

Type	Promotor		Exon		Intron		Untranslated	
	SOD 1	Alsin	SOD1 *	Alsin	SOD 1	Alsin	SOD1	Alsin
Substitution	0	0	93	1	2	0	0	0
Deletion	0	0	4	6	0	0	0	0
Insertion	0	0	3	0	0	0	0	
Compound mutation	0	0	1 (1)	0	0	0	0	0
Polymorphism	0	0	5	0	0	0	0	1

*: SOD1 mutations are located in exon 1 (n=19), exon 2 (n=13), exon 3 (n=8), exon 4 (n=38), exon 5 (n=27) and in introns (n=2)

Most of the SOD1 mutations are substitutions resulting in missense mutations (preserved reading frame) [6]. Additionally, exonic insertions, and exonic deletions have been described, which all result in a stop-codon (nonsense-mutation) (table 3) [5]. Only eight mutations in exon 3, which contains the active site, have been reported (table 3). Penetrance may be incomplete and complicated by age dependence [78]. Usually, SOD1 mutations occur in the heterozygous form. In rare cases homozygosity has been reported, like in northern Scandinavia, southern France, southern Italy, Germany and North America [7,68]. Why homozygosity for the D90A mutation is associated with a milder phenotype than heterozygosity is assumed due to a genetic factor, which ameliorates the effect of the D90A mutation in the homozygous but not in the heterozygous form [7].

D) Effects of Mutant SOD1

The effect of a mutation on the protein function is determined by the position and type of the amino-acid exchange. Some mutations lead to a reduction of the copper and zinc content of the enzyme, some to reduced thermostability, some to reduced enzyme activity, and some to molecules, similar to those of the wild-type gene, without a significant reduction of the enzyme activity. SOD1 mutations cluster in regions influencing the architectural integrity of the enzyme [79]. Characterization of β-barrel and dimer interface revealed reduced stability and drastically increased aggregation propensity [79]. These defects promote the formation of filamentous aggregates [79]. Since the active channel of mutant SOD1 is slightly larger than that of wild-type SOD1, H_2O_2 has access to the active site of the enzyme. The resulting hydroxyl radical may react with a histidine of the active site, thereby inactivating the enzyme [5]. SOD1 folding dynamics and aggregation propensity seems to be altered by non-native disulfide bond formation [60,80]. In the G93A SOD1 mutant mouse motor neuron excitability is increased, which may contribute to the pathogenesis of the disease [81]. There are also indications that SOD1 mutations alter α-amino-3-hydroxy-5-methyl-n-isoxazol-proprionacid (AMPA) function, resulting in increased vulnerability of motor neurons to glutamatergic excitotoxicity [82].

E) Phenotype of SOD1 Mutants

FALS patients with SOD1 mutations are clinically hardly different from FALS-patients without a SOD1 mutation. By contrast, phenotypes of the various SOD1 mutations differ considerably with regard to disease onset, severity, progression and prognosis (table 4). FALS phenotypes due to the C146A SOD1 mutation can be variable even between siblings of a single family [83]. Disease onset for patients with SOD1-mutations is on the average 46.9 years and for non-SOD1-mutations 50.5 years [84]. The earliest onset has been reported for the L106V mutation with a mean of 35.5 years. The latest onset was found for the I113T mutation with 58.9 years (table 4). The I113T mutation is also the one, which is the most frequent among SALS patients. It is speculated, that in case of a late onset, most of those carrying the mutation die before manifestation of the disease and are thus erroneously diagnosed as SALS. However, there are also SOD1 mutations in SALS patients with early onset (table 4).

The A4V and A4T mutations are associated with an aggressive FALS type with a survival time of less than 1.5 years [85]. Also the H48Q mutation (strongly conserved region) results in a severe phenotype with quick progression and a survival time of 8 month on the average [67,86,87]. On the contrary, the H46R mutation (strongly conserved region) is associated with slow progression and an average life expectancy of 18 years. Slow progression over 10-15 years is also reported for the E21G, G37R, G41D, D90A, G93C, G93V, I104F, L144S, L144F, and I151T mutations [20]. Usually, the onset is late in patients with initially bulbar manifestations. Patients with bulbar-onset are older at onset, whereas the G37R and the L38V mutation predict early onset. An early onset is also described for the G37R and L38V mutations. Early onset is not automatically associated with short survival. There are SOD1 mutations, which result in predominant affection of the lower motor neuron (e.g. A4V mutation), which show female predominance, and low penetrance (table 4). The mutations D90A and D96N are transmitted via a dominant as well as recessive trait (table 4)

[6,88]. The autosomal recessive D90A SOD1 mutant ALS in northern Sweden and Finland is found as a polymorphism in up to 3% of clinically unaffected individuals. Homozygous patients complain about painful muscle spasms and lower limb paresthesias with difficulty with micturition and may additionally present with typical ALS signs [58]. Though SOD1 function is completely preserved in these patients, it is associated with an ALS phenotype with favorable prognosis [88]. Confirmation of a common ancestor of all FALS families with the D90A mutation and the less severe manifestations for the homozygous compared to the heterozygous state, indicate that there are other genetic influences, which modify the effect of SOD1 mutations. Recently FALS patients with the recessive SOD1 D90A and also the recessive D96N mutation (compound heterozygosity) have been described [5].

Table 4. Phenotype variation of SOD1 mutations [4,7]

Predominant clinical feature	SOD1 mutation
Early onset	G37R, L38V, H46R, H80A, G85R, L106V
Late onset	I113T
Slow progression	E21G, G37R, G41D, H46R, D90A, G93A, G93V, G93C, I104F, I113T, I151T, L144S, L144F
Rapid progression	A4T, A4V, H48Q, N86S, L106V, V148G
Short survival	A4V
Long survival	G37R, G41D, H46R, G93A
Bulbar onset	A4V, L8O, D76Y, D90A, V148I, I151T
Predominant affection of the 2. motor neuron	A4V, H80A, L84V, D101N
Female predominance	G41D
Associated with dementia	D76T
Prolonged central motor conduction time	K12A, D76Y, D90A
Low penetrance	D90A, I113T
Hundred percent penetrance by age 70	L38V, E100G, I113T
Dominant and recessive transmission	D90A, D96N
Reduced capacity to bind copper	H46R, H48Q
Occurrence in SALS	H80A, D90A
Non-penetrance	V4G, G16S, G21L, A76T, A101A, I113T
Neurofibrillary inclusions	A4V, H48Q, I113T

F) Testing for SOD1 Mutations

To test for SOD1 mutations DNA is extracted from blood lymphocytes. Afterwards, the five exons of the SOD1 gene are amplified by PCR. PCR products then undergo single strand conformation polymorphism or heteroduplex mutational analysis [26]. Subsequent sequence analysis may identify point mutations, which can be confirmed by restriction digest [26].

FALS2

In 17 Tunisian families with a number of consanguineous couples, a FALS type was described with juvenile onset, autosomal recessive trait, and linkage to a 1.7cM long region on chromosome 2q33-35, which contains 5 different genes [89]. Initially, the candidate gene proposed was that for the aldehyde-oxidase, based on its location within the tissues, linkage-data and its role in the metabolism of free radicals. Meanwhile mutations in the alsin gene have been identified as causative for FALS2 (table 2) [11,13,90].

A) Alsin Gene/Gene Product

The alsin gene comprises 34 exons and encodes for alsin, a putative GTPase regulator. Alsin exists as 2 alternative splice variants, a long variant, consisting of 6394 nucleotides, and a short variant, which consists of 2651 nucleotides. The alsin protein contains two guanine-nucleotide-exchange factor (GEF) domains (regulator of chromosome condensation (RCC1)-like domain (RLD, RanGEF) and vacuolar protein sorting 9 (VPS9, Rab5GEF) domain, the Dbl homology domain, the pleckstrin homology (DH/PH) domain, and two membrane occupation and recognition plexus (MORN) motifs [2,11,91,92].

B) Alsin Function

The physiological function of alsin is yet unknown. However, there are indications that it is involved in the microtubule assembly, in the endosomal dynamics, in signaling cascades, in the membrane transport and in the organization of the cytoskeleton [11,92]. Alsin seems to play an important role in the JNK/SAPK pathway, which itself is involved in neuroprotection [93]. The carboxy-terminus of alsin, carrying the VPS9 domain, mediates not only the activation of the small GTPase Rab5 via a guanine-nucleotide exchanging reaction, but also the endosomal localization of alsin, while the amino-terminal half, containing RLD, acts suppressive in its membranous localization [92]. Furthermore, the DH/PH domain in the middle portion of alsin enhances the VPS9 domain-mediated endosome fusion. Ectopically expressed ALS2 protein localizes with Rab5 and early endosome antigen-1 onto early endosomal compartments and stimulates the enlargements of endosomes in cultured cortical neurons [92]. Altogether, alsin seems to be implicated in the endosomal dynamics. Perturbation of endosomal dynamics due to loss of alsin activity might underlie neuronal dysfunction and degeneration in ALS [92].

C) Alsin Mutations

So far 7 mutations (6 deletions and a single splice-site mutation) have been detected, which are associated with a FALS phenotype [94]. The deletion 261 del A in codon 46 causes disruption of the reading frame and generates a truncated protein [12]. The deletion 1548 del AG in codon 475 also results in a frame shift, which generates a stop codon [11]. The deletion 3742 del A in exon 22 results in a stop codon at position 1206 aa. The deletion del GTTTCCCCCA in exon 6 results in a frame shift and thus stop-codon at position 483 aa. The deletion 2660 del AT in exon 13 results in a frame shift and ultimately stop-codon, 12 codons after the deletion site at the at position 858 aa. The deletion 1130 del AT in exon 4 also results in a frame shift and lastly stop-codon at position 335 aa [11,90]. Deletions in the alsin gene are made responsible also for familial, juvenile, primary lateral sclerosis [13]. Alsin mutations are predicted to cause loss of alsin protein function [91]. In addition to FALS, alsin mutations also cause various types of hereditary spastic paraplegia [90]. In a study on autosomal recessive FALS in Japan single-nucleotide polymorphisms in non-coding regions of the ALS2 gene were found (table 3) [91].

D) Phenotype of Alsin Mutations

FALS2 has its onset in the 1. or 2. decade (on the average in the 12. year), and takes a slow, progressive course. Clinically, 3 types were initially delineated: Type 1, the most prevalent of the three types, is characterized by weakness and wasting in spastic muscles. Type 1 has been recently mapped to chromosome 15q15.1-q21.1 (FALS5). Type 2 is characterized by spasticity only in the lower limbs. Type 2 is an intermediate type between ALS and hereditary spastic paraplegia [7]. Type 3 is characterized by spasticity predominantly in the face and the upper limbs. Type 3 represents the real FALS2 and the causative gene has been recently mapped to chromosome 2q33-35.

FALS3

In a single big European family with classical ALS phenotype, linkage analysis located the defective gene to a locus on chromosome 18q21 (table 2) [6,95,96].

FALS4

In a single, extended Anglo-American family with autosomal dominant FALS with juvenile onset, complete penetrance, slow progression, without bulbar involvement, and normal lifespan, linkage with a locus on chromosome 9q34 within an interval of 5cM has been demonstrated [97]. The disease affected four family members. FALS4 starts on the average at age 17 years and shows slow progression of distal limb amyotrophy and upper motor neuron signs. Bulbar symptoms are absent. The disorder may go along with dementia (table 2) [5,6].

FALS5

In one of the 17 Tunisian families with presumed type 1 of FALS2, genome-wide linkage analysis revealed linkage with a locus on chromosome 15q15.1-q21.1 [89]. This locus was also detected in four other families from Europe and South Asia. Missing linkage in three further families with autosomal recessive FALS indicates that heterogeneity of autosomal recessive FALS is even broader than so far assumed [5]. FALS5 is presumably the most common recessive type of FALS and has been identified in a number of ethnic groups meanwhile (table 2) [5,6].

FALS6

Genome-wide linkage analysis in 16 families from Boston and Chicago (>700 FALS cases) mapped the defective gene to chromosome 9q21-q22. The region extends over approximately 17cM [98]. In addition to features of classical ALS the phenotype includes fronto-temporal dementia (table 2) [98].

FALS7

In another single family with a classical ALS phenotype linkage to a locus on chromosome 16q12.1-q12.2 was detected (table 2) [95,99].

FALS8

When screening 16 FALS families without a SOD1 or alsin mutation, linkage to a locus on chromosome 10 was found in one of these families (table 2) [100].

FALS 9

In a single, large American pedigree with typical clinical and neuropathological ALS features, X-linked, dominant transmission was described. The causative gene has yet to be found [101]. This finding may be of relevance since the sex ratio women/men of FALS is higher than that of SALS [5,8]. There is an earlier onset by 5-10 years in men (table 2) [100].

FALS 10

Recent findings have shown that ALS may be also due to mutations in the tau gene on chromosome 17q21 [102]. Mutations in the tau gene affect the alternative splicing of exon 10, resulting in an excess of four-repeat tau isoforms [6]. These isoforms presumably result in reduced binding of tau to axonal microtubuls. The first description of a tauopathy with ALS was that of patients with behavioral disorder, speech disturbance, memory decline, Parkinson symptoms and amyotrophy [6]. Neuropathologically FALS10 shows neurofilamentous deposits (neurofibrillary tangles) build up of tau-protein without senile plaques. The pattern of neurofibrillary tangle tau-protein is isoform and similar to that in Alzheimer's disease [19]. Tauopathies other than FALS10 are the fronto-temporal dementia, Pick's disease, the corticobasal degeneration, and the familial progressive supranuclear palsy [6].

Other syndromes, in which ALS is a feature of a multisystem disorder and is associated with Parkinson syndrome or dementia are the ALS syndromes of Guam, Papua-New Guinea, Guadeloupe, Kii, and of the Amish community (table 5) [6,19,103]. Though Guam ALS syndrome, locally known as "bodig" (Parkinsonism and dementia predominate) or "lytico"

(ALS predominates) is associated with ingestion of cycad plants, there are also a number of familial cases [104]. Bodig cases are neuropathologically characterized by the extensive occurrence of neurofibrillar tangles, which are surrounded by reactive microglia and astrocytes and other inflammatory reactants, suggesting that plaques and tangles generate exacerbating inflammatory responses [104].

Table 5. FALS associated with dementia and/or Parkinsonism

Disorder	Gene/linkage	ALS/amyotrophy	Dementia	Parkinsonism
FALS1	SOD1 (A76T)	+	+	-
FALS4	9q34	+	+	-
FALS6	9q21-q22	+	+	-
FALS10	tau	+	+	-
Guam ALS syndrome	uk, SOD1*	+	+	+
Guadeloupe Parkinson	tau?	+	+	+
Kii ALS	uk	+	+	+
Papua New Guinea	uk	+	+	+
Amish community ALS	uk	+	+	-
Machado-Joseph disease	SCA3	+	-	+

Uk: unknown, *: in 2 of 23 unrelated families.

Candidate Genes

Various genes other than SOD1, alsin or tau are suspected to cause FALS. (table 6). In some of these genes mutations or an association between a gene and the FALS phenotype have been found. In a single family with SALS mutations were identified in the gene for the NFH subunit (table 6). These mutations occur in a region of the protein involved in cross-linking, why normal aggregation may be disrupted [5]. In a single family mutations in the SOD2 gene were reported (table 6). So far, no mutations were found in the SOD3 gene. However, if a FALS mouse carries a SOD1 and a SOD2 mutation, the clinical course is more severe, than if only the SOD1 mutation is present. The association between apolipoprotein E alleles and FALS is uncertain. There are some indications that the APOE ε2 allele is associated with a protective effect, whereas the APOE ε4 allele is associated with a negative effect [5]. Possibly, APOE alleles influence ALS presentation and progression. Recently, the gene encoding vascular endothelial growth factor in ALS patients and mice has been identified as a modifier gene associated with motor neuron degeneration [69]. Also LIF could act as a modifier gene, which together with other genetic predisposition might lead to FALS [105]. In a study on 66 FALS patients, 177 SALS patients and 14 patients with sporadic pure lower motor neuron features, mutations have been found only in the latter group. A number of genes has been suggested to confer a greater risk for the development of FALS, which include: Deletions or insertions in the ICSP domain of NFH [8,106]; Point mutations and deletions in the mitochondrial DNA [107]; ribonucleic acid (RNA)-processing errors in the glutamate transporter EAAT2 (excitatory amino-acid carrier 2) [108,109]; An abnormal copy number of the survival motor neuron (SMN) gene [23]; Deletions in the NAIP gene [110]. Since the multifunctional DNA repair enzyme, encoded by the apurinic/apurimidinic exonuclease (APEX nuclease) gene, is reduced in the frontal cortex of SALS patients, it is quite likely that also APEX contributes to the etiology of FALS [5].

Table 6. Susceptibility genes and association with phenotype [6,7]

Gene product	Gene	Locus	AP*	Reference
Neurofilament heavy chain	NFH	22q12.2	yes	[174]
Neurofilament light chain	NFL	8p21	yes	[131,161,175]
Peripherin	PRPH	12q12-13	yes	[176,177]
Glutamate transporter	EAAT2	11p13-12	yes	[108,178]
Glutamate receptor	AMPA	5p33	yes	[179]
P450 debrisoquine hydroxylase	Cyp2D6	22q13.1	yes	[180]
Apurinic apyrimidinic endonuclease	APEX nuclease	14q11.2-12	yes	[181]
Respiratory chain enzymes	COX	mtDNA	yes	[175,182]
Dynactin p150	Glued	2p13	yes	[183]
Neuronal apoptosis inhibitory polypeptide	NAIP	5 tel	yes	[58,183]
Neuron specific kinesin heavy chain	KHC	2	yes	[184]
IL2 receptor β-chain	IL-2β	22q12.1-2	yes	[185]
Leukemia inhibitory factor	LIF	22q12.1-2	yes	[105]
Vascular endothelial growth factor	VEGF	6p12	yes	[69]
Apolipoprotein E ε4 allele	ApoE ε4	19q13.2	yes	[186,187]
Manganese superoxide dismutase	SOD2	6q25	yes	[188]
Survival motor neuron	SMN	5q13	yes	[189]
Ciliary neurotrophic factor	CNTF	11q12.2	no	[190]
Presenilin	PSEN2	1	no	[191]
Alpha-synnuclein (persyn)	Persyn	10q23.2-q23.3	no	[192,193]
Parkin	Parkin	6q25.2-27	no	[194]
Hexosaminidase A	HEXA	15q23	no	[195]
Copper chaperone for SOD1	CCS	11	no	[146]
Bulbospinal muscular atrophy	BSMA	X	no	[58]
Catalase	CAS1	2	no	[196]
Dynein	Dynein	7q11.23	no	[174]

AP: association with ALS phenotype.

Additionally, the frequent occurrence of polymorphisms in the gene for the APEX nuclease in SALS patients indicates that other genes play a pathogenic role in FALS. Other genes susceptible to be involved in the pathogenesis of FALS are those for NFL, peripherin, the AMPA-receptor, the debrisoquine hydroxylase, dynactin, kinesin heavy chain, and the interleukin-2 β-chain (table 6). Genes excluded as disease modifiers of the FALS phenotype are listed in table 6.

Pathomechanisms

How SOD1, alsin, tau or other mutations exhibit their deleterious effect on motor neurons is still not fully understood. SOD1 mutations result in over-activity (gain-of-function) rather than reduced SOD1 activity (loss-of-function), depending on the type of SOD1 mutation. Over- or under-activity of wild-type SOD1, however, is not sufficient for the development of an ALS phenotype in transgenic mice (table 5). SOD1 knockout mice do not develop motor neuron disease. On the contrary, mice over-expressing mutant SOD1 develop late onset motor neuron degeneration [8]. Accordingly, FALS seems to be caused by the acquisition of an adverse toxic property of mutant SOD1 rather than reduced SOD1 activity [5]. Among various mechanisms postulated to explain how mutant SOD1 causes motor neuron degeneration, two hypotheses predominate the actual discussion: the oligomerization-hypothesis and the oxidative stress hypothesis (figure 1).

SOD1 Oligomerization

The SOD1 oligomerization hypothesis assumes that SOD1 mutations lead to impaired protein folding, solubility, or degradation and consequently to oligomerization of mutant SOD1 to high molecular aggregates (SOD1 aggregation) [111]. The amyloid-like filaments and nanotubes arise through extensive interactions between loop and β-barrel elements of neighboring SOD1 molecules and manifest as axonal inclusion [79]. Indeed, metal-deficient, pathogenic SOD1 mutant proteins crystallize in three different crystal forms, all of which reveal higher order assemblies of aligned β-sheets. The increased protein/protein interaction between dimers is explained by a conformation change of the protein in the sense of an opening of the β-barrel [100,112], leading to higher-order arrays [113]. That these aggregates remain soluble, heat-shock proteins are required, which are indeed up-regulated in motor neurons of FALS patients. It has been speculated that the attempt to remove the SOD1 aggregates from the cell exhausts motor neurons. If SOD1 proteins within the aggregates are shortened, if they are going to be oxidized, demetallized or covalently modified, remains speculative [60,70]. Within motor neurons aggregates lead to obstruction of the axonal transport, to protein degradation, and apoptosis [114]. SOD1 aggregates can be found in upper as well as lower motor neurons [115].

Oxidative Stress

Definition

Oxidative stress is defined as strain on cellular function induced by ROS, which derive from the oxygen metabolism (figure 1) [66]. H_2O_2 and O_2^- can give rise to OH^- through the

Fenton respectively Haber-Weis reaction, while O_2^- can generate $OONO^-$ through reaction with NO. ROS can induce lethal cellular damage through oxidation and peroxidation of proteins, lipids and nuclear acids. Up to 10% of the oxygen used by tissues is converted to ROS [61]. SOD1, catalase and glutathion peroxidase are the crucial components of the cellular defense against oxidative stress, because of their conversion of ROS into more innocent molecules. Vitamin C and α-tocopherol (vitamin E) also have a protective effect. Detoxification of ROS is a vital function of each cell. This is particularly the case for motor neurons, which are more sensitive to oxidative stress than other cells. Motor neurons have a high energy demand, which is almost exclusively covered by mitochondrial oxidative phosphorylation, which in turn increases oxidative stress. Since ROS are extremely toxic, it becomes self-explanatory why a single mutation in genes responsible for the complex framework of production and removal of ROS can have such deleterious consequences as in FALS [70,116,117,118]. ROS have also been implicated in ageing, since over-expression of wild-type SOD1 and application of SOD1 or catalase mimetics dramatically extend life span in Drosophila and C. elegans [119,120]. Generally, oxidative damage, particularly of cerebral DNA, increases with age [121,122].

Activity of Mutant SOD1

According to the oxidative stress hypothesis mutant SOD1 has various negative effects: 1. Mutant SOD1 insufficiently catalyzes the degradation of ROS (loss-of-function, reduction of radical scavenger capacity), which in turn damage substrates essential for the viability of motor neurons. On the average the SOD1 activity is reduced by 50% (20-60%) in FALS patients, but normal in SALS patients and FALS patients without SOD1 mutations [5,123]. Arguments against motor neuron death due to loss of SOD1 function are: SOD1 a) Mutations do not result in the absence of the enzyme, suggesting that SOD1 needs to be present to cause disease. b) Some SOD1 mutations cause disease despite intact enzyme function. c) Transgenic mice over-expressing human mutant SOD1 develop disease in spite of normal endogenous SOD1 function [66]. 2. Mutant SOD1 becomes overactive and increases its oxidative activity (gain-of-function), resulting in excessive production of hydrogen peroxide (increased H_2O_2 turn-over), which is rapidly degradated to the more toxic hydroxyl radical [5,116], and in increased protein/protein interaction [116]. A further indicator for a gain-of function of SOD1 mutants is the finding that apoptosis is inhibited in neurons over-expressing wild-type SOD1, whereas FALS mutants promote apoptosis [124]. 3. Mutant SOD1 has a dominant negative effect, which means that it can also impair the function of the normal enzyme from the wild-type allele [5]. 4. Mutant SOD1 reverses its physiological function such, that $O2^-$ arises from H_2O_2 [5,61,64,125,126,127,128]. Presumably, this is because H_2O_2 has access to the active site of the enzyme due to conformational changes of the mutated enzyme. When hydrogen-peroxide (H_2O_2) interacts with the active site of SOD1 O_2^- is generated, which either damages amino-acid residues at the active site, inactivating the enzyme (self-oxidative pathway) or oxidizes substrates exogenous to the active site (external oxidative pathway) [113]. The hydroxyl radical, the most toxic of the ROS is not generated by an enzymatic reaction, but results from slowly decomposition of H_2O_2, a reaction, which is catalyzed by Fe++. 5. Mutant SOD1 has a greater copper-dependent peroxidase activity than wild-type SOD1, leading to increased oxidative stress, oxidation of essential substrates, and subsequent cellular damage.[8,66]. 6. Mutant SOD1 is highly susceptible to glycation, which could enhance oxidative stress in FALS [129]. 7. Mutant SOD1 leads to inhibition of the ubiquitine-proteasome pathway and consecutively motor neuron death [128].

Arguments for the oxidative hypothesis are that antioxidants like vitamin C and vitamin E have a beneficial effect in transgenic SOD1 mice and in cell cultures, and that deficiency of vitamin E may result in neurological symptoms. However, clinical trials with a selection of ROS scavengening antioxidants, did not have a beneficial effect in ALS patients. These negative results may be due to under-dosing, inappropriate selection of patients, wrong choice of the antioxidant, or that the complex biochemistry of ROS does not lend to such treatment [5]. Whether oxidative damage contributes pathogenically to motor neuron degeneration, or whether it is an epiphenomenon of motor neuron death, is unclear [66], Possibly, the role of oxidative stress in the pathogenesis of FALS is just a secondary one [66]. Oxidative stress is not specific for ALS but occurs in various other neurodegenerative diseases. However, this does not necessarily mean that oxidative stress is pathogenically irrelevant. Oxidative stress may be part of a final common pathway, through which motor neuron degeneration evolves [66].

Protein Nitrozilation

Mutant SOD1 not only shows a pro-oxidant activity but also supports the cross-talk between ROS and nitric oxide synthetase (NOS) via the proteasome pathway [130]. The superoxide-anion (O_2^-) spontaneously (non-enzymatically) reacts with NO at a rate three times faster than the SOD1 reaction, whereby peroxynitrite ($ONOO^-$) is generated. NO itself is generated by NOS, which is calcium dependent, thus prone to glutamate excitotoxicity [8]. Accordingly, those SOD1 mutations, which increase the production of O_2^-, also increase the $ONOO^-$ production. Toxicity of peroynitrite occurs by lipid peroxidation, sulfhydryl oxidation, generation of hydroxyl radicals, and nitration of phenole residues [4]. Peroxynitrite also induces DNA strand breaks and the frustrate attempt to repair these breaks by poly-ADP ribosyl-polymerase leads to NAD and ATP depletion, apoptosis and cell death [4].

The reaction of $ONOO^-$ with tyrosin residues is catalized by SOD1. Nitrozylation of tyrosin results in 3-nitro-tyrosin, which is elevated up to 7 times in ALS patients. Targets of such protein nitrozylation are the NFs. Since NFL has 40 tyrosin molecules it presumably acts as a scavenger for reactive nitrating molecules. Co-localization of NF aggregates with SOD1 and NOS in the brain of FALS and SALS patients supports the hypothesis that nitrated tyrosin residues impair phosphorylation and assembly of NFs. A further argument is the reduction of mRNA for NFL in motor neurons of ALS patients [8]. Impaired NF phosphorylation may lead to NF accumulation, affection of the axonal transport and progressive motor neuron death (figure 1).

Arguments against the nitrozylation hypothesis are that SOD1 G93A transgenic mice without the NOS gene do not live longer than those with the NOS gene, that the cortex of SOD G93A transgenic mice contains normal levels but reduced activity of NOS, that some studies did not find measurable levels of nitro-tyrosin on NF subunits [5], and that administration of NOS inhibitors does not alter the disease course in SOD1 G93A mice [4].

Neurofilaments

Accumulation of NFs in the pericaryon and the proximal parts of the axon are the most frequently observed neuropathologic abnormalities in FALS and SALS patients [4,131]. Whether NF accumulation is due to the primary pathogenic process or just a byproduct of another process is under debate [5,8]. Disregarding this ongoing area of uncertainties and research, the disease course appears to be influenced by the degree of NF expression and the interaction between various other filament proteins. NFs are the key module of the axonal cytoskeleton and the axonal transport. Their expression and interaction is crucial for the cell function. An intact cytoskeleton is the prerequisite for proper shape and function of the up to 1 m long axons of anterior horn cells. Their concentration within an axon is high. The initial cytoskeletal network of neurons consists of nestin, peripherin, vinculin and α-internexin, which are gradually replaced by NFs. During this transition to mature neurons, the initial components of the cytoskeleton form homo- and hetero-polymers with NFs [4].

NF aggregation in motor neurons of ALS patients raised the suspicion that mutations in the NF genes might be causative. Investigations concerning this hypothesis by Figlewicz et al. revealed deletions in the NFH gene [106]. The tail of the NFH consists of a repetitive lysine-serin-proline (LSP) motif. In five unrelated SALS patients deletions were found within this LSP repeat domain. Four of these patients had the same 3bp deletion [106]. Another three deletions in this region have been recently described [8]. Interestingly, 22 of the included FALS patients additionally had SOD1 mutations. However, there was no association between SOD1 genotype, HF-genotype, and phenotype. In a single SALS case with classical ALS features, Tomkins et al. found a 84bp insertion containing four LSP repeat motifs [132]. It has been estimated that one percent of the ALS patients carries a NFH mutation [6,8], representing a risk factor for the development of ALS. Since other studies on SALS patients could not demonstrate any NFH gene mutation, it is quite likely that NFH gene mutations are only rarely the primary defect in FALS or SALS [7].

The potential importance of NFs in the pathogenesis of FALS is underscored by the marked NF pathology in FALS patients with the A4V, D48Q, and I113T mutation [7]. A further argument for a role of NFs in the pathogenesis of ALS is that through phosphorylation of NFs by the cyclin-dependent kinase 5 (cdk5), the same epitopes are generated as those found in NF accumulations in ALS patients [133]. In addition, cdk5 is present in some of the accumulations and is found in affected motor neurons in association with lipofuscin, a protein associated with oxidative stress and ageing [8]. Down-regulation of cdk5 activity leads to motor neuron degeneration. Associated with lipofuscin is B-cell lymphoma-2 (bcl-2), a protector against apoptosis. However, over-expression of bcl-2 in transgenic mice mutant for the NFL gene did not protect neurons from degeneration [134]. A further argument for the NF hypothesis is that accumulation of NFs induces axonal degeneration in ALS mouse models (table 7).

Table 7. Animal models of FALS [5]

Animal	Gene	Mutation	SOD1 activity	Clinical manifestations	Reference
Mouse	SOD1	G93A	Reduced?	Motor neuron disease	[197]
Mouse	SOD1	G86R	Normal	Motor neuron disease	[198]
Mouse	SOD1	G37R	Adverse*	Motor neuron disease	[199]
Mouse	SOD1 injury	Knock-out	Absent	No ALS, increased vulnerability to axonal	[200]
Yeast	SOD1	Knock out	Absent	Dissociated SOD1 activity	[124]
Mouse	NFL	Substitution	Uk	Motor neuron degeneration	[201]

Uk: unknown, NFL: neurofilament light chain, *: adverse property by the mutant enzyme, rather than elevation or loss of SOD1 activity.

Further evidence for the involvement of NFs in the pathogenesis of ALS comes from the finding that NFs are modified by advanced glycation end products (AGE), which itself have a cytotoxic effect [8,87,135,136]. AGEs result from a non-enzymatic reaction of sugars with biological molecules, resulting in irreversible glycation [8]. Because of their stability, NFs are particularly prone to this process. The lysine residues of the KSP multi-phosphorylation repeat domain and the O-glycation site at the N-terminus, essential for the interaction of NFs with each other, are particularly vulnerable to this type of glycation. AGE products are removed by binding to AGE-receptors, which presumably produce oxidative stress. SOD1 co-aggregates with AGE-NFs [137].

Recent findings showed that the phosphorylation state of NFH from ALS patients is normal, suggesting that post-translational modifications are unlikely to cause NF-aggregation [4]. By using the RNAse protection assay and real time reverse transcriptase-PCR, Ge et al. observed significant elevations of NF mRNA in ALS [131]. They also observed that trans-acting NFL destabilizing elements are selectively suppressed in ALS homogenates, resulting in increased stability and level of light NF mRNA [131]. Evidence for involvement of NFs in the pathogenesis of FALS comes also from the finding that peripherin, which normally binds to NFL, interacts with the NFM and NFH subunits, creating a disorganized NF network and NF aggregation, leading to motor neuron death [138]. An abnormal NF network occurs also if peripherin is increased and if NFL is decreased [8]. Arguments against the NF hypothesis are that in NFL -/- and NFH/lacZ mice an intact NF structure is not required for mutant SOD1-dependent motor neuron death.

Glutamate Excitotoxicity

Glutamate-Receptors

Glutamate, the most abundant excitatory neurotransmitter of the central nervous system (CNS), can be neurotoxic in isolation [4]. Glutamate is released from presynaptic vesicles by a Ca++-dependent mechanism. Glutamate activates two specific types of post-synaptic receptors, ionotropic (ligand-gated) and metabotropic receptors. Among the ionotropic receptors 3 subtypes are differentiated (kainate, N-methyl-D-aspartate (NMDA) and AMPA-receptors, consisting of 4 subunits (GluR1-4). There are also three types of metabotropic receptors, build up of a total of 8 subunits. Stimulation of glutamate-receptors initiates a cascade of events, like calcium influx and sodium influx (figure 1), which consequently leads to intracellular edema, and activates processes, by which ROS are released. Following uptake, glutamate is either transaminated to form glutamine or is metabolized to α-keto-glutarate, which both serve as precursors of the glutamate synthesis. AMPA stimulation also activates NOS-generating pathways. NOS produce NO, which together with superoxide binds to peroxynitrite (figure 1).

Glutamate excitotoxicity has been implicated as a major pathophysiologic mechanism in SALS. Arguments for the pathogenic role of glutamate are, that CSF glutamate is increased up to threefold in 80% of the ALS patients compared with controls [4] and that exposure of spinal cord cultures to glutamate results in selective motor neuron loss [139]. In other studies glutamate was increased in the CSF in only 30% of the patients [8]. By contrast, expression level and proportion of GluR2 mRNA in motor neurons is the lowest among various neurons, and does not differ from controls, implying that selective reduction of the GluR2 subunit cannot explain AMPA-receptor mediated neurotoxicity [140].

Glutamate Carriers

Another effect of SOD1 mutations may be an increased vulnerability towards excitotoxic mechanisms through selective inactivation of the glutamate transport [6]. To prevent excitotoxicity (neurotoxicity) from excessive extracellular glutamate, it is of crucial importance that presynaptically released glutamate is discarded from the synaptic cleft to the surrounding astrocytes. For this transport, three glutamate transporters, EAAT1, GLT1 (rat glial glutamate transporter, in human beings EAAT2) and GLAST (rat glial glutamate and aspartate transporter) are available. EAAT1 is neuron-specific, whereas GLT1 and GLAST are solely expressed in astrocytes. In 60-70% of ALS patients GLT1 and EAAT1 are decreased by 35-95% in the cortex and spinal cord. Reduction of GLT1 is predominantly found in SOD1 mutants. Despite impaired function, mRNA levels of the three glutamate carriers are not decreased in ALS patients, suggesting that impairment of glutamate carriers occurs on the translational or post-translational level [5]. Interestingly, EAAT2 and GLT1 mRNA is aberrant in approximately two thirds of FALS and SALS patients [108]. Aberrant transcripts, however, may be also found in normal controls. Aberrant EAAT2 mRNA possibly results from a defect RNA processing - various transcripts reduce expression of EAAT2 - or from mutations in the EAAT2 gene. However, only in a single patient a missense mutation in the EAAT2 gene, which alters a glycation site, has been detected. Additionally, the functional significance of this mutation remains unclear. Thus the EAAT2 gene mutation does not explain the high level of aberrant EAAT2 mRNA. In another study no EAAT2 mutations were found at all, suggesting that genomic mutations in the EAAT2 gene are rare causes of ALS [7].

The exact mechanism, which leads to impaired glutamate transporter activity and protein localization, and RNA-stability, has not been fully elucidated yet [141]. Glutamate-carriers are also directly damaged by oxidative stress. In transgenic mice with the A4V and I113T mutation, oxidative reactions, triggered by hydrogen peroxide and mutant SOD1, inactivate EAAT2 [109]. Inactivation of EAAT2 results in motor neuron death, suggesting that SOD1 mutations mediate toxicity through an excitotoxic mechanism [8]. This hypothesis is substantiated by findings in transgenic SOD1 G93A mice, which exhibited increased sensitivity to glutamate, possibly through decreased glutamate transporter activity [8]. Glutamate transporters may be impaired in ALS also through modification by 4-hydroxynonenal (HNE), a product of membrane lipid peroxidation. Interestingly, HNE is detoxified differently by the ApoE ε2, ε3, and ε4 allele. ApoE ε4 has the least capacity to neutralize HNE.

Further arguments for the glutamate-hypothesis of ALS are, that the glutamate analogue β-N-oxalyl-L-α,β-di-amino-proprionate (β-ODAP and BOAA) seems to induce upper motor neuron lesion in lathyrism and that β-methylamino-L-alanine (BMAA) is implicated in the Guam ALS syndrome. The discrepancy between quick reaction of the glutamate-receptors and the slow decline of motor neurons is explained by chronic triggering of the calcium release or by a modifying effect of EAAT2-expressing astrocytes. This is in line with damage of astrocytes and consecutive reduction of GLT1 and neurodegeneration in some SOD1 mutants [8,87,135,142].

Microglial Activation

Proliferation and activation of microglia is a prominent histological feature of ALS and there is considerable experimental evidence that microglial activation plays a role in motor neuron degeneration [4]. In G93A SOD1 transgenic mice there is up-regulation of pro-inflammatory factors in the pre-symptomatic phase and prominent and sustained microglial response throughout disease progression [143,144]. This is associated with an increased level of COX-2 mRNA and protein and an increase in PGE2. Furthermore, it has been reported that aluminum can reverse motor neuron degeneration by inhibiting microglial activation and microglial-mediated cell death [145]. Effects of microglial activation are up-regulation of NOS, increased generation of ROS and glutamate, and activation of IL-1, resulting in further astrocytes activation and upregulation of COX-2 and PGE2 [4].

Copper and Zinc Toxicity

Each SOD1 subunit contains one atom Cu++ and Zn++. Most SOD1 mutations do not seem to result in the exposure of its copper and zinc molecules towards other molecules. However, some SOD1 mutations go along with conformational changes through which copper is exposed at the active site [8]. Accordingly, copper chelates (trientine) improved the survival of isolated SOD1 G93A motor neurons by 46% [91]. Since free copper is neurotoxic, the amount of free copper is physiologically maintained at less than one atom per cell, by means of the copper chaperone for SOD1 (CCS). CCS co-localizes with SOD1 in healthy and ALS motor neurons and directly inserts copper into the apo-enzyme [8]. SOD1 and CCS are highly homologous concerning the conserved region, which is responsible for the homodimerization of SOD1. This region contains many Cu++ and Zn++ ligands, but also most of the SOD1 mutations. In the SOD1 mutations H46R and H48Q copper is completely absent, because the corresponding ligands, which link SOD1 to CCS, are also missing. Presumably, the attempt of CCS to install copper fails in these mutants, why copper ions are released. An argument for an interaction of SOD1 and CCS is the co-localization of SOD1 and CCS in FALS patients and that CCS null mice have normal SOD1 levels but reduced SOD1 activity [5]. However, in a study on FALS patients no linkage to the human CCS gene on chromosome 11 could be demonstrated [5,143,146].

In mutant SOD1, insertion of copper and zinc into the proper sites is impaired, but more pronounced for copper than zinc, why the copper/zinc ratio is reduced. Impaired metal binding of mutant SOD1 may thus be the common effect of all SOD1 mutations [8]. Conformation change of mutant SOD1 results in reduced capacity to buffer neurotoxic copper and zinc. Since mutant SOD1 has a reduced affinity to zinc compared to that of NFs, zinc is removed from SOD1 to NFs. This may result in reduced O_2^- scavenging and increased catalyzation of tyrosin nitration by $ONOO^-$. Depending on its amount of copper and zinc, SOD1 mutants can be divided into a group, which carries levels of copper and zinc similar to that of wild-type and into a second group, in which levels of copper and zinc are markedly decreased [60]. In the second group of SOD1 mutants misfolding of the zinc site has been observed. SOD1 mutants of the second group are poorly metalated with zinc and copper, being primed for aggregation without further modification. By contrast, SOD1 mutants of the first group undergo site-specific oxidative damage, compromising the ability of these mutants to bind metal ions and converting them to forms prone to aggregation [60]. A further indication for involvement of metal ions in the development of ALS is the increased immunoreactivity of metallothionin in ALS. Metallthionin is involved in the homeostasis and detoxification of metal-ions, particularly zinc, and in the scavangening of ROS [5].

Mitochondrial Damage and Apoptosis

Another possible effect of SOD1 mutations is dysfunction and disruption of mitochondria [4,6]. This is substantiated by presynaptic accumulation of abnormally shaped and structured mitochondria in motor nerve terminals, reduced cytochrome oxidase activity, and increased complex I or II activity [4,147]. Mitochondrial disruption may be due to oxidative damage. Particularly mitochondrial DNA (mtDNA) is vulnerable to oxidative stress. This is because mtDNA is not only characterized by a 10 times higher mutation rate compared to nuclear DNA, but additionally has no effective repair-mechanism and no histones. Since the CNS carries a particularly high amount of ROS, CNS mitochondria are particularly exposed towards oxidative stress. Oxidative stress-induced damage of mtDNA, proteins and phospholipids increases with age. Oxidative damage of mitochondria leads to mitochondrial mutations and reduced activity or respiratory chain enzymes, in particular cytochrome c oxidase and succinat-dehydrogenase. Mitochondrial damage also leads to altered calcium homeostasis, resulting in increased cytochrome c release [4].

Generally, cell death may be either due to necrosis or apoptosis. Necrosis is a passive type of cell death due to a stimulus alterating cell metabolism, typified by the presence of clusters of degenerating neurons and associated with an inflammatory response. Apoptosis is energy-dependent and a more active pathway, defined as programmed cell death, triggered by a single stimulus, which initiates a cascade of well-recognized reactions [5]. Apoptosis tends to affect individual cells without an inflammatory response and is characterized by blebbing of the cell membrane [4]. Death of motor neurons, observed in ALS is apoptotic. Stimulation of apoptosis requires the activation of caspases. There are 2 primary pathways of caspase activation: by cell death-receptors of the TNF-family (Fas/CD95, type-1 TNF-receptor, death-receptor 3), or by intracellular stimuli from dysfunctional mitochondria (mtDNA damage, ceramide generation), leading to the release of cytochrome c. There are proteins, which have an anti-apoptotic effect (bcl-2, bcl-x_L, a1, mcl-1, boo), some, which have an apoptotic effect (bax, bcl-x_S, bak, mtd), and some, which combine both effects (bad, bik, hrk, bim, blk).

Other proteins involved in apoptosis are, carboxy-fullerenes, interleukin-1β-converting enzyme (ICE, caspase I), SOD1, p53, MAP-kinases (c-Jun, p38), anti-apoptotic transcription factors (AP-1, NF-κB), and prostate apoptosis response-4 protein (par4). Over-expression of bcl-2, bax and carboxy-fullerenes, and inhibition of caspase I, or wild-type SOD1 respectively, have a cell protective effect. ICE, on the contrary, is apoptotic. Without additional oxidative stress, mutant SOD1 is not capable to activate ICE. If SOD1 mutants also activate the p53 cascade, is controversially discussed. At least par-4 is over-expressed in the spinal cord of ALS patients [4,148]. There is also increased expression of the death-receptor Fas/CD95 [149], redistribution of bax and bak, caspase-3 activation and increased p53 expression in ALS [150]. Another marker of apoptosis identified in ALS tissue is the Le^Y antigen. There are also elevated levels of bcl-2 mRNA, and bax mRNA in ALS lumbar spine.

Autoimmunity and Inflammation

After detection of antibodies against various calcium channels in SALS, an immunological basis of ALS was proposed. Although there may be a role for antibodies in the pathogenesis of ALS, it is rather unlikely that they are responsible for the primary pathogenic process [5]. However, reactive microglia and astrocytes are abundant in pathologically affected areas of human ALS. These may release pro-inflammatory molecules, which propagate the neurodegenerative process. Also the role of anti-Fas antibodies, which are elevated in FALS, SALS and Parkinson's disease, remains to be elucidated [32].

Growth Factors

Growth factors were proposed to have an essential pathogenic role in the development of ALS, because motor neuron death can be prevented by application of neurotrophic factors, because insulin growth factor binding proteins are significantly increased in the serum of ALS patients, because insulin-growth-factor-1 and insulin are decreased in these patients, and because mutations in the gene encoding for LIF, a potent survival factor of motor neurons, have been found in ALS patients [5].

Infections

The role of viral infections in the pathogenesis of ALS remains controversial. In some studies it was not possible to cultivate viruses from CNS tissues of ALS patients. By contrast, other studies report on indications for a viral involvement in the pathogenesis of FALS. They found enterovirus-RNA-sequences in 88% of SALS patients and increased activity of the reverse transcriptase in SALS patients [5,151].

Environmental Factors

There are indications that aluminum and food toxins play a role in the pathogenesis of SALS. An argument for this hypothesis is that abstention from cycad plants, which are particularly consumed on the Marian islands, resulted in a marked decline in the incidence of endemic Guam ALS syndrome [5,141,142,152].

Further Suspected Pathomechanisms

Investigating protein expression in a cell-culture model of FALS by a proteasomic approach, seven up-regulated (arginine succinate synthase, arginine succinate lyase, neuronal nitric oxide synthase, RNA binding protein 3, peroxiredoxin 1, proteasome subunit b5, glutathione S-transferase (GST) alpha2) and seven down-regulated proteins (GST mu1, GST mu2, GST mu5, GST mux, GST piB, leukotrien B12, 12-hydroxy-dehydrogenase, proteasome subunit b5i) were detected [116]. These findings provided further evidence for involvement of alterations in the antoxidant defense, proteasome function, and nitric oxide metabolism in the pathogenesis of FALS. Furthermore, recent studies on transgenic mice showed, that the toxic effect of SOD1 mutations may be caused by reduced activity of calcineurin, an enzyme regulating neuronal excitability by controlling the activity of ion channels and the release of neurotransmitter [153]. Expression of FALS in neuroblastoma cell lines induced calcineurin-dependent activation of nuclear factor-kappa B (NF-κB) [154]. In neuroblastoma hybrid cells, expressing the SOD1 G93A mutation, a defect in neurite outgrowth was described, being attributed to a cytoskeletal defect [155]. Recent data also indicate a role for connective tissue growth factor (CTGF) in the complex reactive process, which is associated with motor neuron degeneration. The dramatically increased CTGF levels in astrocytes of the ventral horns suggest a role for CTGF in the mechanisms underlying astroglyosis in ALS [156]. Recent research also points to involvement of down-regulated cdk5 activity in the pathogenesis of mutant SOD1-mediated diseases [157].

Pathoklisis (Selective Vulnerability)

Why mutations in different genes all result in the degeneration of motor neurons and a similar phenotype is unknown. Elucidation of the physiological function of these genes may contribute to the clarification of the pathogenic consequences of these mutations. It is also unclear why motor neurons are selectively affected in FALS patients, although SOD1 and alsin are ubiquitously distributed proteins. Possible causes of selective vulnerability of motor neurons in ALS include: motor neurons have a particularly high energy demand and thus a particularly high mitochondrial activity with extensive oxidative stress; AMPA-receptors are particularly permeable in motor neurons; Ca++-binding proteins parvalbumin and calbindin D28k are reduced in motor neurons or are not expressed at all; NFs accumulate particularly in motor neurons, impairing the axonal transport and the sprouting of axons; abnormal collagen is produced [141]. Most likely, a combination of the above mentioned factors is responsible for the selectivity of the anterior horn cell affection. However, there are also indications that cell death is not restricted to motor neurons, but only pretended by the usually short survival time. After prolonged survival the disease process additionally affects also sensory fibers, fibers of the spino-rubral tracts, vegetative fibers and fibers of the frontal cortex.

Therapy

Approved Therapy

Since there is still no causal treatment of FALS, which can prevent disease progression, therapy is largely supportive [8]. Supportive measures include physiotherapy to prevent muscle contractions and joint stiffness, devices to maintain mobility and independence (ankle-foot orthoses, head supports, mobile arm supports, bathroom aids) and drugs or other measures for the relief of distressing symptoms, such as spasticity (baclofen, tizanidine, dantrolene), cramps (vitamin E, magnesium, quinine sulfate, low dose diazepam, carbamazepine, phenytoin), fatigue (pyridostigmine), depression and pseudobulbar affect (serotonin reuptake inhibitors, amitriptyline), sialhorrea (hyoscine transdermal patches, atropin, scopolamine, dimenhydramine, glycopyrolate, amitriptyline, portable suction devices, beta-blockers or carbocysteine to reduce viscosity, low dose parotid irradiation if drugs fail), constipation (review medication, adequate fluid intake, bulk-forming or osmotic laxatives, glycerol suppositories), and pain (physiotherapy, opioids opiates) [158,159].

Riluzole (2x50mg), a glutamate-antagonist, which impedes the presynaptic release of glutamate, and which represents the only approved remedy for ALS, prolongs the survival time of SALS patients by some months [160]. Symptomatic therapy with analgesics and antispastics respectively, in reasonable dosages is indicated in case of pain in unstable joints or in case of extensive spasticity with sudden cramping or sleep disturbances. In case of sleep disorders, treatment should be directed towards the cause of insomnia (respiratory insufficiency, anxiety, depression, cramps, inability to change position). If there are pronounced bulbar symptoms and absent swallowing function, implantation of a percutaneous gastroenterostomia is indicated. Those FALS types, which are associated with Parkinson symptoms, may profit from a treatment with anti-Parkinson medication. Decarboxylase-inhibitors are the treatment of choice in cases associated with dementia [4,158].

The management of respiratory complications include early recognition and treatment of aspirate pneumonia with antibiotics, chest physiotherapy, postural drainage to clear secretions, sleeping in upright position, sublingual benzodiazepines for severe anxiety and dyspnea, and small doses of opiates to ease breathlessness in terminal stages. The possibility of non-invasive positive-pressure supportive respiratory therapy or complete mechanical ventilation should be discussed with the patient and his relatives already as soon as the diagnosis is established [55,141,161,162]. A valuable screening test to establish the need of a non-invasive ventilation is nocturnal pulse-oximetry [163]. Interventions for respiratory failure should be seen in the context of the wishes, needs and expectations of those affected by the disease [4,158].

Ineffective Therapy

Antioxidants like vitamin E and polyphenoles were only of limited effect in the treatment of FALS [164]. A beneficial effect from vitamin E, has been demonstrated only in transgenic SOD1 mice and in cell cultures [5]. Topiramate, even in doses of 800 mg/day did not have a beneficial effect on the disease course [84]. Intrathecal administration of recombinant human SOD1 did not result in a benefit in two patients with FALS [165]. Gabapentine did not slow the decline of muscle strength or pulmonary function in 204 ALS patients [166]. Lamotrigine (100 mg/day) reduced the frequency of fasciculations but was otherwise ineffective [166]. Other ineffective drugs were L-threonine, guanidine, branched-chain amino-acids, dextrometorphan, L-DOPA, L-deprenyl, amantadine, gangliosides, N-acetylcystein, reduced glutathion, coenzyme Q, creatine, physostigmin, pyridostigmin, diaminopyridine, tetra-hydro-amino-acridine, Ca++-channel-blockers (verapamil, nifedipine, nimodipine), intravenous immunoglobulins, corticosteroids, azathioprin, α-interferon, high-dose cyclophosphamide, plasmapheresis, total lymphoid irradiation, thyreotropin releasing-factor, ciliary neurotrophic factor, glial cell-derived neurotrophic factor, brain-derived neurotrophic factor (BDNF), insulin-like growth factor, tilorone, and modified snake venom [4].

Promising, Experimental Therapy

Some beneficial effects (delayed onset, prolonged survival, impaired function) were observed with modified catalase, given subcutaneously, the copper chelate D-penicillamine, trientine, ascorbate, lysine acetylsalicylate, and blocking of caspase I by blocking N-benzyl-oxy-carbonyl-Val-Asp-fluoro-methyl-ketone (zVAD-fmk) [58]. Administration of the AMPA antagonist LY300164 resulted in a non-statistical trend towards slower deterioration of muscle power than those receiving placebo. Also the AMPA-receptor antagonist NBQX prolonged survival in a transgenic mouse model of ALS [167]. Ultra-high dosages of methyl-cobalamin resulted in an increased compound muscle action potential in 12 patients [166]. In a small phase II trial, xaliproden, which has neurotrophic and neuroprotective properties, yielded promising results in one of two primary endpoints and positive trends [166]. Employment of recombinant adeno-associated virus to deliver bcl-2 to spinal cord motor neurons of FALS transgenic mice prevented from cell degeneration and motor deficits [168]. Treatment of FALS motor neurons with par-4 antisense oligonucleotides prevented oxidative stress-induced apoptosis and reversed the resulting mitochondrial dysfunction [5,35]. Administration of serotonin-precursor 5-hydroxy-tryptophan to SOD1 G93A mice led to improved locomotor function and survival [115]. A potential therapeutic approach may be also the inhibition of CCS or the disruption of the SOD1/CCS interaction to prevent copper-mediated toxicity [5]. Procystein has been recently shown to increase intracellular glutathion levels [169]. Administration of minocycline, a second generation tetracycline and caspase 1 and 3 inhibitor, and celecoxib, a ROS scavenger and inhibitor of cyclo-oxigenase, delayed motor neuron dysfunction in transgenic SOD1 mice [93]. Pentoxyfylline, a phosphodiesterase inhibitor, which is used in the treatment of peripheral vascular disease, has been identified as a potential therapeutic target for ALS through screening in transgenic SOD1 mice. Treatment of mice with the vascular endothelial growth factor (VEGF) stimulated survival of motor neurons under stress conditions [69]. Most interestingly, wild-type non-neuronal cells extend survival of SOD1 motor neuron cells [170]. Systemic administration of LIF in the G93A SOD1 mouse model resulted in subtle beneficial behavioral changes, like better grip strength and delayed onset of motor impairment [171]. If carboxy-fullerenes (block glutamate-receptor-mediated excitotoxicity), β2-mimetics like clenbuterol, nitromidazole (inhibitor of NOS), L-carnitine, copper chelation, inhibition of janus kinase-3, or bcl-2 over-expression, have a therapeutic benefit, is not sufficiently investigated [166]. Pramipexol, which has been shown to reduce oxidative stress, reduces 3-hydroxy-bencoic acid, a reliable marker of increased free radical activation in SALS patients [172]. A prospective, future therapeutic option may be gene therapy, like stem cell therapy [173].

Genetic Counseling

Sufficient genetic counseling requires thorough data about the individual disease expression, number of offsprings, cause of death, and data of at least 4 subsequent generations. Additionally, the diagnosis of FALS needs to be a definite one. In case of autosomal recessive FALS with a penetrance of 100% the likelihood for FALS to have been transmitted to the F1 generation is 50%. In case of reduced penetrance, genetic counseling becomes unreliable. If the pedigree is incomplete, the risk to develop FALS amounts to that between the normal population (1/1000) and 50%. If the disease is present only in a single generation, this may indicate SALS or an autosomal recessive form. The risk in such a family to be homozygous is 25%. The actual risk, however, is also dependent on age and penetrance. Presymptomatic genetic testing is feasible, but should be carried out only in individuals at risk from families with proven FALS and FALS with high penetrance. First or second-degree relatives of FALS patients should be tested only in case of the SOD1 D90A mutation, which can be found also in SALS patients. Also SALS patients homozygous for the D90A SOD1 mutation should undergo presymptomatic genetic screening [7].

Conclusions and Future Perspectives

Since the first descriptions of FALS more than 150 years ago, a lot of progress has been made, concerning the elucidation of the pathogenic background of the disease. Since 1993 mutations in several genes (SOD1, alsin, tau) have been detected. Current evidence indicates that motor neuron death in ALS reflects a complex interplay between genetic factors, oxidative stress, toxic activation of SOD1 aggregates, glutamate-receptors and damage to critical proteins. The pathogenic importance of these factors may vary in different subgroups of patients. The development of adequate cellular and animal models for defining the precise molecular targets affected by these mechanisms will allow the development of therapies, which target the specific molecular damage in ALS motor neurons. Another main goal of future FALS research will be the detection of further defective genes. Detection of such genes would not only facilitate the detection of affected and suspected individuals, but would also elucidate the underlying pathogenic background of such mutations. Based upon such new insights effective therapies may evolve. One among various such therapies could be over-expression of wild-type SOD1 in FALS patients with heterozygous SOD1 mutations [55]. Despite intensive research and scientific effort, FALS remains a major diagnostic, therapeutic, and research challenge.

References

[1] Andersen PM, Sims KB, Xin WW, Kiely R, O'Neill G, Ravits J, Pioro E, Harati Y, Brower RD, Levine JS, Heinicke HU, Seltzer W, Boss M, Brown RH Jr. Sixteen novel mutations in the Cu/Zn superoxide dismutase gene in amyotrophic lateral sclerosis: a decade of discoveries, defects and disputes. *Amyotroph Lateral Scler Other Motor Neuron Disord* 2003; 4: 62-73.

[2] Strong M, Rosenfeld J. Amyotrophic lateral sclerosis: A review of current concepts. *Amyotroph Lateral Scler Other Motor Neuron Disord* 2003; 4: 136-143.

[3] Swash M, Desai J. Motor neuron disease: classification and nomenclature. *Amyotroph Lateral Scler Other Motor Neuron Disord* 2000; 1: 105-112.

[4] Strong MJ. The basic aspects of therapeutics in amyotrophic lateral sclerosis. *Pharmacol Ther* 2003; 98: 379-414.

[5] Hand CK, Rouleau GA. Familial amyotrophic lateral sclerosis. *Muscle Nerve* 2002; 25: 135-159.

[6] Majoor-Krakauer D, Willems PJ, Hofman A. Genetic epidemiology of amyotrophic lateral sclerosis. *Clin Genet* 2003; 63: 83-101.

[7] Brown RH, Meininger V, Swash M (eds.). *Amyotrophic lateral sclerosis*. Martin Dunitz, London, 2000

[8] Al-Chalabi A, Leigh PN. Recent advances in amyotrophic lateral sclerosis. *Curr Opinion Neurol* 2000; 13: 397-405

[9] Siddique T, Figlewicz DA, Pericak-Vance MA, Haines JL, Rouleau G, Jeffers AJ, Sapp P, Hung WY, Bebout J, McKenna-Yasek D, et al. Linkage of a gene causing familial

amyotrophic lateral sclerosis to chromosome 21 and evidence of genetic-locus heterogeneity. *N Engl J Med* 1991; 324: 1381-1384.

[10] Rosen DR, Siddique T, Patterson D, Figlewicz DA, Sapp P, Hentati A, Donaldson D, Goto J, O'Regan JP, Deng HX. Mutations in Cu/Zn superoxide dismutase gene are associated with familial amyotrophic lateral sclerosis. *Nature* 1993; 362: 59-62.

[11] Hadano S, Hand CK, Osuga H, Yanagisawa Y, Otomo A, Devon RS, Miyamoto N, Showguchi-Miyata J, Okada Y, Singaraja R, Figlewicz DA, Kwiatkowski T, Hosler BA, Sagie T, Skaug J, Nasir J, Brown RH Jr, Scherer SW, Rouleau GA, Hayden MR, Ikeda JE. A gene encoding a putative GTPase regulator is mutated in familial amyotrophic lateral sclerosis 2. *Nat Genet* 2001; 29: 166-173.

[12] Hadano S, Yanagisawa Y, Skaug J, Fichter K, Nasir J, Martindale D, Koop BF, Scherer SW, Nicholson DW, Rouleau GA, Ikeda J, Hayden MR. Cloning and characterization of three novel genes, ALS2CR1, ALS2CR2, and ALS2CR3, in the juvenile amyotrophic lateral sclerosis (ALS2) critical region at chromosome 2q33-q34: candidate genes for ALS2. *Genomics* 2001; 71: 200-213.

[13] Yang Y, Hentati A, Deng HX, Dabbagh O, Sasaki T, Hirano M, Hung WY, Ouahchi K, Yan J, Azim AC, Cole N, Gascon G, Yagmour A, Ben-Hamida M, Pericak-Vance M, Hentati F, Siddique T. The gene encoding alsin, a protein with three guanine-nucleotide exchange factor domains, is mutated in a form of recessive amyotrophic lateral sclerosis. *Nat Genet* 2001; 29: 160-165.

[14] Hu MT, Ellis CM, Al-Chalabi A, Leigh PN, Shaw CE. Flail arm syndrome: a distinctive variant of amyotrophic lateral sclerosis. *J Neurol Neurosurg Psychiatry* 1998; 65: 950-951.

[15] Carri MT, Ferri A, Cozzolino M, Calabrese L, Rotilio G. Neurodegeneration in amyotrophic lateral sclerosis: the role of oxidative stress and altered homeostasis of metals. *Brain Res Bull* 2003; 61: 365-374.

[16] Govoni V, Granieri E, Capone J, Manconi M, Casetta I. Incidence of amyotrophic lateral sclerosis in the local health district of Ferrara, Italy, 1964-1998. *Neuroepidemiology* 2003; 22: 229-234.

[17] Mandrioli J, Faglioni P, Merelli E, Sola P. The epidemiology of ALS in Modena, Italy. *Neurology* 2003; 60: 683-689.

[18] Okumura H. Epidemiological and clinical patterns of western pacific amyotrophic lateral sclerosis (ALS) in Guam and sporadic ALS in Rochester, Minnesota, U.S.A. and Hokkaido, Japan: a comparative study. *Hokkaido Igaku Zasshi* 2003; 78: 187-195.

[19] Kuzuhara S. Amyotrophic lateral sclerosis-parkinsonism-dementia complex of the Kii peninsula of Japan. *Rinsho Shinkeigaku* 2002; 42: 1073-1076.

[20] Arisato T, Okubo R, Arata H, Abe K, Fukada K, Sakoda S, Shimizu A, Gin XH, Izumo S, Osame M, Nakagawa M. Clinical and pathological studies of familial amyotrophic lateral sclerosis (FALS) with SOD1 H46R mutation in large Japanese families. *Acta Neuropathol* 2003; 106: 561-568.

[21] Watanabe Y, Kato S, Adachi Y, Nakashima K. Frameshift, nonsense and non amino acid altering mutations in SOD1 in familial ALS: report of a Japanese pedigree and literature review. *Amyotroph Lateral Scler Other Motor Neuron Disord* 2000; 1: 251-258.

[22] Malaspina A, Alimonti D, Poloni TE, Ceroni M. Disease clustering: the example of ALS, PD, dementia and hereditary ataxias in Italy. *Funct Neurol* 2002; 17: 177-182.

[23] Corcia P, Khoris J, Couratier P, Mayeux-Portas V, Bieth E, De Toffol B, Autret A, Muh JP, Andres C, Camu W. SMN1 gene study in three families in which ALS and spinal muscular atrophy co-exist. *Neurology* 2002; 59: 1464-1466.

[24] Gourie-Devi M, Nalini A, Sandhya S. Early or late appearance of "dropped head syndrome" in amyotrophic lateral sclerosis. *J Neurol Neurosurg Psychiatry* 2003; 74: 683-686.

[25] Scelsa SN, Yakubov B, Salzman SH. Dyspnea-fasciculation syndrome: early respiratory failure in ALS with minimal motor signs. *Amyotroph Lateral Scler Other Motor Neuron Disord* 2002; 3: 239-243.

[26] Alexander MD, Traynor BJ, Miller N, Corr B, Frost E, McQuaid S, Brett FM, Green A, Hardiman O. "True" sporadic ALS associated with a novel SOD-1 mutation. *Ann Neurol* 2002; 52: 680-683.

[27] Kobayashi M, Ikeda K, Kinoshita M, Iwasaki Y. Amyotrophic lateral sclerosis with supranuclear ophthalmoplegia and rigidity. *Neurol Res* 1999; 21: 661-664.

[28] Lomen-Hoerth C, Anderson T, Miller B. The overlap of amyotrophic lateral sclerosis and frontotemporal dementia. *Neurology* 2002; 59: 1077-1079.

[29] Mantovan MC, Baggio L, Dalla Barba G, Smith P, Pegoraro E, Soraru' G, Bonometto P, Angelini C. Memory deficits and retrieval processes in ALS. *Eur J Neurol* 2003; 10: 221-227.

[30] Toyoshima Y, Piao YS, Tan CF, Morita M, Tanaka M, Oyanagi K, Okamoto K, Takahashi H. Pathological involvement of the motor neuron system and hippocampal formation in motor neuron disease-inclusion dementia. *Acta Neuropathol (Berl)* 2003; 106: 50-56.

[31] Mizutani K, Oka N, Kusunoki S, Kaji R, Kanda M, Akiguchi I, Shibasaki H. Amyotrophic lateral sclerosis with IgM antibody against gangliosides GM2 and GD2. *Intern Med* 2003; 42: 277-280.

[32] Sengun IS, Appel SH. Serum anti-Fas antibody levels in amyotrophic lateral sclerosis. *J Neuroimmunol* 2003; 142: 137-140.

[33] Yi FH, Lautrette C, Vermot-Desroches C, Bordessoule D, Couratier P, Wijdenes J, Preud'homme JL, Jauberteau MO. In vitro induction of neuronal apoptosis by anti-Fas antibody-containing sera from amyotrophic lateral sclerosis patients. *J Neuroimmunol* 2000; 109: 211-220.

[34] Chad DA. Electrodiagnostic approach to the patient with suspected motor neuron disease. *Neurol Clin* 2002; 20: 527-555.

[35] Eisen A. Clinical electrophysiology of the upper and lower motor neuron in amyotrophic lateral sclerosis. *Semin Neurol* 2001; 21: 141-154.

[36] Krivickas LS. Amyotrophic lateral sclerosis and other motor neuron diseases. *Phys Med Rehabil Clin N Am* 2003; 14: 327-345.

[37] Finsterer J, Fuglsang-Frederiksen A, Mamoli B. Needle EMG of the tongue: motor unit action potential versus peak ratio analysis in limb and bulbar onset amyotrophic lateral sclerosis. *J Neurol Neurosurg Psychiatry* 1997; 63: 175-180.

[38] Finsterer J, Erdorf M, Mamoli B, Fuglsang-Frederiksen A. Needle electromyography of bulbar muscles in patients with amyotrophic lateral sclerosis: evidence of subclinical involvement. *Neurology* 1998; 51: 1417-1422.

[39] Mills KR. The natural history of central motor abnormalities in amyotrophic lateral sclerosis. *Brain* 2003; 126: 2558-2566.

[40] Zanette G, Tamburin S, Manganotti P, Refatti N, Forgione A, Rizzuto N. Different mechanisms contribute to motor cortex hyperexcitability in amyotrophic lateral sclerosis. *Clin Neurophysiol* 2002; 113: 1688-1697.

[41] Ellis CM, Simmons A, Dawson JM, Williams SC, Leigh PN. Distinct hyperintense MRI signal changes in the corticospinal tracts of a patient with motor neuron disease. *Amyotroph Lateral Scler Other Motor Neuron Disord* 1999; 1: 41-44.

[42] Pohl C, Block W, Karitzky J, Traber F, Schmidt S, Grothe C, Lamerichs R, Schild H, Klockgether T. Proton magnetic resonance spectroscopy of the motor cortex in 70 patients with amyotrophic lateral sclerosis. *Arch Neurol* 2001; 58: 729-735.

[43] Przedborski S, Dhawan V, Donaldson DM, Murphy PL, McKenna-Yasek D, Mandel FS, Brown RH Jr, Eidelberg D. Nigrostriatal dopaminergic function in familial amyotrophic lateral sclerosis patients with and without copper/zinc superoxide dismutase mutations. *Neurology* 1996; 47: 1546-1551.

[44] Karlsborg M, Andersen EB, Wiinberg N, Gredal O, Jorgensen L, Mehlsen J. Sympathetic dysfunction of central origin in patients with ALS. *Eur J Neurol* 2003; 10: 229-234.

[45] Hishikawa N, Niwa J, Doyu M, Ito T, Ishigaki S, Hashizume Y, Sobue G. Dorfin localizes to the ubiquitylated inclusions in Parkinson's disease, dementia with Lewy bodies, multiple system atrophy, and amyotrophic lateral sclerosis. *Am J Pathol* 2003; 163: 609-619.

[46] Rabin BA, Griffin JW, Crain BJ, Scavina M, Chance PF, Cornblath DR. Autosomal dominant juvenile amyotrophic lateral sclerosis. *Brain* 1999; 122: 1539-1550.

[47] Kato S, Funakoshi H, Nakamura T, Kato M, Nakano I, Hirano A, Ohama E. Expression of hepatocyte growth factor and c-Met in the anterior horn cells of the spinal cord in the patients with amyotrophic lateral sclerosis (ALS): immunohistochemical studies on sporadic ALS and familial ALS with superoxide dismutase 1 gene mutation. *Acta Neuropathol (Berl)* 2003; 106: 112-120.

[48] Kikuchi H, Yamada T, Furuya H, Doh-ura K, Ohyagi Y, Iwaki T, Kira J. Involvement of cathepsin B in the motor neuron degeneration of amyotrophic lateral sclerosis. *Acta Neuropathol (Berl)* 2003; 105: 462-468.

[49] Caparros-Lefebvre D, Sergeant N, Lees A, Camuzat A, Daniel S, Lannuzel A, Brice A, Tolosa E, Delacourte A, Duyckaerts C. Guadeloupean parkinsonism: a cluster of progressive supranuclear palsy-like tauopathy. *Brain* 2002; 125: 801-811.

[50] Traynor BJ, Codd MB, Corr B, Forde C, Frost E, Hardiman O. Amyotrophic lateral sclerosis mimic syndromes: a population-based study. *Arch Neurol* 2000; 57: 109-113.

[51] Bclsh JM. ALS diagnostic criteria of El Escorial Revisited: do they meet the needs of clinicians as well as researchers? *Amyotroph Lateral Scler Other Motor Neuron Disord* 2000; 1(suppl 1): S57-S60.

[52] Miller RG, Munsat TL, Swash M, Brooks BR. Consensus guidelines for the design and implementation of clinical trials in ALS. World Federation of Neurology committee on Research. *J Neurol Sci* 1999; 169: 2-12.

[53] Traynor BJ, Codd MB, Corr B, Forde C, Frost E, Hardiman OM. Clinical features of amyotrophic lateral sclerosis according to the El Escorial and Airlie House diagnostic criteria: A population-based study. *Arch Neurol* 2000; 57: 1171-1176.

[54] Michael poon's shrine of neurology. Modified version of the formal ElEscorial criteria. http://www.angelfire.com/retro/michaelpoon168/el_escorial_criteria_for_MND,htm

[55] Patel SA, Maragakis NJ. Amyotrophic lateral sclerosis: pathogenesis, differential diagnoses, and potential interventions. *J Spinal Cord Med* 2002; 25: 262-273.

[56] Finsterer J. Mitochondriopathy as a differential diagnosis of amyotrophic lateral sclerosis. *Amyotroph Lateral Scler Other Motor Neuron Disord* 2002; 3: 219-224.

[57] Ceroni M, Curti D, Alimonti D. Amyotrophic lateral sclerosis and SOD1 gene: an overview. *Funct Neurol* 2001; 16(suppl 4): 171-180.

[58] Orrell RW, Figlewicz DA. Clinical implications of the genetics of ALS and other motor neuron diseases. *Neurology* 2001; 57: 9-17.

[59] Strange RW, Antonyuk S, Hough MA, Doucette PA, Rodriguez JA, Hart PJ, Hayward LJ, Valentine JS, Hasnain SS. The structure of holo and metal-deficient wild-type human Cu, Zn superoxide dismutase and its relevance to familial amyotrophic lateral clerosis. *J Mol Biol* 2003; 328: 877-871.

[60] Valentine JS, Hart PJ. Misfolded CuZnSOD and amyotrophic lateral sclerosis. *Proc Natl Acad Sci USA* 2003; 100: 3617-3622.

[61] Noor R, Mittal S, Iqbal J. Superoxide dismutase - applications and relevance to human diseases. *Med Sci Monit* 2002; 8: RA210-215.

[62] Inoue M, Sato EF, Nishikawa M, Park AM, Kira Y, Imada I, Utsumi K. Cross talk of nitric oxide, oxygen radicals, and superoxide dismutase regulates the energy metabolism and cell death and determines the fates of aerobic life. *Antioxid Redox Signal* 2003; 5: 475-484.

[63] Hough MA, Hasnain SS. Structure of fully reduced bovine copper zinc superoxide dismutase at 1.15 A. Structure (Camb) 2003; 11: 937-946.

[64] Gaudette M, Hirano M, Siddique T. Current status of SOD1 mutations in familial amyotrophic lateral sclerosis. *Amyotroph Lateral Scler Other Motor Neuron Disord* 2000; 1: 83-89.

[65] Beckman JS, Carson M, Smith CD, Koppenol WH. ALS, SOD and peroxynitrite. *Nature* 1993; 364: 584.

[66] Robberecht W. Oxidative stress in amyotrophic lateral sclerosis. *J Neurol* 2000; 247 (suppl 1): I1-6.

[67] Orrell RW. Amyotrophic lateral sclerosis: copper/zinc superoxide dismutase (SOD1) gene mutations. *Neuromuscul Disord* 2000; 10: 63-68.

[68] Andersen PM, Forsgren L, Binzer M, Nilsson P, Ala-Hurula V, Keranen ML, Bergmark L, Saarinen A, Haltia T, Tarvainen I, Kinnunen E, Udd B, Marklund SL. Autosomal recessive adult-onset amyotrophic lateral sclerosis associated with homozygosity for Asp90Ala CuZn-superoxide dismutase mutation. A clinical and genealogical study of 36 patients. *Brain* 1996; 119: 1153-1172.

[69] Lambrechts D, Storkebaum E, Morimoto M, Del-Favero J, Desmet F, Marklund SL, Wyns S, Thijs V, Andersson J, van Marion I, Al-Chalabi A, Bornes S, Musson R, Hansen V, Beckman L, Adolfsson R, Pall HS, Prats H, Vermeire S, Rutgeerts P, Katayama S, Awata T, Leigh N, Lang-Lazdunski L, Dewerchin M, Shaw C, Moons L, Vlietinck R, Morrison KE, Robberecht W, Van Broeckhoven C, Collen D, Andersen PM, Carmeliet P. VEGF is a modifier of amyotrophic lateral sclerosis in mice and humans and protects motoneurons against ischemic death. *Nat Genet* 2003; 34: 383-394.

[70] Valentine JS. Do oxidatively modified proteins cause ALS? *Free Radic Biol Med* 2002; 33: 1314-1320.

[71] Alsod.org. The als online database for mutations in als related genes. www.alsod.org,

[72] Cardoso RM, Thayer MM, DiDonato M, Lo TP, Bruns CK, Getzoff ED, Tainer JA. Insights into Lou Gehrig's disease from the structure and instability of the A4V mutant of human Cu,Zn superoxide dismutase. *J Mol Biol* 2002; 324: 247-256.

[73] Ishigaki S, Niwa J, Ando Y, Yoshihara T, Sawada K, Doyu M, Yamamoto M, Kato K, Yotsumoto Y, Sobue G. Differentially expressed genes in sporadic amyotrophic lateral sclerosis spinal cords - screening by molecular indexing and subsequent cDNA microarray analysis. *FEBS Lett* 2002; 531: 354-358.

[74] Kato S, Takikawa M, Nakashima K, Hirano A, Cleveland DW, Kusaka H, Shibata N, Kato M, Nakano I, Ohama E. New consensus research on neuropathological aspects of familial amyotrophic lateral sclerosis with superoxide dismutase 1 (SOD1) gene mutations: inclusions containing SOD1 in neurons and astrocytes. *Amyotroph Lateral Scler Other Motor Neuron Disord* 2000; 1: 163-184.

[75] Lindberg MJ, Tibell L, Oliveberg M. Common denominator of Cu/Zn superoxide dismutase mutants associated with amyotrophic lateral sclerosis: Decreased stability of the apo state. *Proc Natl Acad Sci USA* 2002; 99: 16607-16612

[76] Parton MJ, Broom W, Andersen PM, Al-Chalabi A, Nigel Leigh P, Powell JF, Shaw CE. D90A-SOD1 mediated amyotrophic lateral sclerosis: a single founder for all cases with evidence for a cis-acting disease modifier in the recessive haplotype. *Hum Mutat* 2002; 20: 473.

[77] Xu Z. Mechanism and treatment of motoneuron degeneration in ALS: what have SOD1 mutants told us? *Amyotroph Lateral Scler Other Motor Neuron Disord* 2000; 1: 225-234.

[78] Rezania K, Yan J, Dellefave L, Deng HX, Siddique N, Pascuzzi RT, Siddique T, Roos RP. A rare Cu/Zn superoxide dismutase mutation causing familial amyotrophic lateral sclerosis with variable age of onset, incomplete penetrance and a sensory neuropathy. *Amyotroph Lateral Scler Other Motor Neuron Disord* 2003; 4: 162-166.

[79] DiDonato M, Craig L, Huff ME, Thayer MM, Cardoso RM, Kassmann CJ, Lo TP, Bruns CK, Powers ET, Kelly JW, Getzoff ED, Tainer JA. ALS mutants of human superoxide dismutase form fibrous aggregates via framework destabilization. *J Mol Biol* 2003; 332: 601-615.

[80] Khare SD, Ding F, Dokholyan NV. Folding of Cu, Zn Superoxide Dismutase and Familial Amyotrophic Lateral Sclerosis. *J Mol Biol* 2003; 334: 515-525.

[81] Pieri M, Albo F, Gaetti C, Spalloni A, Bengtson CP, Longone P, Cavalcanti S, Zona C. Altered excitability of motor neurons in a transgenic mouse model of familial amyotrophic lateral sclerosis. *Neurosci Lett* 2003; 351: 153-156.

[82] Pieri M, Gaetti C, Spalloni A, Cavalcanti S, Mercuri N, Bernardi G, Longone P, Zona C. alpha-amino-3-hydroxy-5-methyl-isoxazole-4-propionate receptors in spinal cord motor neurons are altered in transgenic mice overexpressing human Cu,Zn superoxide dismutase (Gly(93)-->Ala) mutation. *Neuroscience* 2003; 122: 47-58.

[83] Ito K, Uchiyama T, Fukutake T, Arai K, Kanesaka T, Hattori T. Different clinical phenotypes of siblings with familial amyotrophic lateral sclerosis showing Cys146Arg point mutation of superoxide dismutase 1 gene. *Rinsho Shinkeigaku* 2002; 42: 175-177.

[84] Cudkowicz ME, Shefner JM, Schoenfeld DA, Brown Jr RH Jr, Johnson H, Qureshi M, Jacobs M, Rothstein JD, Appel SH, Pascuzzi RM, Heiman-Patterson TD, Donofrio PD, David WS, Russell JA, Tandan R, Pioro EP, Felice KJ, Rosenfeld J, Mandler RN, Sachs GM, Bradley WG, Raynor EM, Baquis GD, Belsh JM, Novella S, Goldstein J, Hulihan J. A randomized, placebo-controlled trial of topiramate in amyotrophic lateral sclerosis. *Neurology* 2003; 61: 456-464.

[85] Aksoy H, Dean G, Elian M, Deng HX, Deng G, Juneja T, Storey E, McKinlay Gardner RJ, Jacob RL, Laing NG, Siddique T. A4T mutation in the SOD1 gene causing familial amyotrophic lateral sclerosis. *Neuroepidemiology* 2003; 22: 235-238.

[86] Radunovic A, Leigh PN. ALSODatabase: database of SOD1 (and other) gene mutations in ALS on the Internet. European FALS Group and ALSOD Consortium. *Amyotroph Lateral Scler Other Motor Neuron Disord* 1999; 1: 45-49.

[87] Shaw CE, al-Chalabi A, Leigh N. Progress in the pathogenesis of amyotrophic lateral sclerosis. *Curr Neurol Neurosci Rep* 2001; 1: 69-76.

[88] Mancuso M, Filosto M, Naini A, Rocchi A, Del Corona A, Sartucci F, Siciliano G, Murri L. A screening for superoxide dismutase-1 D90A mutation in Italian patients with sporadic amyotrophic lateral sclerosis. *Amyotroph Lateral Scler Other Motor Neuron Disord* 2002; 3: 215-218.

[89] Ben Hamida M, Hentati F, Ben Hamida C. Juvenile amyotrophic lateral sclerosis. Study of 43 cases. *Bull Acad Natl Med* 1992; 176: 213-219;

[90] Eymard-Pierre E, Lesca G, Dollet S, Santorelli FM, di Capua M, Bertini E, Boespflug-Tanguy O. Infantile-onset ascending hereditary spastic paralysis is associated with mutations in the alsin gene. *Am J Hum Genet* 2002; 71: 518-527.

[91] Nagano S, Fujii Y, Yamamoto T, Taniyama M, Fukada K, Yanagihara T, Sakoda S. The efficacy of trientine or ascorbate alone compared to that of the combined treatment with these two agents in familial amyotrophic lateral sclerosis model mice. *Exp Neurol* 2003; 179: 176-180.

[92] Otomo A, Hadano S, Okada T, Mizumura H, Kunita R, Nishijima H, Showguchi-Miyata J, Yanagisawa Y, Kohiki E, Suga E, Yasuda M, Osuga H, Nishimoto T, Narumiya S, Ikeda JE. ALS2, a novel guanine nucleotide exchange factor for the small GTPase Rab5, is implicated in endosomal dynamics. *Hum Mol Genet* 2003; 12: 1671-1687.

[93] Zhu X, Perry G, Smith MA. Amyotrophic lateral sclerosis: a novel hypothesis involving a gained 'loss of function' in the JNK/SAPK pathway. *Redox Rep* 2003; 8: 129-133.

[94] Devon RS, Helm JR, Rouleau GA, Leitner Y, Lerman-Sagie T, Lev D, Hayden MR. The first nonsense mutation in alsin results in a homogeneous phenotype of infantile-onset ascending spastic paralysis with bulbar involvement in two siblings. *Clin Genet* 2003; 64: 210-215.

[95] Ruddy DM, Parton MJ, Al-Chalabi A, Lewis CM, Vance C, Smith BN, Leigh PN,Powell JF, Siddique T, Meyjes EP, Baas F, de Jong V, Shaw CE. Two families with familial amyotrophic lateral sclerosis are linked to a novel locus on chromosome 16q. *Am J Hum Genet* 2003; 73: 390-396.

[96] Hand CK, Khoris J, Salachas F, Gros-Louis F, Lopes AA, Mayeux-Portas V, Brewer CG, Brown RH Jr, Meininger V, Camu W, Rouleau GA. A novel locus for familial amyotrophic lateral sclerosis, on chromosome 18q. *Am J Hum Genet* 2002; 70: 251-256.

[97] Chance PF, Rabin BA, Ryan SG, Ding Y, Scavina M, Crain B, Griffin JW, Cornblath DR. Linkage of the gene for an autosomal dominant form of juvenile amyotrophic lateral sclerosis to chromosome 9q34. *Am J Hum Genet* 1998; 62: 633-640.

[98] Hosler BA, Siddique T, Sapp PC, Sailor W, Huang MC, Hossain A, Daube JR,Nance M, Fan C, Kaplan J, Hung WY, McKenna-Yasek D, Haines JL, Pericak-Vance MA, Horvitz HR, Brown RH Jr. Linkage of familial amyotrophic lateral sclerosis with frontotemporal dementia to chromosome 9q21-q22. *JAMA* 2000; 284: 1664-1669.

[99] Abalkhail H, Mitchell J, Habgood J, Orrell R, de Belleroche J. A new familial amyotrophic lateral sclerosis locus on chromosome 16q12.1-16q12.2. *Am J Hum Genet* 2003; 73: 383-389.

[100] Sapp PC, Hosler BA, McKenna-Yasek D, Chin W, Gann A, Genise H, Gorenstein J, Huang M, Sailer W, Scheffler M, Valesky M, Haines JL, Pericak-Vance M, Siddique T, Horvitz HR, Brown RH Jr. Identification of two novel loci for dominantly inherited familial amyotrophic lateral sclerosis. *Am J Hum Genet* 2003; 73: 397-403.

[101] Siddique T, Pericak-Vance MA, Caliendo J, Hong ST, Hung WY, Kaplan J, McKenna-Yasek D, Rimmler JB, Sapp P, Saunders AM, Scott WK, Siddique N, Haines JL, Brown RH. Lack of association between apolipoprotein E genotype and sporadic amyotrophic lateral sclerosis. *Neurogenetics* 1998; 1: 213-216.

[102] Hulette CM, Pericak-Vance MA, Roses AD, Schmechel DE, Yamaoka LH, Gaskell PC, Welsh-Bohmer KA, Crowther RA, Spillantini MG. Neuropathological features of frontotemporal dementia and parkinsonism linked to chromosome 17q21-22 (FTDP-17): Duke Family 1684. *J Neuropathol Exp Neurol* 1999; 58: 859-866.

[103] Kowalska A, Konagaya M, Sakai M, Hashizume Y, Tabira T. Familial amyotrophic lateral sclerosis and parkinsonism-dementia complex - tauopathy without mutations in the tau gene? *Folia Neuropathol* 2003; 41: 59-64.

[104] McGeer PL, Schwab C, McGeer EG, Haddock RL, Steele JC. Familial nature and continuing morbidity of the amyotrophic lateral sclerosis-parkinsonism dementia complex of Guam. *Neurology* 1997; 49: 400-409.

[105] Giess R, Beck M, Goetz R, Nitsch RM, Toyka KV, Sendtner M. Potential role of LIF as a modifier gene in the pathogenesis of amyotrophic lateral sclerosis. *Neurology* 2000; 54: 1003-1005.

[106] Figlewicz DA, Krizus A, Martinoli MG, Meininger V, Dib M, Rouleau GA, Julien JP. Variants of the heavy neurofilament subunit are associated with the development of amyotrophic lateral sclerosis. *Hum Mol Genet* 1994; 3: 1757-1761.

[107] Borthwick GM, Johnson MA, Ince PG, Shaw PJ, Turnbull DM. Mitochondrial enzyme activity in amyotrophic lateral sclerosis: implications for the role of mitochondria in neuronal cell death. *Ann Neurol* 1999;46:787-790.

[108] Lin CL, Bristol LA, Jin L, Dykes-Hoberg M, Crawford T, Clawson L, Rothstein JD. Aberrant RNA processing in a neurodegenerative disease: the cause for absent EAAT2, a glutamate transporter, in amyotrophic lateral sclerosis. *Neuron* 1998; 20: 589-602.

[109] Trotti D, Rolfs A, Danbolt NC, Brown RH Jr, Hediger MA. SOD1 mutants linked to amyotrophic lateral sclerosis selectively inactivate a glial glutamate transporter. *Nat Neurosci* 1999; 2: 427-433.

[110] Jackson M, Morrison KE, Al-Chalabi A, Bakker M, Leigh PN. Analysis of chromosome 5q13 genes in amyotrophic lateral sclerosis: homozygous NAIP deletion in a sporadic case. *Ann Neurol* 1996; 39: 796-800.

[111] Durham HD, Roy J, Dong L, Figlewicz DA. Aggregation of mutant Cu/Zn superoxide dismutase proteins in a culture model of ALS. *J Neuropathol Exp Neurol* 1997; 56: 523-530.

[112] Stathopulos PB, Rumfeldt JA, Scholz GA, Irani RA, Frey HE, Hallewell RA, Lepock JR, Meiering EM. Cu/Zn superoxide dismutase mutants associated with amyotrophic lateral sclerosis show enhanced formation of aggregates in vitro. *Proc Natl Acad Sci USA* 2003; 100: 7021-7026.

[113] Elam JS, Taylor AB, Strange R, Antonyuk S, Doucette PA, Rodriguez JA, Hasnain SS, Hayward LJ, Valentine JS, Yeates TO, Hart PJ. Amyloid-like filaments and water-filled nanotubes formed by SOD1 mutant proteins linked to familial ALS. *Nat Struct Biol* 2003; 10: 461-467.

[114] Valentine JS. Do oxidatively modified proteins cause ALS? *Free Radic Biol Med* 2002; 33: 1314-20.

[115] Turner BJ, Lopes EC, Cheema SS. Neuromuscular accumulation of mutant superoxide dismutase 1 aggregates in a transgenic mouse model of familial amyotrophic lateral sclerosis. *Neurosci Lett* 2003; 350: 132-136.

[116] Allen S, Heath PR, Kirby J, Wharton SB, Cookson MR, Menzies FM, Banks RE, Shaw PJ. Analysis of the cytosolic proteome in a cell-culture model of familial amyotrophic lateral sclerosis reveals alterations to the proteasome, antioxidant defences and nitric oxide synthetic pathways. *J Biol Chem* 2003; 278: 6371-6383.

[117] Echaniz-Laguna A, Zoll J, Ribera F, Tranchant C, Warter JM, Lonsdorfer J, Lampert E. Mitochondrial respiratory chain function in skeletal muscle of ALS patients. *Ann Neurol* 2002; 52: 623-627.

[118] Jung C, Higgins CM, Xu Z. Mitochondrial electron transport chain complex dysfunction in a transgenic mouse model for amyotrophic lateral sclerosis. *J Neurochem* 2002; 83: 535-545.

[119] Parkes TL, Elia AJ, Dickinson D, Hilliker AJ, Phillips JP, Boulianne GL. Extension of Drosophila lifespan by overexpression of human SOD1 in motorneurons. *Nat Genet* 1998; 19: 171-174.

[120] Melov S, Ravenscroft J, Malik S, Gill MS, Walker DW, Clayton PE,Wallace DC, Malfroy B, Doctrow SR, Lithgow GJ. Extension of life-span with superoxide dismutase/catalase mimetics. *Science* 2000; 289: 1567-1569.

[121] Mecocci P, Polidori MC, Ingegni T, Cherubini A, Chionne F, Cecchetti R, Senin U. Oxidative damage to DNA in lymphocytes from AD patients. *Neurology* 1998; 51: 1014-1017.

[122] Simpson EP, Yen AA, Appel SH. Oxidative Stress: a common denominator in the pathogenesis of amyotrophic lateral sclerosis. *Curr Opin Rheumatol* 2003; 15: 730-736.

[123] Rosen DR, Bowling AC, Patterson D, Usdin TB, Sapp P, Mezey E, McKenna-Yasek D, O'Regan J, Rahmani Z, Ferrante RJ. A frequent ala 4 to val superoxide dismutase-1 mutation is associated with a rapidly progressive familial amyotrophic lateral sclerosis. *Hum Mol Genet* 1994; 3: 981-987.

[124] Rabizadeh S, Gralla EB, Borchelt DR, Gwinn R, Valentine JS, Sisodia S, Wong P, Lee M, Hahn H, Bredesen DE. Mutations associated with amyotrophic lateral sclerosis convert superoxide dismutase from an antiapoptotic gene to a proapoptotic gene: studies in yeast and neural cells. *Proc Natl Acad Sci USA* 1995; 92: 3024-3028.

[125] Liochev SI, Fridovich I. Reversal of the superoxide dismutase reaction revisited. *Free Radic Biol Med* 2003; 34: 908-910.

[126] Ranganathan S, Bowser R. The 12th International Symposium on ALS/MND: scientific advancements in amyotrophic lateral sclerosis. November 18-20, 2001, Oakland, Calif. *Brain Pathol* 2002; 12: 511-514.

[127] Tiwari A, Hayward LJ. Familial ALS mutants of Cu/Zn superoxide dismutase are susceptible to disulfide reduction. *J Biol Chem* 2003; 278: 5954-5992.

[128] Urushitani M, Kurisu J, Tsukita K, Takahashi R. Proteasomal inhibition by misfolded mutant superoxide dismutase 1 induces selective motor neuron death in familial amyotrophic lateral sclerosis. *J Neurochem* 2002; 83: 1030-1042.

[129] Takamiya R, Takahashi M, Myint T, Park YS, Miyazawa N, Endo T, Fujiwara N, Sakiyama H, Misonou Y, Miyamoto Y, Fujii J, Taniguchi N. Glycation proceeds faster in mutated Cu, Zn-superoxide dismutases related to familial amyotrophic lateral sclerosis. *FASEB J* 2003; 17: 938-940.

[130] Aquilano K, Rotilio G, Ciriolo MR. Proteasome activation and nNOS down-regulation in neuroblastoma cells expressing a Cu,Zn superoxide dismutase mutant involved in familial ALS. *J Neurochem* 2003; 85: 1324-1335.

[131] Ge WW, Leystra-Lantz C, Wen W, Strong MJ. Selective loss of trans-acting instability determinants of neurofilament mRNA in amyotrophic lateral sclerosis spinal cord. *J Biol Chem* 2003; 278: 26558-26563.

[132] Tomkins J, Usher P, Slade JY, Ince PG, Curtis A, Bushby K, Shaw PJ. Novel insertion in the KSP region of the neurofilament heavy gene in amyotrophic lateral sclerosis *(ALS) Neuroreport* 1998; 9: 3967-3970.

[133] Bajaj NP, al-Sarraj ST, Leigh PN, Anderson V, Miller CC. Cyclin dependent kinase-5 (CDK-5) phosphorylates neurofilament heavy (NF-H) chain to generate epitopes for

antibodies that label neurofilament accumulations in amyotrophic lateral sclerosis (ALS) and is present in affected motor neurons in ALS. *Prog Neuropsychopharmacol Biol Psychiatry* 1999; 23: 833-850.

[134] Houseweart MK, Cleveland DW. Bcl-2 overexpression does not protect neurons from mutant neurofilament-mediated motor neuron degeneration. *J Neurosci* 1999; 19: 6446-6456.

[135] Cluskey S, Ramsden DB. Mechanisms of neurodegeneration in amyotrophic lateral sclerosis. *Mol Pathol* 2001; 54: 386-392.

[136] Farah CA, Nguyen MD, Julien JP, Leclerc N. Altered levels and distribution of microtubule-associated proteins before disease onset in a mouse model of amyotrophic lateral sclerosis. *J Neurochem* 2003; 84: 77-86.

[137] Chou SM, Han CY, Wang HS, Vlassara H, Bucala R. A receptor for advanced glycosylation endproducts (AGEs) is colocalized with neurofilament-bound AGEs and SOD1 in motoneurons of ALS: immunohistochemical study. *J Neurol Sci* 1999; 169: 87-92.

[138] Beaulieu JM, Nguyen MD, Julien JP. Late onset death of motor neurons in mice overexpressing wild-type peripherin. *J Cell Biol* 1999; 147: 531-544.

[139] Spreux-Varoquaux O, Bensimon G, Lacomblez L, Salachas F, Pradat PF, Le Forestier N, Marouan A, Dib M, Meininger V. Glutamate levels in cerebrospinal fluid in amyotrophic lateral sclerosis: a reappraisal using a new HPLC method with coulometric detection in a large cohort of patients. *J Neurol Sci* 2002; 193: 73-78.

[140] Kawahara Y, Kwak S, Sun H, Ito K, Hashida H, Aizawa H, Jeong SY, Kanazawa I. Human spinal motoneurons express low relative abundance of GluR2 mRNA: an implication for excitotoxicity in ALS. *J Neurochem* 2003; 85: 680-689.

[141] Ludolph AC, Meyer T, Riepe MW. The role of excitotoxicity in ALS – what is the evidence. *J Neurol* 2000; 247 (suppl 1): 7-16.

[142] Heath PR, Shaw PJ. Update on the glutamatergic neurotransmitter system and the role of excitotoxicity in amyotrophic lateral sclerosis. Muscle Nerve 2002; 26: 438-458.

[143] Elliott JL. Zinc and copper in the pathogenesis of amyotrophic lateral sclerosis. *Prog Neuropsychopharmacol Biol Psychiatry* 2001; 25: 1169-1185.

[144] Hall ED, Oostveen JA, Gurney ME. Relationship of microglial and astrocytic activation to disease onset and progression in a transgenic model of familial ALS. *Glia* 1998; 23: 249-256.

[145] He BP, Wen W, Strong MJ. Activated microglia (BV-2) facilitation of TNF-alpha-mediated motor neuron death in vitro. *J Neuroimmunol* 2002; 128: 31-28.

[146] Orlacchio A, Kawarai T, Massaro AM, St George-Hyslop PH, Sorbi S. Absence of linkage between familial amyotrophic lateral sclerosis and copper chaperone for the superoxide dismutase gene locus in two Italian pedigrees. *Neurosci Lett* 2000; 285: 83-86.

[147] Higgins CM, Jung C, Xu Z. ALS-associated mutant SOD1G93A causes mitochondrial vacuolation by expansion of the intermembrane space and by involvement of SOD1 aggregation and peroxisomes. *BMC Neurosci* 2003; 4: 16.

[148] Sathasivam S, Ince PG, Shaw PJ. Apoptosis in amyotrophic lateral sclerosis: a review of the evidence. *Neuropathol Appl Neurobiol* 2001; 27: 257-274.

[149] de la Monte SM, Sohn YK, Ganju N, Wands JR. P53- and CD95-associated apoptosis in neurodegenerative diseases. *Lab Invest* 1998; 78: 401-411.

[150] Martin LJ, Price AC, Kaiser A, Shaikh AY, Liu Z. Mechanisms for neuronal degeneration in amyotrophic lateral sclerosis and in models of motor neuron death (Review). *Int J Mol Med* 2000; 5: 3-13..

[151] McGeer PL, McGeer EG. Inflammatory processes in amyotrophic lateral sclerosis. *Muscle Nerve* 2002; 26: 459-470.

[152] Chen KM, Craig UK, Lee CT, Haddock R. Cycad neurotoxin, consumption of flying foxes, and ALS/PDC disease in Guam. *Neurology* 2002; 59: 1664-1665.

[153] Ferri A, Gabbianelli R, Casciati A, Celsi F, Rotilio G, Carri MT. Oxidative inactivation of calcineurin by Cu,Zn superoxide dismutase G93A, a mutant typical of familial amyotrophic lateral sclerosis. *J Neurochem* 2001; 79: 531-538.

[154] Casciati A, Ferri A, Cozzolino M, Celsi F, Nencini M, Rotilio G, Carri MT. Oxidative modulation of nuclear factor-kappaB in human cells expressing mutant fALS-typical superoxide dismutases. *J Neurochem* 2002; 83: 1019-1029.

[155] Lee KW, Kim HJ, Sung JJ, Park KS, Kim M. Defective neurite outgrowth in aphidicolin/cAMP-induced motor neurons expressing mutant Cu/Zn superoxide dismutase. *Int J Dev Neurosci* 2002; 20: 521-526.

[156] Spliet WG, Aronica E, Ramkema M, Aten J, Troost D. Increased expression of connective tissue growth factor in amyotrophic lateral sclerosis human spinal cord. *Acta Neuropathol (Berl).* 2003; 106: 449-457.

[157] Patzke H, Tsai LH. Cdk5 sinks into ALS. Trends Neurosci 2002; 25: 8-10.

[158] Brockington A, Shaw P. Developments in the treatment of motor neuron disease. *ACNR* 2003; 3: 13-19.

[159] Kirkinezos IG, Hernandez D, Bradley WG, Moraes CT. Regular exercise is beneficial to a mouse model of amyotrophic lateral sclerosis. *Ann Neurol* 2003;53:804-807.

[160] Bensimon G, Lacomblez L, Meininger V. A controlled trial of riluzole in amyotrophic lateral sclerosis. ALS/Riluzole Study Group. *N Engl J Med* 1994; 330: 585-591.

[161] Xu Z, Cork LC, Griffin JW, Cleveland DW. Increased expression of neurofilament subunit NF-L produces morphological alterations that resemble the pathology of human motor neuron disease. *Cell* 1993; 73: 23-33.

[162] Jackson M, Llado J, Rothstein JD. Therapeutic developments in the treatment of amyotrophic lateral sclerosis. *Expert Opin Investig Drugs* 2002; 11: 1343-1364.

[163] Pinto A, de Carvalho M, Evangelista T, Lopes A, Sales-Luis L. Nocturnal pulse oximetry: a new approach to establish the appropriate time for non-invasive ventilation in ALS patients. *Amyotroph Lateral Scler Other Motor Neuron Disord* 2003; 4: 31-35.

[164] Di Matteo V, Esposito E. Biochemical and therapeutic effects of antioxidants in the treatment of Alzheimer's disease, Parkinson's disease, and amyotrophic lateral sclerosis. *Curr Drug Target CNS Neurol Disord* 2003; 2: 95-107.

[165] Cudkowicz ME, Warren L, Francis JW, Lloyd KJ, Friedlander RM, Borges LF,Kassem N, Munsat TL, Brown RH Jr. Intrathecal administration of recombinant human superoxide dismutase 1 in amyotrophic lateral sclerosis: a preliminary safety and pharmacokinetic study. *Neurology* 1997; 49: 213-222.

[166] Murray B, Mitsumoto H. *Drug therapy in amyotrophic lateral sclerosis. In: Pourmand H, Harati Y* (eds). Advances in Neurology. Volume 88. Neuromuscular disorders. Lippincott Williams and Wilkins 2002; 63-82

[167] Van Damme P, Leyssen M, Callewaert G, Robberecht W, Van Den Bosch L. The AMPA receptor antagonist NBQX prolongs survival in a transgenic mouse model of amyotrophic lateral sclerosis. *Neurosci Lett* 2003; 343: 81-84.

[168] Azzouz M, Hottinger A, Paterna JC, Zurn AD, Aebischer P, Bueler H. Increased motoneuron survival and improved neuromuscular function in transgenic ALS mice after intraspinal injection of an adeno-associated virus encoding Bcl-2. *Hum Mol Genet* 2000; 9: 803-811.

[169] Cudkowicz ME, Sexton PM, Ellis T, Hayden DL, Gwilt PR, Whalen J, Brown RH Jr. The pharmacokinetics and pharmaco-dynamics of Procysteine in amyotrophic lateral sclerosis. *Neurology* 1999; 52: 1492-1494.

[170] Clement AM, Nguyen MD, Roberts EA, Garcia ML, Boillee S, Rule M, McMahon AP,Doucette W, Siwek D, Ferrante RJ, Brown RH Jr, Julien JP, Goldstein LS,Cleveland DW. Wild-type nonneuronal cells extend survival of SOD1 mutant motor neurons in ALS mice. *Science* 2003; 302: 113-117.

[171] Azari MF, Lopes EC, Stubna C, Turner BJ, Zang D, Nicola NA, Kurek JB, Cheema SS. Behavioural and anatomical effects of systemically administered leukemia inhibitory factor in the SOD1(G93A G1H) mouse model of familial amyotrophic lateral sclerosis. *Brain Res* 2003; 982: 92-97.

[172] Pattee GL, Post GR, Gerber RE, Bennett JP Jr. Reduction of oxidative stress in amyotrophic lateral sclerosis following pramipexole treatment. *Amyotroph Lateral Scler Other Motor Neuron Disord* 2003; 4: 90-95.

[173] Dib M. Amyotrophic lateral sclerosis: progress and prospects for treatment. *Drugs* 2003; 63: 289-310.

[174] Ahmad-Annuar A, Shah P, Hafezparast M, Hummerich H, Witherden AS, Morrison KE, Shaw PJ, Kirby J, Warner TT, Crosby A, Proukakis C, Wilkinson P, Orrell RW,Bradley L, Martin JE, Fisher EM. No association with common Caucasian genotypes in exons 8, 13 and 14 of the human cytoplasmic dynein heavy chain gene (DNCHC1) and familial motor neuron disorders. *Amyotroph Lateral Scler Other Motor Neuron Disord* 2003; 4: 150-157.

[175] Menzies FM, Grierson AJ, Cookson MR, Heath PR, Tomkins J, Figlewicz DA, Ince PG, Shaw PJ. Selective loss of neurofilament expression in Cu/Zn superoxide dismutase (SOD1) linked amyotrophic lateral sclerosis. *J Neurochem* 2002; 82: 1118-1128.

[176] Beaulieu JM, Julien JP. Peripherin-mediated death of motor neurons rescued by overexpression of neurofilament NF-H proteins. J Neurochem 2003; 85: 248-256.

[177] Lariviere RC, Beaulieu JM, Nguyen MD, Julien JP. Peripherin is not a contributing factor to motor neuron disease in a mouse model of amyotrophic lateral sclerosis caused by mutant superoxide dismutase. *Neurobiol Dis* 2003; 13: 158-166.

[178] Guo H, Lai L, Butchbach ME, Stockinger MP, Shan X, Bishop GA, Lin CL. Increased expression of the glial glutamate transporter EAAT2 modulates excitotoxicity and

delays the onset but not the outcome of ALS in mice. *Hum Mol Genet* 2003; 12: 2519-2532.

[179] Carriedo SG, Yin HZ, Weiss JH. Motor neurons are selectively vulnerable to AMPA/kainate receptor-mediated injury in vitro. *J Neurosci* 1996; 16: 4069-4079.

[180] Siddons MA, Pickering-Brown SM, Mann DM, Owen F, Cooper PN. Debrisoquine hydroxylase gene polymorphism frequencies in patients with amyotrophic lateral sclerosis. *Neurosci Lett* 1996; 208: 65-68.

[181] Shaikh AY, Martin LJ. DNA base-excision repair enzyme apurinic/apyrimidinic endonuclease/redox factor-1 is increased and competent in the brain and spinal cord of individuals with amyotrophic lateral sclerosis. *Neuromolecular Med* 2002; 2: 47-60.

[182] Kikuchi H, Furuta A, Nishioka K, Suzuki SO, Nakabeppu Y, Iwaki T. Impairment of mitochondrial DNA repair enzymes against accumulation of 8-oxo-guanine in the spinal motor neurons of amyotrophic lateral sclerosis. *Acta Neuropathol (Berl)* 2002; 103: 408-414.

[183] LaMonte BH, Wallace KE, Holloway BA, Shelly SS, Ascano J, Tokito M, Van Winkle T, Howland DS, Holzbaur EL. Disruption of dynein/dynactin inhibits axonal transport in motor neurons causing late-onset progressive degeneration. *Neuron* 2002; 34: 715-727.

[184] Warita H, Itoyama Y, Abe K. Selective impairment of fast anterograde axonal transport in the peripheral nerves of asymptomatic transgenic mice with a G93A mutant SOD1 gene. *Brain Res* 1999; 819: 120-131.

[185] Panzara MA, Gussoni E, Begovich AB, Murray RS, Zang YQ, Appel SH, Steinman L, Zhang J. T cell receptor BV gene rearrangements in the spinal cords and cerebrospinal fluid of patients with amyotrophic lateral sclerosis. *Neurobiol Dis* 1999; 6: 392-405.

[186] Smith RG, Haverkamp LJ, Case S, Appel V, Appel SH. Apolipoprotein E epsilon 4 in bulbar-onset motor neuron disease. *Lancet* 1996; 348: 334-335.

[187] Mui S, Rebeck GW, McKenna-Yasek D, Hyman BT, Brown RH Jr. Apolipoprotein E epsilon 4 allele is not associated with earlier age at onset in amyotrophic lateral sclerosis. *Ann Neurol* 1995; 38: 460-463.

[188] Tomkins J, Banner SJ, McDermott CJ, Shaw PJ. Mutation screening of manganese superoxide dismutase in amyotrophic lateral sclerosis. *Neuroreport* 2001; 12: 2319-2322.

[189] Orrell RW, Habgood JJ, de Belleroche JS, Lane RJ. The relationship of spinal muscular atrophy to motor neuron disease: investigation of SMN and NAIP gene deletions in sporadic and familial ALS. *J Neurol Sci* 1997; 145: 55-61.

[190] Giess R, Holtmann B, Braga M, Grimm T, Muller-Myhsok B, Toyka KV, Sendtner M. Early onset of severe familial amyotrophic lateral sclerosis with a SOD-1 mutation: potential impact of CNTF as a candidate modifier gene.*Am J Hum Genet* 2002; 70: 1277-1286.

[191] Panas M, Karadima G, Kalfakis N, Psarrou O, Floroskoufi P, Kladi A, Petersen MB, Vassilopoulos D. Genotyping of presenilin-1 polymorphism in amyotrophic lateral sclerosis. *J Neurol* 2000; 247: 940-942.

[192] Flowers JM, Leigh PN, Davies AM, Ninkina NN, Buchman VL, Vaughan J, Wood NW,Powell JF. Mutations in the gene encoding human persyn are not associated with

amyotrophic lateral sclerosis or familial Parkinson's disease. *Neurosci Lett* 1999; 274: 21-24.

[193] Crawford TO, Skolasky RL Jr. The relationship of SMN to amyotrophic lateral sclerosis. *Ann Neurol* 2002; 52: 857-861.

[194] Hyun DH, Lee M, Halliwell B, Jenner P. Proteasomal inhibition causes the formation of protein aggregates containing a wide range of proteins, including nitrated proteins. *J Neurochem* 2003; 86: 363-373.

[195] Drory VE, Birnbaum M, Peleg L, Goldman B, Korczyn AD. Hexosaminidase A deficiency is an uncommon cause of a syndrome mimicking amyotrophic lateral sclerosis. *Muscle Nerve* 2003; 28: 109-112.

[196] Herpers BL, Schrama LH, Kaal EC, Joosten EA, Dop Bar PR. Microinjection of catalase cDNA prevents hydrogen peroxide-induced motoneuron death. *Neuroreport* 1999; 10: 2647-2650.

[197] Gurney ME. The use of transgenic mouse models of amyotrophic lateral sclerosis in preclinical drug studies. J Neurol Sci 1997; 152 (suppl 1): S67-73.

[198] Ripps ME, Huntley GW, Hof PR, Morrison JH, Gordon JW. Transgenic mice expressing an altered murine superoxide dismutase gene provide an animal model of amyotrophic lateral sclerosis. *Proc Natl Acad Sci USA* 1995; 92: 689-693.

[199] Wong PC, Pardo CA, Borchelt DR, Lee MK, Copeland NG, Jenkins NA, Sisodia SS, Cleveland DW, Price DL. An adverse property of a familial ALS-linked SOD1 mutation causes motor neuron disease characterized by vacuolar degeneration of mitochondria. *Neuron* 1995; 14: 1105-1116.

[200] Reaume AG, Elliott JL, Hoffman EK, Kowall NW, Ferrante RJ, Siwek DF, Wilcox HM, Flood DG, Beal MF, Brown RH Jr, Scott RW, Snider WD. Motor neurons in Cu/Zn superoxide dismutase-deficient mice develop normally but exhibit enhanced cell death after axonal injury. *Nat Genet* 1996; 13: 43-47.

[201] Lee MK, Marszalek JR, Cleveland DW. A mutant neurofilament subunit causes massive, selective motor neuron death: implications for the pathogenesis of human motor neuron disease. *Neuron* 1994; 13: 975-988.

In: Amyotrophic Lateral Sclerosis: New Research
Editor: Christine A. Murray, pp. 49-70 ISBN 1-59454-179-5

Chapter II

The Lesson We Can Learn from Familial ALS Patients Carrying a SOD1 Mutation

Cristina Cereda[1,2,*], Manuel Corato[1,2], Dario Alimonti[1,2] and Mauro Ceroni[1,2,3]

[1]Neurological Science Dept University of Pavia, Italy.
[2]Experimental Neurobiology Lab IRCCS "Neurological Foundation C. Mondino", Pavia, Italy.
[3]Neurological Dept Polyclinic of Monza, Italy.

Abstract

Amyotrophic Lateral Sclerosis (ALS) is a neurodegenerative disease causing progressive death of the motor neurons in both brain cortex and spinal cord. Twenty per cent of ALS familial cases (fALS) are caused by a mutation in the SOD1 gene.

The SOD1 gene is located in the short arm of human chromosome 21 and consists of 5 exons encoding for 153 amino acids. More than 100 mutations have been identified that are spred in all parts of the SOD1 gene; the majority of them are missense mutations but there are both insertions and deletions. Two mutations, in 126 and 141 codons, define a signal stop that produces a shorter protein. Mutations have been found also in intronic parts of the gene in two ALS cases. All mutations behave as autosomal dominant traits except for the D90A and the L84F, that exist in both dominant and recessive forms.

Attempts to correlate genotype with phenotype demonstrated that prediction of disease severity based on age of onset and disease duration on the basis of the single SOD1 mutation remains uncertain. Some mutations are associated with early onset (L38V, G37S), while others are associated with particularly short (A4V) or relatively long (D100G) disease duration. Mutations in SOD1 gene were also found in ALS patients with no family history. Subjects with SOD1 mutations (L84F, L144F and D76V) that did not develop the disease were reported. Epidemiological data underline that, in some

* Correspondence concerning this article should be addressed to: Cristina Cereda, Lab of Experimental Neurobiology, Neurologic Institute IRCCS C. Mondino, v. Brodolini, 7, 27028, S. Martino Siccomario, Pavia, Italy; Phone: +39-0382-556963; Fax: +39-0382-556615; e-mail: cristina.cereda@mondino.it

cases, a mutation is present only in a single population: A4T mutation in the Japanese population, D76V in the hispanic one, the L144F mutation in several patients coming from Slavic regions (Yugoslavia, Croatia). Correlation between sex, regional disease onset, age of onset and SOD1 gene mutations have not been found. SOD1 mutations have been divided in three groups considering the three-dimensional structure of the wt protein. One group of mutations occurs within the dimer interface (A4V), while another group is positioned in loop regions at the end of beta strands (G93A). Mutant proteins falling into these two groups appear to have full SOD1 activity and biophysical properties similar to the wt SOD1 protein. The third group of mutations is located near the metal binding site, in particular the protein region that binds copper ion. These mutant proteins (H46R, H48Q) carry little amount of copper or zinc and have biophysical properties quite different from the wt SOD1 protein.

In fALS carrying a SOD1 mutation the mutated protein is the cause for the development of ALS. In fALS various mutated SOD1 proteins show unaltered enzymatic activity, thus suggesting that the mutations in SOD1 gene may act causing a toxic "gain of function" in SOD1 rather than a loss of function. In fALS SOD1 accumulates within the cytoplasm of the motor neurons. Similarly in sporadic ALS, intracellular aggregates in motor neurons have been found, possibly containing SOD1. As ALS, several other neurodegenerative disorders, like Alzheimer's disease, Parkinson's disease and prion diseases, are characterized by the accumulation of specific proteins in the brain areas in which neuronal loss occurs. The majority of neurodegenerative disorders have both familial and sporadic presentation and the gene involved in the familial form encodes for the protein that accumulates in both familial and sporadic form. Moreover, the mutated proteins may function normally, but tend to accumulate in a conformation that hampers degradation (amyloid). While the specific features of each disorder is related to the affected neuronal population and to the protein involved, the common aspect relies in the mechanisms of cell death. In fact, many experimental data demonstrate that in neurodegenerative disorders a common apoptotic mechanism causes the neuronal death through the activation of different factors (such as cdk5, Apaf-1 and JNK) belonging to the same pathway.

We think that the neuronal cell peculiar condition of being unable to replicate is of fundamental importance in understanding neurodegeneration. In the CNS the condition of permanent neuronal cells throughout the individual life span exists only by the strict interaction between neurons and glial cells. In ALS peripheral blood cells express mutated SOD1 and display alterations in mitochondrial metabolism and calcium homeostasis, but they show no degeneration. In our hypothesis neurodegenerative diseases are the expression of a general difficulty in degradation of misfolded proteins that are toxic to the cell. Whereas replicating tissues can resolve such problem by replacing itscellular components, nervous tissue can not. This is the reason why only neurons contain the aggregated protein. This could also explain why neurodegeneration and aging are so closely related.

Keywords: Amyotrophic Lateral Sclerosis (ALS) – Familial ALS (FALS) - Superoxide Dismutase 1 (SOD1) – aggregates

1. Introduction

Amyotrophic Lateral Sclerosis (ALS) is a progressive neurodegenerative disorder affecting lower motor neurons in the spinal cord ventral horns and in the brainstem and upper motor neurons in the motor cortex. Clinically ALS is characterized by varying degrees of spasticity, weakness, wasting and atrophy of limb muscles. The muscles controlling speech, swallowing and breathing are also involved. Respiratory failure is normally the cause of death in the last stage of the disease[1]. Current therapies have only a very limited effect on disease progression.

2. Epidemiology

Worldwide ALS prevalence is estimated to be about 4 to 6 per 100,000, with an annual incidence of 0.4 to 2.2 per 100,000[2]. ALS appears to be homogeneously widespread with the exception of some disease foci where its seems to have a remarkably higher concentration of cases and to occur in a sort of mixed neurological phenotypes referred to as Amyotrophic Lateral Sclerosis and Parkinson-dementia complex (ALS/PDC)[3].

3. Familial ALS

ALS was first described over 134 years ago by Charcot as a sporadic form[4]. Mulder and Kurland have recognized the inherited form of the disease in 1955 in a comprehensive study[5]. The majority of ALS patients are sporadic (SALS), while familial cases comprise about 5-10% of all cases (FALS). Transmission is usually autosomal dominant, but a few recessive cases have been reported[6,7]. Due to the severity of this neurological disorder, most FALS cases throughout the world belong to small families with few affected members. This feature makes the allele-genotyping studies, which rely on a consistent number of sufficiently extended pedigrees, rather difficult to perform. In a number of families showing a dominant transmission of the disease and with structures suitable for allele genotyping, linkage analysis studies have identified a disease-locus in a defined region on chromosome 21q, which contains the gene that encodes a cytosolic Cu/Zn-binding Superoxide Dismutase (SOD1)[8]. In 1993 several SOD1 gene missense point mutations were firstly reported in FALS families[9]. Subsequent studies carried out on British[10] and American[11] FALS families have shown that SOD1 gene mutations accounts for about 20% of cases of inherited ALS. A higher rate of SOD1 gene mutation (about 40%) has been reported among Japanese families[12,13]. Since the first description of SOD1 mutated FALS families, over 100 mutations in SOD1 gene have been identified. In the following years linkage analyses helped to disclose a few other disease-related loci. In 2001, Yang et al.[14] and Hadano et al.[15] identified a gene located at 2q33 that is mutated in a rare recessive form of juvenile ALS.

The hereditary forms of ALS are divided in two groups, respectively adult onset and childhood/juvenile onset forms. The first group comprises five dominant transmission forms:

ALS-1, corresponding to cases with autosomal dominant transmission linked to SOD1 gene on chromosome 21q22.1[16]; ALS-3, with autosomal dominant transmission linked to chromosome 18q21[17]; ALS-6, an autosomal dominant form linked to chromosome 16q12[18]; ALS-7, with autosomal dominant transmission linked to chromosome 20p[19]; a X-linked ALS variant with predominance in man was reported in 1998, but further descriptions are lacking[20].

The second group includes both dominant and recessive forms: ALS-2, an autosomal recessive form with childhood onset and long survival, linked to mutation in a gene discovered in 2001 which is located on chromosome 2q33.2 and encodes for a protein called "alsin"[14]; ALS-4, an autosomal dominant form with juvenile onset and slow progression, linked to chromosome 9q34[21]; ALS-5, the most common of the ALS recessive forms, which has childhood onset and is linked to chromosome 15q15.1-q21.1[22].

4. SOD1 Gene and Protein

SOD1 mutations represent the only known cause of ALS development. In spite of the low percentage of ALS cases linked to mutations in SOD1 gene (less than 2% of all cases), the discovery of SOD1 mutations in FALS families had an enormous importance, giving us the first opportunity to investigate ALS pathogenesis starting from a known cause. Since 1993, many studies demonstrated the involvement of SOD1 protein and/or mechanisms related to SOD1 function and oxidative damage in the development of both familial and sporadic ALS. SOD1 gene and SOD1 protein became the most studied factor in the research on ALS aetiology.

There are three isoforms of superoxide dismutase in humans: cytosolic Cu/Zn SOD (SOD1), mithocondrial Mn SOD (SOD2) and extracellular SOD (SOD3). SOD1, SOD2 and SOD3 are ubiquitary enzymes, which inactivate the superoxide radical ($O_2^{\cdot -}$) generated as a by-product of normal and aberrant metabolic reactions. SOD enzymes convert $O_2^{\cdot -}$ into hydrogen peroxide (H_2O_2) and oxygen (O_2). In turn, the H_2O_2 is converted to H_2O by the action of glutatione peroxidase or catalase. The genes encoding for each isoenzyme are respectively located on chromosomes 21q22[23], 6q27[24] and 4p.

The SOD1 gene is located on the long arm of chromosome 21 (21q22.11) and is present as a single copy per haploid genome spanning 11kb of chromosomal DNA. Four distinct human SOD1-related sequences have been isolated from genomic DNA and characterized as pseudogenes not residing on chromosome 21[23]. SOD1 gene contains five rather small exons, coding for 153 amino acids, and four introns[25].

The dominant structural feature of Cu,Zn SuperOxi-Dismutase (SOD1) protein is an 8-stranded barrel of antiparallel beta-pleated sheet. There is one very short helical section and two long loops of non repetitive structure. The Cu and Zn are bound between the loops and one side of the beta barrel with a common histidine ligand (H63). The Cu has four histidine ligands (H46, 48, 63, 120) in a somewhat distorted square plane, and the Zn has three histidines (H63, 71, 80) and an aspartate (D83) in approximately tetrahedral arrangement. Aspartate at the 124 position is very important to correct geometry of the metal ligand sites[26].

The active protein is a 32kDa homodimer containing two copper and zinc atoms. The two subunits have essentially the same conformation and have an extensive contact area that mainly involves hydrophobic side chain interactions in the b-barrel structure[26].

SOD1 protein activity consists in neutralizing free radicals, which are normally produced within the cells and are toxic to biological systems. A SOD1 impairment leads to the generation of an excess of superoxide radicals and therefore to formation of reactive oxygen species (ROS), such as hydroxyl radicals OH^- and peroxynitrite $ONOO^-$. ROS are a potential source of damage to DNA, lipids, membranes and proteins. Oxidative stress is characterized by the imbalance between the intracellular production of free oxygen radicals and anti-oxidant defence mechanisms. Due to the discovery of SOD1 gene alterations in 20% of FALS cases, oxidative stress is considered a key element in ALS pathogenesis[27]. Despite the implication of oxidative stress in the pathogenesis of ALS and the importance of SOD1 function in balancing oxidative metabolism are evident, the exact mechanisms by which SOD1 dysfunction promotes neuronal damage in ALS remain unclear. A definite explanation of how SOD1 mutations can lead to the selective motoneuronal death in FALS has not yet been found. The most simple hypothesis is the loss of protection from free oxygen radicals due to an altered SOD1 function. Nevertheless, many experimental data, such as the finding of an unaltered enzymatic activity in the majority of mutated SOD1, are in contrast with this hypothesis. For this reason, it is likely that SOD1 mutations may exert their pathogenic effect conferring a toxic activity to the altered protein.

More than 100 SOD1 mutations have been described in all the five exons[28]. So far 19 mutations were found in exon 1, 13 in exon two, 8 in exon three, 38 in exon four and 27 in exon five. Two mutations, in 126[29] and 141[30] codons, define a signal stop that produces a shorter protein.

The majority of mutations are single base pair substitutions but a two base pair substitution in exon 1 has been described[31]. Also many deletions[30,32,33] and insertion[34,35,10] have been reported.

Interestingly, a single base pair substitution was found also in intron one[36] and four[37]. Five single substitutions are translated in polymorphisms[32,34,35]. The precious tool about the mutational SOD1 data is http://alsod.org site were several known mutations with the related clinical features and geographic localization are listed.

5. Population Data

Familial ALS cases have widespread and uniform world-wide prevalence, lacking racial and geographic predisposition. The number of SOD1 gene mutations among the British[10], American[11] and Japanese[12] families appears to be significantly higher compared to data of continental European studies. In fact the data in French[38], German[39] and Italian[40] populations reveal the lower degree of mutation.

Epidemiological data, also, underline that, in some cases, a mutation is present only in a single population: A4T[41] and C146R[42] mutations in the Japanese population , D76V[43] in the Hispanic one, the G12R mutation in the Italian population[44,45]. An additional genetic factor has been hypothesized to explain the different people distribution of SOD1 mutations.

This molecular abnormality may play a specific role in each ethnic group according to its genetic background[11].

6. Genotype- Phenotype Correlation

A number of reports of SOD1 gene mutations in familial ALS cases failed to disclose a clear association between a mutation and a specific clinical phenotype. In our opinion, a definitive genotypic-phenotypic correlation in ALS cannot yet be drawn. However, few SOD1 gene point mutations are linked to a specific clinical pattern, including age of onset, disease duration and site of disease presentation[46,47]. In fact phenotype differences are found among diverse amino acid substitutions occurring in the same codon. G93A and G93R mutations are associated respectively to a wide variability within families in disease duration and to mild form of the disease[9,48]. Moreover, the same mutation may lead to similar clinical patterns: for example A4V and H46R mutations demonstrate a consistent disease duration in all affected individuals whereas clinical pattern at onset may vary[49]. Instead the same pattern has been reported in families harbouring the L84F SOD1 gene mutation: clinical picture at onset is monomorphic in all affected individuals, whereas age of onset and disease duration vary considerably even within the same family[50]. The phenotypic heterogeneity has important implications and a substantial impact in the construction of a correct strategy of genetic counselling of individuals carrying a mutated SOD1 gene. It is difficult to provide advice to individual patients regarding disease prognosis based on the finding of a specific mutation as well as it is hard to approach a family environment where clear indications about life expectancy and disease progression are expected[46].

a. The Ala 4 Val (A4V) Mutation

The A4V mutation, initially reported in North America[51], is the most frequently occurring SOD1 gene point mutation in ALS. This mutation occurs in a low conserved site of the SOD1 gene [26,51]. Theoretically, it might be a residue of minor importance for the normal enzyme function. Nevertheless, the A4V mutation is associated to a rapid disease progression. The clinical features related to A4V mutation are as follows:

a. The age at onset varies between 55 years and 68 years in a large family originated from Central Sweden[35] or between 21 and 78 with a mean of 47.8 +/- 13.3 years in another report comprising 27 families from North America[11,51]. There is a substantial variation of the age at onset in the affected individuals belonging to families sharing this same mutation.
b. Symptoms and site of disease presentation vary from case to case. Within the same family the disease can begin from the upper limbs or from the lower limbs, or can initially affect the bulbar function[11]. The progression to the other muscular

districts does not follow an identical pattern. Dysarthria, dyspnoea, tongue atrophy with fasciculations, facial muscles palsy can appear as the first sign or at the end of the disease.

c. All patients apparently show only lower motor neurone impairment with wasting, weakness and atrophy and decreased or absent deep tendon reflexes. No pathological reflexes are present.

d. The A4V mutation is found in patients with very poor survival and a rapidly progressive form of the disease. The duration of the disease from onset to death is also variable but generally less than 2 years[52].

b. The Ile 113 Thr (I113T) Mutation

The second most common mutation in the SOD1 gene is the Ile113Thr, found in Britain[53,54], North America[55], Australia, and New Zealand families. Studies on a common founder for these families scattered all over the world but possibly linked by the same molecular abnormality have identified a possible common ancestor of Scottish origin who underwent the mutational event few centuries ago[54].

The Ile113Thr mutation has been also reported in apparently sporadic ALS cases in Scotland[53]. This could be related to the SOD1 gene mutation low penetrance or to high rate of occurrence of new mutation events or to an uncompleted/non-detailed assessment of family history in these individuals.

Ile113Thr mutation is likely to disrupt dimeric interaction of the enzyme and to produce a severe clinical form. A marked heterogeneity of the ALS clinical pattern in the Ile113Thr-mutated individuals has been reported including the coexistence in the same pedigree of patients with a rapidly progressive course and patients with a mild form of ALS[8]. The disease duration is comprised between 3 and 20 years. In spite of the high variability the ALS patients with the Ile113Thr seem to share a particularly advanced age of onset (58.9 +/- 12.6) among FALS-SOD1 related individuals[11].

c. The Leu 84 Phe (L84F) Mutation

The mutation is located in the sequence encoding for the active channel of the SOD1 enzyme. The L84F mutation can indirectly destabilise the copper ligand His46 (one of the four His residues, which stabilise the enzyme centre: His46, His48, His63, His120), affecting enzyme structure and possibly resulting in a defective packing of the molecule[26].

We have described three separate kindreds of familial ALS originated from a small Italian region[50]. Each pedigree showed only one living affected individual. The three pedigrees appeared to be unrelated. Following a detailed family history investigation dating back to the XIX century, we were unable to disclose a common origin for the three pedigrees. Molecular investigations led to the identification of the same L84F point mutation in the SOD1 gene in all affected individuals. The three families combine a total of 28 affected subjects spanning six generations with an autosomal dominant inheritance. The disease shows high penetrance which is 90% by the age of 70. The age of onset ranges between 20 and 69 years. The mean age of onset over the last four generations is 42.8 ± 11.3 years. A significantly younger age of onset ($p<0.05$) is present when generation III (mean onset age 51.5 ± 8.4) is compared to generation V (mean onset age 33 ± 10). This observation might be in keeping with a certain degree of generational anticipation, but the number of affected individuals spanning the generations is not sufficient to draw any statistically significant conclusion. The duration of the illness varies between 1.5 and 12 years with a mean of 4.8 ± 2.7 years. There is no gender prevalence. The age of onset and the duration of the illness vary considerably within the three families. In all affected individuals the clinical picture shows a predominant lower motor neuron involvement and a pattern of ascending progression of the disease. Clinical manifestations begin in the lower limbs, then spread to the upper limbs and subsequently to the bulbar muscles[50].

Shaw has described a small family with 2 affected members carrying the L84F mutation whose clinical features resemble those in the families reported by us[28]. Age of onset was respectively 55 years in the father and 45 years in the daughter. Both developed progressive muscle weakness, beginning in the legs and spreading to the upper limbs. Disease duration was 5 years in the father.

Abe and colleagues reported a Japanese family bearing a mutation in the same L84 codon with substitution of leucine for valine in the SOD1 gene[56]. They described 5 affected members distributed on three generations. Mean age at onset is 53.8 +/- 15.3 years. The disease first affects the hands manifesting with weakness and atrophy. Disease progression is rapid spreading to the 4 limbs and to the bulbar muscles and leading to death in 1.6 +/- 0.5 years.

These findings suggest that mutations in the same codon leading to a different amino acid substitution have specific clinical patterns.

d. The Codon 93

The Gly93 codon located in exon 4 seems to be particularly vulnerable, since six different amino acid substitutions have been reported in this position (G93C[9], G93R[48], G93S, G93D, G93A[9], G93V). The introduction of amino acid with side chains at position 93 is critical for the stability of the protein backbone conformation[26]. The clinical course of ALS patients bearing a SOD1 gene mutation with a change in the Gly93 position shows a high degree of variability depending on the type of amino acid substitution. Gly93Cys[9] and Gly93Asp[48] mutations are associated to a long survival with a similar mean duration of the disease: respectively 10.1 +/- 6.2 years and 10.5 +/- 5.5 years. Conversely, the Gly93Ala substitution gives rise to a shorter survival (2.2 +/- 1.5 years)[11].

A marked variability in disease duration (2 to 12 years) within and among FALS families carrying the Gly93Arg SOD1 mutation has been reported[10].

Mutations occurring in codon Gly93 show no clear correlation between a specific mutation and disease duration or age of onset, hence it is difficult to provide advice to individual patients on disease prognosis based on the detection of a specific mutation.

e. The Asp 90 Ala (D90A) Mutation

If the association between a SOD1 gene mutation and the phenotypic appearance in affected individuals is still not well known, at least in one case the molecular abnormality in SOD1 gene seems to exert a dose-dependent effect on clinical pattern according to the homozygous or heterozygous nature of the mutation. In the Scandinavian population the D90A mutation was shown to determine ALS only in homozygous individuals[57], whereas the heterozygous carriers of this mutation showed only little or no clinical signs of the disease[58]. In Belgium, the D90A heterozygous mutation was found in two families with ALS and in one sporadic case with a focal non-progressing ALS suggesting the association of a D90A mutation with an autosomal dominant pattern of inheritance[58].

Assuming that mutated SOD1 acquires a toxic function, a double dose of mutant protein would be expected to result in a more severe disease. However, homozygous patients from recessive D90A families present a mild disease with most individuals living longer than 10 years[57]. Moreover, these recessive FALS patients are characterised by a homogeneous phenotype with predominantly lower motor neuron involvement and lower limb weakness at onset. This finding is unusual since most SOD1 mutated heterozygous familial cases show phenotypic heterogeneity even within the same family. Disease phenotype for the heterozygous D90A families is not homogeneous.

Al-Chalabi identified 28 families with the D90A SOD1 allele, 8 of which have dominant transmission. The two Scandinavian cases had bulbar onset, the UK case had mainly upper motor neuron involvement, while the three Belgian and two French cases showed a variable clinical presentation with intrafamilial heterogeneity and various disease progression patterns[59]. The markedly different behaviour of the D90A mutation in FALS pedigrees of different origin has prompted the search of additional genetic factors which could act in association with the same SOD1 mutation determining a differential phenotypic expression. An haplotype study on both D90A autosomal recessive and autosomal dominant pedigrees (using six highly polymorphic microsatellite markers close to chromosome 21 SOD1 gene location) identified a common founder only in the autosomal recessive FALS suggesting the presence of a co-segregating gene interacting with the SOD1 gene mutation phenotypic expression[16].

Morita and colleagues reported a Japanese family bearing a mutation in the same D90 codon with substitution of aspartate for valine in the SOD1 gene, the D90V mutation[60]. Inheritance pattern is dominant. The clinical picture at onset is similar to the D90A heterozygous mutation and shows a lower limb involvement with an ascending trend. Disease duration is significantly shorter than D90A averaging between 2 and 3 years. Unlike the D90A mutation that demonstrates normal SOD1 activity, the D90V mutation shows reduced SOD1 activity [60].

7. Different Hypotheses About "New Property" of SOD1 Mutant Proteins

A loss of enzymatic activity of SOD1 mutant proteins has been the first hypothesis to explain the correlation between SOD1 mutations and ALS. However, although some FALS mutations may diminish the specific activity or longevity of SOD1 protein, heterodimers of many mutant enzymes retain activity [61]. Moreover even when expressed in excess, mutant subunits do not appear to alter the enzymatic activity or the stability of the wild-type subunits[62]. Studies in mice provide additional data to support the idea that loss of SOD1 enzymatic activity is not the cause of disease. The deletion of SOD1 gene in mice does not lead to developmental defects or does not cause motor neuron disease[63]. In contrast, mice expressing FALS mutant SOD1 proteins (G37R, G93A, G85R) show motor neuron loss, muscle atrophy, paralysis and death independently from the level of SOD1 activity[64,65]. An increased expression of wild-type human SOD1 proteins causes no disease[66]. The inevitable conclusion is that the mutants have acquired one or more toxic properties, irrespective of the amount of SOD1 activity retained.

A number of biochemical and biophysical studies of SOD1 mutant enzymes have been performed in an effort to identify this new toxic property of SOD1 mutated proteins. Some mutated SOD1 proteins have been synthesized starting from genes bearing FALS-related mutations using different types of expression systems: yeast[67], Baculovirus/insect cell expression system[68,69] and E. coli expression system[70,71]. The first two systems have the advantage that the wild-type and mutant human Cu,ZnSOD proteins are properly N-acetylated, whereas in the E. coli expression system they are not. It is not known if the absence of this post-translational modification significantly alters the properties of the wild-type and mutant human Cu,ZnSOD proteins.

Enzymatic activity, polypeptide half-life, resistance to proteolytic degradation and solubility of some SOD1 mutated proteins were tested in COS-1 and mouse neuroblastoma cells in order to understand the basis for the correlation between mutations of SOD1 enzyme and clinical ALS progression[72]. The various mutants showed a remarkable variation degree for activity, polypeptide half-life and resistance to proteolysis. In fact mutations at H46 and H48 dramatically reduce enzymatic activity and present a long half-life; mutations at G85 reduce the affinity of Cu,Zn protein to bind copper[72]. No biochemical characteristic correlates with clinical progression and, probably, the basis for the different life expectancies of patients in different kindreds of SOD1-linked FALS may result from an yet unidentified property of these mutant enzymes or from interaction with other genes[72].

Valentine and co-workers produced a diverse set of human SOD1 variants for biophysical and biochemical analysis using Sf21 insect cell/baculovirus system[73]. Five SOD1 mutants bearing amino acid substitutions located within the β-barrel (A4V, L38V, G41S, D90A, and G93A) were constructed. A4V SOD1, which causes an aggressive form of the disease, was considered because it could potentially disrupt the SOD1 dimer [26]. L38V, G41S, D90A are located within important turns of the β-barrel reducing the flexibility and stability of the loops. Substitution of Gly-93 with any other amino acid will perturb the Leu-38 amino acid and may disrupt the local structure[74].

Six mutants located near the active site (H46R, H48Q, G72S, D76Y, G85R and D124V) were selected because they may alter metal binding or activity. His-48 maintains in position the copper ion and supports the redox reaction between the Cu(I) and Cu(II) forms[67,75]. His-46 and Asp-124 form an extended bridge between the copper and zinc ions bound at His-71.

The G85R mutation destabilises Asp-83 responsible for the geometry of the zinc-ligand site and this interaction may disrupt the local structure[51]. G72S and D76Y were constructed to examine the importance of the zinc-binding loop for the development of the disease..

SOD1 mutants located in the β-barrel (L38V, G41S, D90A and G93A) or involving some loop residues (D76Y) have metal contents comparable with wild-type SOD1. Conversely, A4V mutant exhibits partial copper deficiency and G72S presents partial zinc deficiency compared to wild-type SOD1[73]. Moreover, all these mutants share normal coordination geometry of the Cu,Zn binding sites and full enzymatic activity.

In contrast, most SOD1 mutants bearing substitutions located near the metal binding sites, with the exception of H48Q, contain only low amounts of both copper and zinc ions. Mutation of three residues (His-46, Gly-85 or Asp-124), that participate in important hydrogen bond network, each resulted in the most severe deficiency of both copper and zinc[76]. This second group of mutants presents with SOD1 specific activity and thermal stability lower than wild-type SOD1 protein[77]. In addition, H48Q mutant presents with some differences from the other metal-binding region mutants. H48Q is the only mutant combining high affinity for both copper and zinc and very low enzymatic activity[73]. Spectroscopic characterization of this mutant indicates that the copper site has, probably, a planar geometry of metal ions binding sites more stable than wild-type CuZnSOD1 binding sites. This mutant also appears to have a redox chemistry quite different from other copper-binding mutants[78].

Considering their biochemical and biophysical properties, mutated Cu,ZnSOD proteins have been divided in two distinct groups: wild-type-like mutant proteins and metal-binding-region mutant proteins. SOD1 mutants falling into the first group appear to have full SOD1 activity and biophysical properties similar to wild-type SOD1 protein. Conversely, mutant proteins belonging to the second group have biophysical properties different from wild-type SOD1, such as a reduced ability to carry copper and zinc ions[73]. No biochemical and biophysical property is common to the two different groups of SOD1 mutants. It is possible that the SOD1 mutant proteins can catalyse reactions using substrates different from H_2O_2.

In fact two hypotheses have dominated recent discussions on the mechanism of toxicity of mutant Cu,ZnSOD proteins in ALS: the oxidative damage hypothesis and the oligomerization hypothesis[79,80]. The oxidative damage hypothesis maintains that mutant Cu,ZnSOD proteins can catalyse reactions with abnormal substrates. Dismutation of superoxide radical to H_2O_2 and O_2 requires enzyme-bound copper, which shifts from reduced (Cu^{1+}) to oxidized (Cu^{2+}) form during two asymmetric catalysis steps. SOD1 mutants probably act with aberrant oxidative chemistry and bind abnormal substrates to the active copper site. A first candidate aberrant substrate is hydrogen peroxide, which is the normal end-product of the oxidized form of the enzyme (SOD1-Cu^{2+}). Use of hydrogen peroxide as a substrate by reduced SOD1-Cu^{1+} might produce the extraordinarily reactive hydroxyl radical, thus leading to a cascade of peroxidation[81]. The second candidate aberrant substrate is peroxynitrite ($^{-}$ONOO), which can be spontaneously formed from superoxide and nitric oxide. In presence of ($^{-}$ONOO) the aberrant tyrosine protein nitration can occur with zinc-depleted SOD1 mutants [68]. In fact, these mutants are able to generate in vitro high levels of tyrosine protein nitration[70,71]. Increased levels of markers of oxidative damage have been reported in some strains of SOD1 transgenic mice[83,84], but not in others[85]; similarly, in sporadic[86,87,88] ALS patients increased markers of oxidative stress have been found, yet this is not true for SOD1-mutated FALS patients[87,88].

The oligomerization hypothesis maintains (a) that mutant Cu,ZnSOD proteins are or become misfolded and consequently oligomerize into increasingly high molecular-weight species that ultimately aggregate and end up in proteinaceous inclusions and (b) that the oligomerized or aggregated proteins are, at some stage of their formation, selectively toxic to motor neurons. Cytoplasmic inclusion bodies are a hallmark of motor neuron degeneration in ALS and have been found in tissue from familiar[89] and sporadic[89,90,91] ALS patients, and ALS-SOD1 transgenic mice[92,93]. Similar cytoplasmatic inclusions are observed in cultured COS[94] cells and cultured motor neurons expressing FALS mutant SOD1 genes[95]. Data suggest that many SOD1 mutant proteins (G93A, G85R, G37R) are able to produce aggregates in mice independently upon mutation localization in the SOD1 protein structure[96].

These proteinaceous inclusions share many similarities to aggregates described in the other neurodegenerative diseases[97]: neurofibrillary tangles (NFTs) in Alzheimer's disease[98], Lewy bodies in Parkinson's disease[99] and prion protein particles in Prion diseases[100]. Probably, the same cellular mechanism is involved in the formations of the aggresomes, but a characteristic protein is involved in each neurodegenerative disease.

Proteinaceous inclusions are large and insoluble structures that sediment upon centrifugation at low speeds (5.000Xg) and can even be seen by light microscopy. In ALS they contain Cu,ZnSOD protein as major component, but ubiquitin, neurofilament proteins, copper chaperon for SOD1 (CCS) and Hsp70 have been found too.

What is the role of these hyaline inclusions in the pathogenesis of ALS remains unclear. In particular, recent data suggest that their effect is not toxic to the cell, yet on the contrary they may have a protective role[101]. In fact, in the motor neuron disease of SOD1 transgenic mice, they can be found only at a relatively late stage, coinciding with the motor neuron death[102]. In addition, these inclusions are also present in non-neuronal cells (astrocytes and other glial cells) in which they induce no cellular death or biochemical abnormalities[92,103]. It is possible that these proteinaceous aggregates are the end product of the activation of a defensive mechanism which protects the cells from the unfolded or damaged proteins through the proteasome pathway degradation[101]. The co-precipitation of SOD1 protein with Hsp70, CCS, 20 S subunity of proteasome and ubiquitine in inclusions underlines the involvement of ubiquitin-proteasome system in the pathogenesis of neurodegenerative disease. There are evidences that mutant SOD1 proteins, but not wild-type, are poly-ubiquitinated and degraded by proteasome and that oxidative stress enhances ubiquitination of mutant SOD1[101]. In addition the formation of aggregates is accelerated when proteasome inhibitors are added to block the degradation of the abnormal proteins[104]. Recently, the hyaline inclusions were named aggresome and the process of their formation begins to be understood[105].

The process that leads to the formation of the aggresomes is complicated and, probably, involves many different cellular mechanisms. Inclusions in the cytoplasm are found at the micro tubular organization centre (MTOK or centrosome) and the process initially involves the transport of smaller aggregates along the microtubules from the cell's periphery toward MTOK[106]. Here they are incorporated into the larger aggresomes, where they await degradation by the proteasomes or packaging into larger inclusion bodies[107]. The aggresome may function as a storage compartment that protect cells by temporarily isolating the denatured potentially damaging proteins, until they can be refolded or digested by proteasomes. Recent data suggest that the aggregate formation is a reversible process: the restoration or increase of proteasome function is able to clear and remove already formed SOD1-positive complexes in spinal cord of mutant SOD1 transgenic mice[108].

SOD1 mutant proteins, that do not fold correctly or that are abnormal, are degraded in the ubiquitin-proteasomal pathway. If abnormal SOD1 proteins overcome the degradation capacity of proteasomes, they may aggregate and form ubiquitinated cellular inclusions. This process seems to be closely connected with the pathogenesis of several neurodegenerative diseases, and we think that the neuronal cell peculiar condition of being unable to replicate is of fundamental importance in understanding neurodegeneration. In the CNS the condition of permanent neuronal cells throughout the individual life span exists only by the strict interaction between neurons and glial cells[92].

In sporadic ALS peripheral blood cells express mutated SOD1 and display alterations in mitochondria metabolism and calcium homeostasis, but they show no degeneration[109]. In our hypothesis neurodegenerative diseases are the expression of a general difficulty in degradation of misfolded proteins that are toxic to the cells. Whereas replicating tissues can resolve such problem by replacing damaged cells, nervous tissue can not. This is the reason why only neurons contain the aggregated protein. This could also explain why neurodegeneration and aging are so closely related.

References

[1] Williams DB, Windebank AJ. *Motor neuron disease.* In Dyck pj, Thomas PK, Griffin JW, Low PA, Pouslo JF, eds. Peripheral neuropathy. Philadelphia: WB saunders 1993:1028-1050

[2] Mulder DW, Kurland LT. Motor neuron disease: epidemiologic studies. *Adv Exp Med Biol.* 1987;209:325-332

[3] Wiederholt WC. Neuroepidemiologic research initiatives on Guam: past and present. *Neuroepidemiology.* 1999;18(6):279-91

[4] Charcot JM, Joffroy A. Deux cas d'atrophie musculaire progressive avec lésions de la substance grise et des faisceaux antéro-latéraux de la moelle épinière. *Arch Physiol Neurol Path* 1869 ;2:744-760

[5] Kurland LT, Mulder DW. Epidemiologic investigations of amyotrophic lateral sclerosis. 2. Familial aggregations indicative of dominant inheritance. *Neurology*. 1955 Mar;5(3):182-96

[6] Andersen PM, Nilsson P, Ala-Hurula V, Keranen ML, Tarvainen I, Haltia T, Nilsson L, Binzer M, Forsgren L, Marklund SL. Amyotrophic lateral sclerosis associated with homozygosity for an Asp90Ala mutation in CuZn-superoxide dismutase. *Nat Genet*. 1995 May;10(1):61-6

[7] Hentati A, Bejaoui K, Pericak-Vance MA, Hentati F, Speer MC, Hung WY, Figlewicz DA, Haines J, Rimmler J, Ben Hamida C, et al. Linkage of recessive familial amyotrophic lateral sclerosis to chromosome 2q33-q35. *Nat Genet*. 1994 Jul;7(3):425-8

[8] Siddique T, Nijhawan D, Hentati A. Molecular genetic basis of familial ALS. *Neurology*. 1996 Oct;47(4 Suppl 2):S27-34

[9] Rosen DR, Siddique T, Patterson D, Figlewicz DA, Sapp P, Hentati A, Donaldson D, Goto J, O'Regan JP, Deng HX, et al. Mutations in Cu/Zn superoxide dismutase gene are associated with familial amyotrophic lateral sclerosis. *Nature*. 1993 Mar 4;362(6415):59-62

[10] Orrell RW, Habgood JJ, Gardiner I, King AW, Bowe FA, Hallewell RA, Marklund SL, Greenwood J, Lane RJ, deBelleroche J. Clinical and functional investigation of 10 missense mutations and a novel frameshift insertion mutation of the gene for copper-zinc superoxide dismutase in UK families with amyotrophic lateral sclerosis. *Neurology*. 1997 Mar;48(3):746-51

[11] Cudkowicz ME, McKenna-Yasek D, Sapp PE, Chin W, Geller B, Hayden DL, Schoenfeld DA, Hosler BA, Horvitz HR, Brown RH. Epidemiology of mutations in superoxide dismutase in amyotrophic lateral sclerosis. *Ann Neurol*. 1997 Feb;41(2):210-21

[12] Abe K, Aoki M, Ikeda M, Watanabe M, Hirai S, Itoyama Y. Clinical characteristics of familial amyotrophic lateral sclerosis with Cu/Zn superoxide dismutase gene mutations. *J Neurol Sci*. 1996 Mar;136(1-2):108-16

[13] Watanabe Y, Kuno N, Kono Y, Nanba E, Ohama E, Nakashima K, Takahashi K. Absence of the mutant SOD1 in familial amyotrophic lateral sclerosis (FALS) with two base pair deletion in the SOD1 gene. *Acta Neurol Scand*. 1997 Mar;95(3):167-72

[14] Yang Y, Hentati A, Deng HX, Dabbagh O, Sasaki T, Hirano M, Hung WY, Ouahchi K, Yan J, Azim AC, Cole N, Gascon G, Yagmour A, Ben-Hamida M, Pericak-Vance M, Hentati F, Siddique T. The gene encoding alsin, a protein with three guanine-nucleotide exchange factor domains, is mutated in a form of recessive amyotrophic lateral sclerosis. *Nat Genet*. 2001 Oct;29(2):160-5

[15] Hadano S, Hand CK, Osuga H, Yanagisawa Y, Otomo A, Devon RS, Miyamoto N, Showguchi-Miyata J, Okada Y, Singaraja R, Figlewicz DA, Kwiatkowski T, Hosler BA, Sagie T, Skaug J, Nasir J, Brown RH Jr, Scherer SW, Rouleau GA, Hayden MR, Ikeda JE. A gene encoding a putative GTPase regulator is mutated in familial amyotrophic lateral sclerosis 2. *Nat Genet*. 2001 Oct;29(2):166-73

[16] Figlewicz DA, McInnis MG, Goto J, Haines JL, Warren AC, Krizus A, Khodr N, Brown RH Jr, McKenna-Yasek D, Antonarakis SE, et al. Identification of flanking

markers for the familial amyotrophic lateral sclerosis gene ALS1 on chromosome 21. *J Neurol Sci.* 1994 Jul;124 Suppl:90-5

[17] Hand CK, Khoris J, Salachas F, Gros-Louis F, Lopes AA, Mayeux-Portas V, Brewer CG, Brown RH Jr, Meininger V, Camu W, Rouleau GA. A novel locus for familial amyotrophic lateral sclerosis, on chromosome 18q. *Am J Hum Genet.* 2002 Jan;70(1):251-6. Epub 2001 Nov 09

[18] Ruddy DM, Parton MJ, Al-Chalabi A, Lewis CM, Vance C, Smith BN, Leigh PN, Powell JF, Siddique T, Meyjes EP, Baas F, de Jong V, Shaw CE. Two families with familial amyotrophic lateral sclerosis are linked to a novel locus on chromosome 16q. *Am J Hum Genet.* 2003 Aug;73(2):390-6. Epub 2003 Jul 01

[19] Sapp PC, Hosler BA, McKenna-Yasek D, Chin W, Gann A, Genise H, Gorenstein J, Huang M, Sailer W, Scheffler M, Valesky M, Haines JL, Pericak-Vance M, Siddique T, Horvitz HR, Brown RH Jr. Identification of two novel loci for dominantly inherited familial amyotrophic lateral sclerosis. *Am J Hum Genet.* 2003 Aug;73(2):397-403. Epub 2003 Jul 09

[20] Hand CK, Rouleau GA. Familial amyotrophic lateral sclerosis. *Muscle Nerve.* 2002 Feb;25(2):135-59

[21] Blair IP, Bennett CL, Abel A, Rabin BA, Griffin JW, Fischbeck KH, Cornblath DR, Chance PF. A gene for autosomal dominant juvenile amyotrophic lateral sclerosis (ALS4) localizes to a 500-kb interval on chromosome 9q34. *Neurogenetics.* 2000 Sep;3(1):1-6

[22] Hentati A, Ouahchi K, Pericak-Vance MA, Nijhawan D, Ahmad A, Yang Y, Rimmler J, Hung W, Schlotter B, Ahmed A, Ben Hamida M, Hentati F, Siddique T. Linkage of a commoner form of recessive amyotrophic lateral sclerosis to chromosome 15q15-q22 markers. *Neurogenetics.* 1998 Dec;2(1):55-60

[23] Groner Y, gieman-Hurwitz J, Dafri N, et al. *The human Cu/Zn superoxide dismutase gene family: architecture and expression of the 21-encoded functionel gene and its processed pseudogenes.* In Rotilis G, ed Superoxide and superoxide dismutase in chemystry, biology and medicine. Amsterdam: Elsiever Science Publishers, Biochemical Division, 1986:247-255

[24] Sarto C, Frutiger S, Cappellano F, Sanchez JC, Doro G, Catanzaro F, Hughes GJ, Hochstrasser DF, Mocarelli P. Modified expression of plasma glutathione peroxidase and manganese superoxide dismutase in human renal cell carcinoma. *Electrophoresis.* 1999 Nov;20(17):3458-66

[25] Levanon D, Lieman-Hurwitz J, Dafni N, Wigderson M, Sherman L, Bernstein Y, Laver-Rudich Z, Danciger E, Stein O, Groner Y. Architecture and anatomy of the chromosomal locus in human chromosome 21 encoding the Cu/Zn superoxide dismutase. *EMBO J.* 1985 Jan;4(1):77-84

[26] Richardson J, Thomas KA, Rubin BH, Richardson DC. Crystal structure of bovine Cu,Zn superoxide dismutase at 3 A resolution: chain tracing and metal ligands. *Proc Natl Acad Sci U S A.* 1975 Apr;72(4):1349-53

[27] Radunovic A, Leigh PN. Cu/Zn superoxide dismutase gene mutations in amyotrophic lateral sclerosis: correlation between genotype and clinical features. *J Neurol Neurosurg Psychiatry.* 1996 Dec;61(6):565-72

[28] Shaw CE, Enayat ZE, Chioza BA, Al-Chalabi A, Radunovic A, Powell JF, Leigh PN. Mutations in all five exons of SOD-1 may cause ALS. *Ann Neurol.* 1998 Mar;43(3):390-4

[29] Zu JS, Deng HX, Lo TP, Mitsumoto H, Ahmed MS, Hung WY, Cai ZJ, Tainer JA, Siddique T. Exon 5 encoded domain is not required for the toxic function of mutant SOD1 but essential for the dismutase activity: identification and characterization of two new SOD1 mutations associated with familial amyotrophic lateral sclerosis. *Neurogenetics.* 1997 May;1(1):65-71

[30] Andersen PM, Sims KB, Xin WW, Kiely R, O'Neill G, Ravits J, Pioro E, Harati Y, Brower RD, Levine JS, Heinicke HU, Seltzer W, Boss M, Brown RH Jr. Sixteen novel mutations in the Cu/Zn superoxide dismutase gene in amyotrophic lateral sclerosis: a decade of discoveries, defects and disputes. *Amyotroph Lateral Scler Other Motor Neuron Disord.* 2003 Jun;4(2):62-73

[31] Morita M, Aoki M, Abe K, Hasegawa T, Sakuma R, Onodera Y, Ichikawa N, Nishizawa M, Itoyama Y. A novel two-base mutation in the Cu/Zn superoxide dismutase gene associated with familial amyotrophic lateral sclerosis in Japan. *Neurosci Lett.* 1996 Feb 23;205(2):79-82

[32] Hosler BA, Nicholson GA, Sapp PC, Chin W, Orrell RW, de Belleroche JS, Esteban J, Hayward LJ, Mckenna-Yasek D, Yeung L, Cherryson AK, Dench JE, Wilton SD, Laing NG, Horvitz RH, Brown RH Jr. Three novel mutations and two variants in the gene for Cu/Zn superoxide dismutase in familial amyotrophic lateral sclerosis. *Neuromuscul Disord.* 1996 Oct;6(5):361-6

[33] Pramatarova A, Goto J, Nanba E, Nakashima K, Takahashi K, Takagi A, Kanazawa I, Figlewicz DA, Rouleau GA. A two basepair deletion in the SOD 1 gene causes familial amyotrophic lateral sclerosis. *Hum Mol Genet.* 1994 Nov;3(11):2061-2

[34] Jackson M, Al-Chalabi A, Enayat ZE, Chioza B, Leigh PN, Morrison KE. Copper/zinc superoxide dismutase 1 and sporadic amyotrophic lateral sclerosis: analysis of 155 cases and identification of a novel insertion mutation. *Ann Neurol.* 1997 Nov;42(5):803-7

[35] Andersen PM, Nilsson P, Keranen ML, Forsgren L, Hagglund J, Karlsborg M, Ronnevi LO, Gredal O, Marklund SL. Phenotypic heterogeneity in motor neuron disease patients with CuZn-superoxide dismutase mutations in Scandinavia. *Brain.* 1997 Oct;120 (Pt 10):1723-37

[36] Shaw PJ, Tomkins J, Slade JY, Usher P, Curtis A, Bushby K, Ince PG. CNS tissue Cu/Zn superoxide dismutase (SOD1) mutations in motor neurone disease (MND). *Neuroreport.* 1997 Dec 22;8(18):3923-7

[37] Sapp PC, Rosen DR, Hosler BA, Esteban J, McKenna-Yasek D, O'Regan JP, Horvitz HR, Brown RH Jr. Identification of three novel mutations in the gene for Cu/Zn superoxide dismutase in patients with familial amyotrophic lateral sclerosis. *Neuromuscul Disord.* 1995 Sep;5(5):353-7

[38] Foulard B, Camu W, Dhib M. Genetic analysis of 19 French familial Amyotrophic Lateral Sclerosis. Absence of Cu,Zn Superoxide Dismutase gene mutations. 4th International Symposium on MND/ALS 1993; November 25-27

[39] Bachus R, Claus A, Megow D, Brockmoller J, Porstmann T, Gericke CA, Riepe M, Kuther G, Zierz S, Ludolph AC. Cu,Zn SOD in German families with ALS. *J Neurol Sci.* 1995 May;129 Suppl:93-5

[40] Malaspina A, Zaman R, Mazzini L, Camana C, Poloni E, Curti D, Ceroni M. Heterogeneous distribution of amyotrophic lateral sclerosis patients with SOD-1 gene mutations: preliminary data on an Italian survey. *J Neurol Sci.* 1999 Jan 15;162(2):201-4

[41] Nakano R, Inuzuka T, Kikugawa K, Takahashi H, Sakimura K, Fujii J, Taniguchi N, Tsuji S. Instability of mutant Cu/Zn superoxide dismutase (Ala4Thr) associated with familial amyotrophic lateral sclerosis. *Neurosci Lett.* 1996 Jun 21;211(2):129-31

[42] Ito K, Uchiyama T, Fukutake T, Arai K, Kanesaka T, Hattori T. Different clinical phenotypes of siblings with familial amyotrophic lateral sclerosis showing Cys146Arg point mutation of superoxide dismutase 1 gene. Rinsho Shinkeigaku. 2002 Feb;42(2):175-7

[43] Segovia-Silvestre T, Andreu AL, Vives-Bauza C, Garcia-Arumi E, Cervera C, Gamez J. A novel exon 3 mutation (D76V) in the SOD1 gene associated with slowly progressive ALS. Amyotroph Lateral Scler Other Motor Neuron Disord. 2002 Jun;3(2):69-74

[44] Penco S, Schenone A, Bordo D, Bolognesi M, Abbruzzese M, Bugiani O, Ajmar F, Garre C. A SOD1 gene mutation in a patient with slowly progressing familial ALS. *Neurology.* 1999 Jul 22;53(2):404-6

[45] Gellera C, Castellotti B, Riggio MC, Silani V, Morandi L, Testa D, Casali C, Taroni F, Di Donato S, Zeviani M, Mariotti C. Superoxide dismutase gene mutations in Italian patients with familial and sporadic amyotrophic lateral sclerosis: identification of three novel missense mutations. *Neuromuscul Disord.* 2001 May;11(4):404-10

[46] Alimonti D, Malaspina A, Poloni TE, Ceroni M. Genotype-phenotype correlation in familial amyotrophic lateral sclerosis with SOD1 mutation. *Funct Neurol.* 2000 Jul-Sep;15(3):177-91

[47] Ceroni M, Curti D, Alimonti D. Amyotrophic lateral sclerosis and SOD1 gene: an overview. *Funct Neurol.* 2001;16(4 Suppl):171-80

[48] Elshafey A, Lanyon WG, Connor JM. Identification of a new missense point mutation in exon 4 of the Cu/Zn superoxide dismutase (SOD-1) gene in a family with amyotrophic lateral sclerosis. *Hum Mol Genet.* 1994 Feb;3(2):363-4

[49] Maurelli M, Marchioni E, Bosone D, Boni S, Bolzani W, Cerretano R, Simonetti F, Savoldi F. Familial adult amyotrophic lateral sclerosis: report of cases. *Ital J Neurol Sci.* 1992 Feb;13(1):75-9

[50] Ceroni M, Malaspina A, Poloni TE, Alimonti D, Rognoni F, Habgood J, Imbesi F, Antonelli P, Alfonsi E, Curti D, deBelleroche J. Clustering of ALS patients in central Italy due to the occurrence of the L84F SOD1 gene mutation. *Neurology.* 1999 Sep 22;53(5):1064-71

[51] Deng HX, Hentati A, Tainer JA, Iqbal Z, Cayabyab A, Hung WY, Getzoff ED, Hu P, Herzfeldt B, Roos RP, et al. Amyotrophic lateral sclerosis and structural defects in Cu,Zn superoxide dismutase. *Science.* 1993 Aug 20;261(5124):1047-51

[52] Rosen DR, Bowling AC, Patterson D, Usdin TB, Sapp P, Mezey E, McKenna-Yasek D, O'Regan J, Rahmani Z, Ferrante RJ. A frequent ala 4 to val superoxide dismutase-1 mutation is associated with a rapidly progressive familial amyotrophic lateral sclerosis. *Hum Mol Genet.* 1994 Jun;3(6):981-7

[53] Jones CT, Swingler RJ, Brock DJ. Identification of a novel SOD1 mutation in an apparently sporadic amyotrophic lateral sclerosis patient and the detection of Ile113Thr in three others. *Hum Mol Genet.* 1994 Apr;3(4):649-50

[54] Jones CT, Swingler RJ, Simpson SA, Brock DJ. Superoxide dismutase mutations in an unselected cohort of Scottish amyotrophic lateral sclerosis patients. *J Med Genet.* 1995 Apr;32(4):290-2

[55] Juneja T, Pericak-Vance MA, Laing NG, Dave S, Siddique T. Prognosis in familial amyotrophic lateral sclerosis: progression and survival in patients with glu100gly and ala4val mutations in Cu,Zn superoxide dismutase. *Neurology.* 1997 Jan;48(1):55-7

[56] Aoki M, Abe K, Houi K, Ogasawara M, Matsubara Y, Kobayashi T, Mochio S, Narisawa K, Itoyama Y. Variance of age at onset in a Japanese family with amyotrophic lateral sclerosis associated with a novel Cu/Zn superoxide dismutase mutation. *Ann Neurol.* 1995 May;37(5):676-9

[57] Andersen PM, Forsgren L, Binzer M, Nilsson P, Ala-Hurula V, Keranen ML, Bergmark L, Saarinen A, Haltia T, Tarvainen I, Kinnunen E, Udd B, Marklund SL. Autosomal recessive adult-onset amyotrophic lateral sclerosis associated with homozygosity for Asp90Ala CuZn-superoxide dismutase mutation. A clinical and genealogical study of 36 patients. *Brain.* 1996 Aug;119 (Pt 4):1153-72

[58] Robberecht W, Aguirre T, Van den Bosch L, Tilkin P, Cassiman JJ, Matthijs G. D90A heterozygosity in the SOD1 gene is associated with familial and apparently sporadic amyotrophic lateral sclerosis. : *Neurology.* 1996 Nov;47(5):1336-9

[59] Al-Chalabi A, Andersen PM, Chioza B, Shaw C, Sham PC, Robberecht W, Matthijs G, Camu W, Marklund SL, Forsgren L, Rouleau G, Laing NG, Hurse PV, Siddique T, Leigh PN, Powell JF. Recessive amyotrophic lateral sclerosis families with the D90A SOD1 mutation share a common founder: evidence for a linked protective factor. *Hum Mol Genet.* 1998 Dec;7(13):2045-50

[60] Morita M, Abe K, Takahashi M. A novel mutation Asp90Val in the SOD1 gene associated with Japanese familial ALS. *Eur J Neurol* 1998;(5):389-392

[61] Borchelt DR, Lee MK, Slunt HS, Guarnieri M, Xu ZS, Wong PC, Brown RH Jr, Price DL, Sisodia SS, Cleveland DW. Superoxide dismutase 1 with mutations linked to familial amyotrophic lateral sclerosis possesses significant activity. *Proc Natl Acad Sci U S A.* 1994 Aug 16;91(17):8292-6

[62] Borchelt DR, Guarnieri M, Wong PC, Lee MK, Slunt HS, Xu ZS, Sisodia SS, Price DL, Cleveland DW. Superoxide dismutase 1 subunits with mutations linked to familial amyotrophic lateral sclerosis do not affect wild-type subunit function. *J Biol Chem.* 1995 Feb 17;270(7):3234-8

[63] Reaume AG, Elliott JL, Hoffman EK, Kowall NW, Ferrante RJ, Siwek DF, Wilcox HM, Flood DG, Beal MF, Brown RH Jr, Scott RW, Snider WD. Motor neurons in Cu/Zn superoxide dismutase-deficient mice develop normally but exhibit enhanced cell death after axonal injury. *Nat Genet.* 1996 May;13(1):43-7

[64] Gurney ME, Pu H, Chiu AY, Dal Canto MC, Polchow CY, Alexander DD, Caliendo J, Hentati A, Kwon YW, Deng HX, et al. Motor neuron degeneration in mice that express a human Cu,Zn superoxide dismutase mutation. *Science.* 1994 Jun 17;264(5166):1772-5

[65] Ripps ME, Huntley GW, Hof PR, Morrison JH, Gordon JW. Transgenic mice expressing an altered murine superoxide dismutase gene provide an animal model of amyotrophic lateral sclerosis. *Proc Natl Acad Sci U S A.* 1995 Jan 31;92(3):689-93

[66] Wong PC, Pardo CA, Borchelt DR, Lee MK, Copeland NG, Jenkins NA, Sisodia SS, Cleveland DW, Price DL. An adverse property of a familial ALS-linked SOD1 mutation causes motor neuron disease characterized by vacuolar degeneration of mitochondria. *Neuron.* 1995 Jun;14(6):1105-16

[67] Lyons TJ, Liu H, Goto JJ, Nersissian A, Roe JA, Graden JA, Cafe C, Ellerby LM, Bredesen DE, Gralla EB, Valentine JS. Mutations in copper-zinc superoxide dismutase that cause amyotrophic lateral sclerosis alter the zinc binding site and the redox behavior of the protein. *Proc Natl Acad Sci U S A.* 1996 Oct 29;93(22):12240-4

[68] Fujii J, Myint T, Seo HG, Kayanoki Y, Ikeda Y, Taniguchi N. Characterization of wild-type and amyotrophic lateral sclerosis-related mutant Cu,Zn-superoxide dismutases overproduced in baculovirus-infected insect cells. *J Neurochem.* 1995 Apr;64(4):1456-61

[69] Okado-Matsumoto A, Myint T, Fujii J, Taniguchi N. Gain in functions of mutant Cu,Zn-superoxide dismutases as a causative factor in familial amyotrophic lateral sclerosis: less reactive oxidant formation but high spontaneous aggregation and precipitation. *Free Radic Res.* 2000 Jul;33(1):65-73

[70] Crow JP, Sampson JB, Zhuang Y, Thompson JA, Beckman JS. Decreased zinc affinity of amyotrophic lateral sclerosis-associated superoxide dismutase mutants leads to enhanced catalysis of tyrosine nitration by peroxynitrite. *J Neurochem.* 1997 Nov;69(5):1936-44

[71] Estevez AG, Crow JP, Sampson JB, Reiter C, Zhuang Y, Richardson GJ, Tarpey MM, Barbeito L, Beckman JS. Induction of nitric oxide-dependent apoptosis in motor neurons by zinc-deficient superoxide dismutase. *Science.* 1999 Dec 24;286(5449):2498-500

[72] Ratovitski T, Corson LB, Strain J, Wong P, Cleveland DW, Culotta VC, Borchelt DR. Variation in the biochemical/biophysical properties of mutant superoxide dismutase 1 enzymes and the rate of disease progression in familial amyotrophic lateral sclerosis kindreds. *Hum Mol Genet.* 1999 Aug;8(8):1451-60

[73] Hayward LJ, Rodriguez JA, Kim JW, Tiwari A, Goto JJ, Cabelli DE, Valentine JS, Brown RH Jr. Decreased metallation and activity in subsets of mutant superoxide dismutases associated with familial amyotrophic lateral sclerosis. *J Biol Chem.* 2002 May 3;277(18):15923-31. Epub 2002 Feb 19

[74] Hart PJ, Liu H, Pellegrini M, Nersissian AM, Gralla EB, Valentine JS, Eisenberg D. Subunit asymmetry in the three-dimensional structure of a human CuZnSOD mutant found in familial amyotrophic lateral sclerosis. *Protein Sci.* 1998 Mar;7(3):545-55

[75] Hart PJ, Balbirnie MM, Ogihara NL, Nersissian AM, Weiss MS, Valentine JS, Eisenberg D. A structure-based mechanism for copper-zinc superoxide dismutase. *Biochemistry.* 1999 Feb 16;38(7):2167-78

[76] Goto JJ, Zhu H, Sanchez RJ, Nersissian A, Gralla EB, Valentine JS, Cabelli DE. Loss of in vitro metal ion binding specificity in mutant copper-zinc superoxide dismutases associated with familial amyotrophic lateral sclerosis. *J Biol Chem.* 2000 Jan 14;275(2):1007-14

[77] Rodriguez JA, Valentine JS, Eggers DK, Roe JA, Tiwari A, Brown RH Jr, Hayward LJ. Familial amyotrophic lateral sclerosis-associated mutations decrease the thermal stability of distinctly metallated species of human copper/zinc superoxide dismutase. *J Biol Chem.* 2002 May 3;277(18):15932-7. Epub 2002 Feb 19

[78] Liochev SI, Chen LL, Hallewell RA, Fridovich I. Superoxide-dependent peroxidase activity of H48Q: a superoxide dismutase variant associated with familial amyotrophic lateral sclerosis. *Arch Biochem Biophys.* 1997 Oct 15;346(2):263-8

[79] Valentine JS. Do oxidatively modified proteins cause ALS? *Free Radic Biol Med.* 2002 Nov 15;33(10):1314-20

[80] Cleveland DW, Rothstein JD. From Charcot to Lou Gehrig: deciphering selective motor neuron death in ALS. *Nat Rev Neurosci.* 2001 Nov;2(11):806-19

[81] Wiedau-Pazos M, Goto JJ, Rabizadeh S, Gralla EB, Roe JA, Lee MK, Valentine JS, Bredesen DE. Altered reactivity of superoxide dismutase in familial amyotrophic lateral sclerosis. *Science.* 1996 Jan 26;271(5248):515-8

[82] Beckman JS, Carson M, Smith CD, Koppenol WH. ALS, SOD and peroxynitrite. *Nature.* 1993 Aug 12;364(6438):584

[83] Ferrante RJ, Shinobu LA, Schulz JB, Matthews RT, Thomas CE, Kowall NW, Gurney ME, Beal MF. Increased 3-nitrotyrosine and oxidative damage in mice with a human copper/zinc superoxide dismutase mutation. *Ann Neurol.* 1997 Sep;42(3):326-34

[84] Andrus PK, Fleck TJ, Gurney ME, Hall ED. Protein oxidative damage in a transgenic mouse model of familial amyotrophic lateral sclerosis. *J Neurochem.* 1998 Nov;71(5):2041-8

[85] Bruijn LI, Beal MF, Becher MW, Schulz JB, Wong PC, Price DL, Cleveland DW. Elevated free nitrotyrosine levels, but not protein-bound nitrotyrosine or hydroxyl radicals, throughout amyotrophic lateral sclerosis (ALS)-like disease implicate tyrosine nitration as an aberrant in vivo property of one familial ALS-linked superoxide dismutase 1 mutant. : *Proc Natl Acad Sci U S A.* 1997 Jul 8;94(14):7606-11

[86] Beal MF, Ferrante RJ, Browne SE, Matthews RT, Kowall NW, Brown RH Jr. Increased 3-nitrotyrosine in both sporadic and familial amyotrophic lateral sclerosis. *Ann Neurol.* 1997 Oct;42(4):644-54

[87] Shaw PJ, Ince PG, Falkous G, Mantle D. Oxidative damage to protein in sporadic motor neuron disease spinal cord. *Ann Neurol.* 1995 Oct;38(4):691-5

[88] Bowling AC, Schulz JB, Brown RH Jr, Beal MF. Superoxide dismutase activity, oxidative damage, and mitochondrial energy metabolism in familial and sporadic amyotrophic lateral sclerosis. *J Neurochem.* 1993 Dec;61(6):2322-5

[89] Shibata N, Asayama K, Hirano A, Kobayashi M. Immunohistochemical study on superoxide dismutases in spinal cords from autopsied patients with amyotrophic lateral sclerosis. *Dev Neurosci.* 1996;18(5-6):492-8

[90] Matsumoto S, Kusaka H, Ito H, Shibata N, Asayama T, Imai T. Sporadic amyotrophic lateral sclerosis with dementia and Cu/Zn superoxide dismutase-positive Lewy body-like inclusions. *Clin Neuropathol.* 1996 Jan-Feb;15(1):41-6

[91] Shibata N, Hirano A, Kobayashi M, Sasaki S, Kato T, Matsumoto S, Shiozawa Z, Komori T, Ikemoto A, Umahara T, et al. Cu/Zn superoxide dismutase-like immunoreactivity in Lewy body-like inclusions of sporadic amyotrophic lateral sclerosis. *Neurosci Lett.* 1994 Sep 26;179(1-2):149-52

[92] Bruijn LI, Becher MW, Lee MK, Anderson KL, Jenkins NA, Copeland NG, Sisodia SS, Rothstein JD, Borchelt DR, Price DL, Cleveland DW. ALS-linked SOD1 mutant G85R mediates damage to astrocytes and promotes rapidly progressive disease with SOD1-containing inclusions. *Neuron.* 1997 Feb;18(2):327-38

[93] Bruijn LI, Houseweart MK, Kato S, Anderson KL, Anderson SD, Ohama E, Reaume AG, Scott RW, Cleveland DW. Aggregation and motor neuron toxicity of an ALS-linked SOD1 mutant independent from wild-type SOD1. *Science.* 1998 Sep 18;281(5384):1851-4

[94] Koide T, Igarashi S, Kikugawa K, Nakano R, Inuzuka T, Yamada M, Takahashi H, Tsuji S. Formation of granular cytoplasmic aggregates in COS7 cells expressing mutant Cu/Zn superoxide dismutase associated with familial amyotrophic lateral sclerosis. *Neurosci Lett.* 1998 Nov 20;257(1):29-32

[95] Durham HD, Roy J, Dong L, Figlewicz DA. Aggregation of mutant Cu/Zn superoxide dismutase proteins in a culture model of ALS. *J Neuropathol Exp Neurol.* 1997 May;56(5):523-30

[96] Watanabe M, Dykes-Hoberg M, Culotta VC, Price DL, Wong PC, Rothstein JD. Histological evidence of protein aggregation in mutant SOD1 transgenic mice and in amyotrophic lateral sclerosis neural tissues. *Neurobiol Dis.* 2001 Dec;8(6):933-41

[97] Kaytor MD, Warren ST. Aberrant protein deposition and neurological disease. *J Biol Chem.* 1999 Dec 31;274(53):37507

[98] Tolnay M, Calhoun M, Pham HC, Egensperger R, Probst A. Low amyloid (Abeta) plaque load and relative predominance of diffuse plaques distinguish argyrophilic grain disease from Alzheimer's disease. *Neuropathol Appl Neurobiol.* 1999 Aug;25(4):295-305

[99] Duvoisin RC. Recent advances in the genetics of Parkinson's disease. *Adv Neurol.* 1996;69:33-40

[100] Prusiner SB, Scott MR, DeArmond SJ, Cohen FE. Prion protein biology. *Cell.* 1998 May 1;93(3):337-48

[101] Sherman MY, Goldberg AL. Cellular defenses against unfolded proteins: a cell biologist thinks about neurodegenerative diseases. *Neuron.* 2001 Jan;29(1):15-32

[102] Morrison BM, Morrison JH, Gordon JW. Superoxide dismutase and neurofilament transgenic models of amyotrophic lateral sclerosis. *J Exp Zool.* 1998 Sep-Oct 1;282(1-2):32-47

[103] Stieber A, Gonatas JO, Gonatas NK. Aggregates of mutant protein appear progressively in dendrites, in periaxonal processes of oligodendrocytes, and in neuronal and astrocytic perikarya of mice expressing the SOD1(G93A) mutation of familial amyotrophic lateral sclerosis. : *J Neurol Sci.* 2000 Aug 15;177(2):114-23

[104] Urushitani M, Kurisu J, Tsukita K, Takahashi R. Proteasomal inhibition by misfolded mutant superoxide dismutase 1 induces selective motor neuron death in familial amyotrophic lateral sclerosis. *J Neurochem.* 2002 Dec;83(5):1030-42

[105] Johonson J, Ward C, Kopito R. Aggresomes: a cellular response to misfolded proteins. J Cell Biol. 1998 Dec 28;143(7):1883-98

[106] Garcia-Mata R, Bebok Z, Sorscher EJ, Sztul ES. Characterization and dynamics of aggresome formation by a cytosolic GFP-chimera. *J Cell Biol.* 1999 Sep 20;146(6):1239-54

[107] Johnston JA, Illing ME, Kopito RR. Cytoplasmic dynein/dynactin mediates the assembly of aggresomes. *Cell Motil Cytoskeleton.* 2002 Sep;53(1):26-38

[108] Puttaparthi K, Wojcik C, Rajendran B, DeMartino GN, Elliott JL. Aggregate formation in the spinal cord of mutant SOD1 transgenic mice is reversible and mediated by proteasomes. *J Neurochem.* 2003 Nov;87(4):851-60

[109] Curti D, Malaspina A, Facchetti G, Camana C, Mazzini L, Tosca P, Zerbi F, Ceroni M. Amyotrophic lateral sclerosis: oxidative energy metabolism and calcium homeostasis in peripheral blood lymphocytes. *Neurology.* 1996 Oct;47(4):1060-4

In: Amyotrophic Lateral Sclerosis: New Research
Editor: Christine A. Murray, pp. 71-109
ISBN 1-59454-179-5

Chapter III

Interactions Between Excitotoxicity and Oxidative Stress in ALS: Clues for Pharmacotherapy

Lucio Tremolizzo[1,2], *Gessica Sala*[1], *Laura Brighina*[1,2], *Simone Beretta*[1,2] *and Carlo Ferrarese*[1,2,*]
[1]Department of Neuroscience and Biomedical Technologies, University of Milano-Bicocca,
[2]Department of Neurology, San Gerardo Hospital, Monza, Italy.

Abstract

The current gap between hypothesized pathogenic mechanisms and efficacy of therapeutics in patients affected by amyotrophic lateral sclerosis (ALS) constitutes a major problem, whose solution represents a serious commitment for researchers. ALS pathogenesis can be viewed as the consequence of a complex neurodegenerative process involving neuron-glia interactions. Excitotoxicity, oxidative stress, mitochondrial dysfunction and apoptosis are all putative mechanisms which seem to operate in ALS and might be amenable of pharmacological intervention. Disturbances of glutamatergic transmission are a well-established feature of ALS, documented by increased glutamate levels in cerebrospinal fluid, reduced glutamate transport and downregulation of the excitatory amino acid transporter EAAT2 in the affected areas. Glutamate toxicity in motor neurons is thought to be principally mediated by the GluR2-defective, calcium-permeable AMPA receptors. Moreover, after the demonstration that mutations in the copper/zinc superoxide dismutase (SOD1) gene are associated with familial ALS, oxidative damage was shown in samples from ALS patients. The recent finding that a substantial amount of SOD1 is localized in the mitochondrial intermembrane space has

* Correspondence concerning this article should be addressed to Prof. Carlo Ferrarese, M.D., Ph.D. University of Milano-Bicocca, Department of Neurology - S. Gerardo Hospital, Via Donizetti, 106 – 20052 Monza (MI) – Italy. Phone: +39-039.233.3595; Fax: +39-039.233.2449; E-mail: carlo.ferrarese@unimib.it.

provided a new rationale for the mitochondrial damage occurring in ALS, which is now regarded as an important step in the pathogenesis of the disease. Interestingly, the excitotoxic and oxidative stress theories of ALS are not mutually exclusive and several experimental evidences suggest the existence of a deep interplay between oxidative stress and excitotoxicity. Free radical-mediated damage could sensitize neurons to glutamate-mediated excitotoxic mechanisms and, conversely, the increase in intracellular calcium concentrations that accompanies excitotoxicity can increase free radical production.
Assessing the role of excitotoxicity in each single patient may provide useful indications as far as prognosis and response to therapy. In fact, molecular and biochemical markers of glutamatergic transmission can be easily assessed in peripheral tissues, such as platelets and fibroblasts, which physiologically express the three major glutamate transporters.
In conclusion, considering this crosstalk between excitotoxicity and oxidative stress, it is conceivable that combination therapies or drugs with multiple mechanisms of actions are likely to be the only way forward for ALS therapeutics.

Keywords: Excitotoxicity, Oxidative Stress, ALS Therapy, Peripheral Markers

Introduction

More than a century from the first Charcot's description (1874), amyotrophic lateral sclerosis (ALS) still represents one of the biggest challenges for modern neuroscientists. In fact, although in the last years several important results have been achieved in identifying the pathogenic mechanisms involved in motor neuron death, the derived therapeutic options still lack of efficacy, so that the prognosis of the disease has not changed dramatically (del Aguila et al., 2003).

In front of such a complex conundrum, it is not surprising that a lot of researchers have investigated themes related to the pathogenesis of this disorder, hoping to succeed in finding out the causes responsible for motor neuronal death. Moreover, the failure of therapeutic approaches developed on the basis of data obtained *in vitro* or in animal models of the disease obliges to a careful revision of the underlying pathogenic concepts, strongly supporting the possibility of a synergic interaction between different mechanisms (Rao and Weiss, 2004). In fact, in light of the more recent contributions, the current hypothesis is that ALS pathogenesis derive from the complex interactions among glutamate excitotoxicity, oxidative stress, and possibly other less investigated factors, such as mitochondrial dysfunction, apoptosis, predisposing genetic traits, and environmental xenobiotic exposure (Ferrarese and Beal, 2003; Beretta et al., 2003c). A better understanding of the pathogenic network underlying ALS neurodegeneration surely will prove to have a major impact on the therapeutic strategy for this terrible disease (Brighina et al., 2001), probably suggesting a multiple approach (Traynor et al., 2003b), with the combined use of drugs acting in a synergic way, rather than targeting a specific single dysfunctional mechanism.

Another major problem that needs to be addressed in ALS research, is the lack of suitable models in which testing both pathogenic hypotheses, and novel therapeutic options. In fact, although SOD1 transgenic mice are available and represents useful tools for such purposes (Shibata, 2001), they model the familial form of the disease, while they are probably less indicated for studying the pathogenesis of the much more diffuse sporadic form of ALS. A possible way to bypass this problem may be offered by the recent developments and transformations in our way of approaching to motor neuron disease. As a matter of fact, concepts given for acquired have been recently revised, first of all the postulate of the selectivity of the motor neuronal lesion (Ince et al., 1998; Strong and Rosenfeld, 2003). In fact, accumulating reports clearly show that ALS may be as well considered as a multi-systemic disorder in which motor neurons are affected earlier and more severely (Shaw and Kuncl, 2002). Interestingly, some of the biochemical and molecular alterations reported in central nervous system (CNS) of ALS patients have been subsequently reported also in different peripheral cell types (Ferrarese et al., 2001b; Curti et al., 1996; Aguirre et al., 1998; Vielhaber et al., 1999), suggesting a more widespread dysfunction respect to what was previously thought. Hence, we truly believe that peripheral cells from ALS patients may represent valid models in which testing experimental hypotheses, in spite of the obvious limitations implicit in using non-neural cell types (Beretta et al., 2003a).

More specifically, in this chapter we will review the most recent acquisitions in the field of ALS pathogenesis, focusing on the interactions between the two major mechanisms postulated up to now, namely excitotoxicity and oxidative stress. Moreover, the available therapeutic strategies will be highlighted, especially in relation to the two aforementioned pathogenic mechanisms. In conclusion we will stress the important role played by *ex vivo* cellular models, extremely useful tools for investigating both pathogenesis mechanisms, and novel therapeutic options in ALS patients.

Glutamate Homeostasis Dysfunction in ALS

Glutamate is the major excitatory neurotransmitter in the vertebrate CNS. Since the first reports in the early '60s (Curtis et al., 1959; Curtis and Watkins, 1960), glutamate role as synaptic mediator has been elucidated and the different elements of the glutamatergic system have been described and studied. Moreover, the concept that glutamate, under specific circumstances, could lead neurons to death was formulated since those early years (Lucas and Newhouse, 1957), and the hypothesis that a dysfunction of the glutamatergic homeostasis might be responsible for both acute (Mody and MacDonald, 1995) and chronic neurological disorders (Beal, 1992a; Beal, 1992b; for an exstensive review see Ferrarese and Beal, 2003) was subsequently called "excitotoxicity" (Olney, 1969; Olney, 1989). In this paragraph we will briefly describe the physiological functioning of the glutamatergic system, before reviewing the evidence for its dysfunction in mediating ALS pathogenesis.

The Glutamatergic System: A Brief Overview

Glutamate is a non essential dicarboxylic amino acid ($COOH-CH_2-CH_2-CH-NH_2-COOH$), involved in metabolic pathways and excitatory neurotransmission in both CNS (Cotman et al., 1988), and peripheral tissues (Skerry and Genever, 2001). Glutamate biosynthesis proceeds mainly from transamination of the respective Krebs cycle component, α-ketoglutarate, by the enzyme glutamate dehydrogenase (GD), and from the deamination of glutamine by the enzyme glutaminase. Although other pathways have been described, the latter is probably the more relevant, accounting for more than 50% of the synthesized neurotransmitter throughout the CNS. Glutamate, packed in secretory vesicles by apposite transporters (VGLUT-1, -2, and -3, see Hisano, 2003), is released from pre-synaptic cells in response to depolarization and crosses the synaptic cleft activating specific receptors present in the post-synaptic density (PSD) specialized region of the post-synaptic neurons. In order to terminate the excitatory signal, glutamate is then removed from the synaptic cleft by means of specific transporter molecules, located both on neurons and astrocytes surrounding the synapses. Astrocytic glutamate is then converted into glutamine, and subsequently shuttled back to neurons where it is converted into the neurotransmitter by glutaminase, closing the so-called glutamate-glutamine cycle (Torgner and Kvamme, 1990; Broer and Brookes, 2001).

A short description of glutamate receptors and transporters follows in light of the crucial role played by these molecules in controlling glutamate homeostasis and therefore, possibly, in mediating neuronal death by excitotoxicity in ALS.

Glutamate Receptors

Glutamate receptors may be classified as ligand-gated structures coupled to either mono- and/or divalent ion permeable pores (also know as ionotropic), or to G proteins (a.k.a. metabotropic), responsible for the intracellular transduction of the message. About 30 genes for different glutamate receptor subunits have been identified up to now, and accumulating evidences show that it is the differential arrangement of these subunits to determine which the functional profile of the receptors is. Considering the number of possible permutations, this determines the hypothetical availability of a considerable variety of different receptor molecules, a data perfectly fitting with the evidence of a tightly regulated regional (both inside, and outside the CNS) and ontogenetic specificity of the glutamate signaling machinery.

Ionotropic receptors may be further sub-classified in NMDA and AMPA/Kainate receptors in function of the specific agonistic molecules by which they are activated.

NMDA receptors are sensitive to both glutamate, and the co-agonist glycine, and they display an unusual profile for ligand-gated ion channels (Heath and Shaw, 2002). In fact, the ionic pore displays a high permeability to divalent cations and is blocked by a magnesium ion, a mechanism that is strongly voltage dependent (Daw et al., 1993). This propriety, as we will show, is crucial in the so-called "secondary" excitotoxicity, in which monovalent cation influx through AMPA/Kainate receptors determines the removal of the Mg^{2+} block from NMDA receptors, with consequent receptor activation and calcium entry, even in presence of glutamate concentrations within the physiologic range (Massieu and Garcia, 1998). Other agents can modulate NMDA activity, such as polyamines (Williams, 1997), zinc (Li et al., 2003), and, interestingly, oxidative stress products (Lipton et al., 1994). NMDA permeability to calcium ions is crucial to understand the role of these receptors in the pathogenesis of neurological disorders, including ALS. In fact calcium homoeostasis is central in the cellular dysfunction that eventually kills neurons, starting several calcium-dependent enzymatic cascades leading to neuronal damage and death (Mattson, 2003b).

On the other hand, AMPA/Kainate receptors are generally regarded as permeable to monovalent cations only, such as sodium and potassium. They are often defined as non-NMDA receptors due to the difficulty to obtain a clear functional distinction between them. Contrariwise to NMDA molecules, they display very fast activity profiles, but they may be as well associated to neuronal dysfunction through membrane depolarization and alteration of the energetic homeostasis. Among the different subunits, GluR2 is particularly interesting because with its presence confers to the receptor impermeability to calcium entry. In fact, AMPA receptors lacking GluR2 subunits have been shown to be highly permeable to calcium ions, potentially determining a perturbation of the intracellular homeostasis of this ion, activating pathways such as the arachidonic acid cascade (Lazarewicz et al., 1988), or the nitric oxide synthesis (Garthwaite et al., 1989), with important implications for the survival of the cell. Interestingly the permeability of the receptor molecules to divalent cations is determined by the post-transcriptional editing within the second transmemebrane domain of the GluR2 AMPA subunit. Here, in position 586, there is normally a glutamine (Q) residue, coded by a CAG triplet, which may be transformed by the enzyme adenosine deaminase into a CIG triplet, coding for an arginine (R) residue (Melcher et al., 1996). Other mechanisms able to determine different functional characteristics of the receptor molecules are a similar adenosine deaminase-mediated transition (R→G) within the exon 13 of the GluR2-4 subunits, and the alternative splicing of a 38 amino acid region within the fourth transmembrane domain, denoted as flip/flop editing. Noteworthy, motor neurons relatively lack of GluR2 AMPA subunits (Shaw et al., 1999; Heath et al., 2002), and this evidence have been pointed out as one of the possible factors underlying their selective vulnerability in ALS (Williams et al., 1997; Shaw and Eggett, 2000).

Metabotropic receptors are membrane-associated G-protein-coupled glutamate receptors that determine the activation of second messenger systems (either hydrolysis of membrane phospholipids, or negative regulation of the adenylate cyclase). They appear to be involved in long-term changes in synaptic strength, modulating both post-synaptic ionotropic response, and pre-synaptic glutamate release functioning as auto-receptors.

Although several of the mechanisms underlying glutamate receptor function, both in CNS (Bredt and Nicoll, 2003; Huettner, 2003; Mori and Mishina, 2003), and peripheral tissues (Skerry and Genever, 2001; Hinoi et al., 2004), have been elucidated, more work is needed to address issues such as the differential regulation of the expression of the receptor molecules, or the better definition of the intracellular transduction cascade systems. In fact, this effort might eventually lead to advancements in our understanding of the mechanisms involved in ALS pathogenesis, and to the possibility of modulating glutamate receptor activity and/or expression as a therapeutic target for treating motor neuron disease.

Glutamate Transporters

Glutamate homeostasis strictly depends on the efficient removal of the neurotransmitter from the synaptic cleft, a function performed by a class of transporters molecules known as excitatory amino acid transporters (or EAATs; for a review see Danbolt, 2001; Beretta et al., 2003b), which includes five members differently expressed throughout the CNS (O'Shea, 2002; Amara and Fontana, 2002): EAAT1 (also known as GLAST in mouse), EAAT2 (a.k.a. GLT1), EAAT3 (a.k.a. EAAC1), EAAT4, and EAAT5. Brain plasma membranes express also another transporter, the glutamate-cystine exchanger (Sato et al., 1999; Flynn and McBean, 2000), which may be implicated in glutamate release (Baker et al., 2002), transporting cystine into cells by using the glutamate transmembrane gradient (Bannai, 1986). Interestingly, brain cells express intracellular glutamate transporters as well (Danbolt et al., 2003), including mitochondrial transporters (Fiermonte et al., 2002) and the class of vesicular glutamate transporters (VGLUTs; for a review see Hisano, 2003) responsible for regulating glutamate packing into secretory structures, in order to release it following depolarization of the pre-synaptic axon terminal.

The role of EAATs consists in tightly regulating the extra-cellular concentration of L-glutamate (they also uptake L- and D-aspartate), in order to maintain it between 1 and 3 μM, both preventing neuronal excitotoxic effects, recycling glutamate to prevent metabolic waste, and securing a high signal to noise ratio (Danbolt et al., 2003). The process of glutamate re-uptake is associated with ion co-transport and is modulated by glutamate itself (Munir et al., 2000; Duan et al., 1999), and other soluble factors such as cytokines (for example TNF-α; see Fine et al., 1996), or oxidative stress products (for example 4-hydroxynonenal; see Keller et al., 1997; Springer et al., 1997).

EAAT1 and EAAT2 are expressed mainly by astrocytes throughout the entire CNS, although EAAT2 is expressed by neurons as well (Chen et al., 2002; Schmitt et al., 2002), surely in early developmental stages (Northington et al., 1999), and this expression is retained at least at the level of the retina (see Rauen et al., 1999). EAAT1 is the major transporter in the cerebellum (Lehre and Danbolt, 1998) and the retina (Rauen et al., 1999), while EAAT2 takes over in the majority of the brain and spinal cord, accounting for the important role played by this molecule in controlling glutamate homeostasis in CNS regions mainly involved in ALS, *i.e.*, cortical motor areas and spinal cord anterior horns. On the other hand, EAAT3 is widely expressed by neurons, especially in hippocampus, cerebellum and basal ganglia (Conti et al., 1998; Rothstein et al., 1994), although its role appears to be secondary, since EAAT3 knock-out mice display normal uptake activity (Peghini et al., 1997), while knocking-out EAAT2 uptake values decrease significantly (Tanaka et al., 1997). EAAT4 and EAAT5 display a very restricted pattern of distribution in adult brain; in fact they are located mainly in the cerebellum (Dehnes et al., 1998) and the retina, respectively.

Interestingly, the different EAAT molecules display a specific pattern of subcellular distribution and may undergo to rapid changes in their expression at the plasma membrane level. Four proteins (Danbolt et al., 2003) have been reported to interact with EAATs, mediating attachment to cytoskeletal structures: Ajuba which binds EAAT2 (Marie et al., 2002), GTRAP3-18 which binds EAAT3 (Lin et al., 2001); GTRAP41, and GTRAP48 which bind EAAT4 (Jackson et al., 2001).

Since 1992, glutamate transporter alterations have been thoroughly investigated as possible causes of both ALS, and other neurodegenerative disorders, after that Rothstein and colleagues showed a decrease in glutamate transport in synaptosomal preparations from ALS patients (Rothstein et al., 1992). Since then, accumulating reports have confirmed a role for

EAATs in mediating excitotoxic neuronal damage in various models, ranging from cell cultures (Mattson, 2003a), to animal models (Mennini and Bendotti, 2003), to *ex vivo* cells obtained from patients (Ferrarese et al., 2001b).

Next paragraph will review the evidence for EAATs involvement in mediating the excitotoxic insult underlying motor neuronal death, before considering the role of oxidative stress products and the possible interplay between these two mechanisms in the pathogenesis of ALS.

Excitoxicity and ALS: What is the Evidence?

The concept of excitotoxicity postulates that increased extracellular concentrations of excitatory neurotransmitters such as glutamate or aspartate, arisen from excessive presynaptic amino acid release or impaired reuptake, can damage postsynaptic cells via an excessive activation of postsynaptic glutamate receptors. Other factors could contribute to the toxicity of glutamate, including the location and the molecular properties of postsynaptic glutamate receptors, the activity of other ion channels, and intracellular mechanisms starting downstream events following glutamate receptor activation. Although the precise details of the molecular mechanisms that lead to glutamate-mediated neuronal injury are still unknown, several pathways have been elucidated that may contribute to toxic effects. These include the activation of multiple enzyme cascades such as calpain, protein kinase C, lipases, phospholipases, endonucleases, the arachidonic acid cascade, xanthine oxidase, and nitric oxide synthesis (Ince et al., 1997). A key step in the excitotoxic process is the disturbance of calcium homeostasis, supported by the calcium-dependency of many of the aforementioned enzyme cascades. Free intracellular calcium levels increase following activation of NMDA receptors, AMPA receptors lacking the GluR2 subunit, or voltage-gated calcium channels (direct or primary excitotoxicity) (Choi, 1988; Miller et al., 1989). If the functional integrity of the postsynaptic cell is altered by a variety of etiological factors, the postsynaptic cell is more vulnerable to this mechanism, which implies that much lower extracellular concentrations of excitatory amino acids are sufficient to initiate the excitotoxic cascade of neuronal death (Henneberry et al., 1989; Ludolph et al., 1993). Since neuronal cells are critically dependent on sufficient supplies of chemical energy, numerous factors may make the cell less capable of maintaining its membrane potential and therefore less resistant to disturbances of ion homeostasis, which may also be induced by physiological levels of excitatory neurotransmitters (indirect or secondary excitotoxicity) (Beal, 1992a). This concept of indirect excitotoxicity may be a contributory mechanism that leads to cell death in chronic neurodegenerative disorders, such as ALS.

Evidence for glutamate contributing to motor neuron degeneration in ALS initially came from several studies that suggested that cerebrospinal fluid glutamate levels are elevated in at least a subgroup of ALS patients (Rothstein et al., 1990; Shaw et al., 1995a), although not all laboratories have replicated this finding (Perry et al., 1990). A similar dichotomy exists in the studies of fasting levels of glutamate in the plasma or serum of ALS patients in comparison with controls. In fact, glutamate plasma levels have been reported to be raised in ALS patients (Plaitakis et al., 1987), although not all studies have confirmed these reports (Camu et al., 1993; Perry et al., 1990; Shaw et al., 1995a), due both to possible heterogeneity in the ALS population regarding to the pathogenic mechanisms involved in motor neuron death, and the metabolic instability of glutamate in biological samples (Ferrarese et al., 1993).

Collectively, these studies seem to indicate a disturbance of glutamate metabolism in ALS, potentially explained by a failure of high-affinity uptake systems. This hypothesis was evaluated and confirmed through the use of membrane preparations of post-mortem tissue from ALS patients, where a significant loss of high-affinity, sodium-dependent glutamate transport was found in ALS with respect to controls (Rothstein et al., 1992). Detailed studies were performed to examine molecular subtypes of glutamate transporters in ALS, revealing that up to 60%to 70% of patients with sporadic ALS have a 30% to 90% loss of the EAAT2 protein, in both motor cortex and spinal cord (Rothstein et al., 1995; Shaw et al., 1994; Fray et al., 1998). Moreover, the loss of EAAT2 appears to be specific to these regions in most but not all patients. Noteworthy, this loss of EAAT2 protein cannot be attributed to cell death since there is no significant astroglial loss in ALS (Rothstein et al., 1995). Northern blotting studies have revealed no difference of EAAT2 mRNA in affected areas of ALS patients, with respect to healthy subjects, suggesting the hypothesis of a post-transcriptional defect, either translational or post-translational (Bristol and Rothstein, 1996). Moreover, except on single report (Trotti et al., 2001), there is currently no evidence that genomic mutation in EAAT2 may be a common cause of ALS (Aoki et al., 1998). Interestingly in the patient reported by Trotti and colleagues, the mutation N206S was shown to reduce in oocyte the glycosylation of EAAT2, reducing its insertion in plasma membrane, decreasing the uptake, and increasing the propensity to reverse the flux (Trotti et al., 2001).

A putative alternative mechanisms for EAAT2 loss in sporadic ALS has been hypothesized, suggesting that abnormal RNA processing of EAAT2 could underlie the decreased expression and function of this protein. In fact, Lin and colleagues (Lin et al., 1998) reported that abnormal intron 7 retention and exon 9 skipping splice variants of EAAT2 were disease-specific to ALS and that the abnormal transcripts could also be detected in CSF. Studies of some of these truncated species indicated that they have a dominant-negative effect on the EAAT2 protein and provide a mechanism for explaining EAAT2 protein loss in patients. However, several other groups have failed to replicate these findings, having demonstrated the presence of these EAAT2 splice variants in the CNS of ALS patients as well as of normal controls (Flowers et al., 2001; Meyer et al., 1999; Nagai et al., 1998; Honig et al., 2000).

Although further studies are required in order to address the issue of EAAT2 selective downregulation in ALS, it is of interest that EAAT2 protein is especially vulnerable to free radicals, resulting in the post-translational inactivation of the transporters (Volterra et al., 1992; Volterra et al., 1994; Trotti et al., 1995; Trotti et al., 1996), strongly pointing to a direct interplay between oxidative stress and excitotoxicity.

However, several issues should be addressed before confirming the role of glutamate homeostasis dysfunction in ALS, and the mechanisms of selective motor neuronal damage must be explained to be plausible. Several characteristics specific of motor neurons have been described that may account for this selectivity (Shaw and Kuncl, 2002). Motor neurons are big cells, with high oxidative demands in order to sustain their metabolism, with consequent possible increased production of free radicals, able to impair glutamate uptake and to modulate glutamate receptor activity. Moreover, the relative lack of GluR2 AMPA subunits has been reported in motor neurons (Williams et al., 1997). As previously described, the latter phenomenon determines increased calcium permeability through AMPA receptors, leading to disruption of calcium intracellular homeostasis, with the already described important functional consequences for the neurons. Additionally, motor neurons relatively lack of calcium-binding proteins, such as parvalbumin and calbindin D28k (Ince et al., 1993), determining a lower capacity of buffering calcium increases in the cytoplasm of these neurons.

Partially sustaining the important role played by excitotoxicity in ALS, are the reports of ALS-like syndromes following the assumption of glutamate-like toxin with the food (Spencer et al., 1991). For example, β-(N)-oxalyl-amino-L-alanine (BOAA) has been strongly implicated in the first motor neuron disorder known as lathyrism, diffused in India among people consuming the peas, *Lathyrus sativus* (Spencer and Schaumburg, 1983). Also β-(N)-methyl-amino-L-alanine (BMAA), contained in the Cycas seeds, has been shown to be a potent excitotoxin, and may be involved in the pathogenesis of ALS-Parkinson-Dementia syndrome, highly diffused in Micronesia among the Chamorro people of the islands of Guam and Rota (Spencer, 1987). Although BMAA role has been questioned during the years, very recently Cox and colleagues (Cox et al., 2003; Banack and Cox, 2003; Cox and Sacks, 2002) have demonstrated that flying foxes, a much appreciated Chamorro's food, may bio-concentrate the toxin, leading to the exposure to very high doses of the substance.

Anti Excitotoxic Therapy: Riluzole and Beyond

Riluzole

Riluzole is thought to act on glutamatergic neurotransmission both by activating a G-protein-dependent process that inhibits glutamate release, and by blocking post-synaptic NMDA glutamate receptors. However, this drug has many effects, including blockade of voltage-dependent sodium channels with subsequent prevention of neuronal depolarization; interaction with potassium, calcium, chloride channels; interference with transporters of neurotransmitters such as GABA, dopamine, acetylcholine, serotonin and D-aspartate. Recently, it has been reported that riluzole also has neurotrophic, antioxidant, antiapoptotic effects and inhibits protein kinase C activation. Anyway, the precise action responsible for its therapeutic effect in ALS is currently unknown and a link between its mechanism of action and the glutamate hypothesis in ALS remains to be demonstrated.

Two prospective, randomized, double-blind, placebo-controlled, clinical trials with riluzole have been conducted in ALS (Bensimon et al., 1994; Lacomblez et al., 1996). The first enrolled 155 patients with definite or probable ALS, from seven French and Belgian hospitals; they received either 100 mg riluzole per day, or placebo for 12 months from the enrollment of the final patient.

The second study enrolled 959 patients from 31 centers in Europe and North America and tested riluzole effect at three different dosages (50 mg-100 mg-150 mg daily). Both trials demonstrated a statistically significant 35% decrease in risk of death or tracheostomy over an

18-month period in patients administered 100 mg/day riluzole compared with placebo. The greatest effect of riluzole was detected after 12 months of treatment. In the second trial, the 100 mg dosage presented the best benefit/risk ratio. There are two interesting differences between these trials: site of onset appeared to condition treatment efficacy in the first study, but not in the second; the first study indicated some slowing of deterioration of muscle strength which was not confirmed by the second study. This latter discrepancy was explained by the drug-related side-effect of asthenia on functional scores. Nevertheless, this symptom was fairly equally distributed in the four treatment groups, including the placebo one, thus possibly constituting a consequence of the disorder.

In conclusion, the progression of ALS may be delayed during treatment with riluzole; no supporting evidence relating to other factors, such as quality of life, was presented to add weight to the trend towards better survival. The limited effect of riluzole might be explained by the fact that it acts at the end of the cascade, when motor neuron damage is practically irreversible. The prolonged survival of transgenic mutant SOD mice treated with riluzole early in the preclinical period and the lack of efficacy after the onset of clinical disease (Gurney et al., 1996) seem to support this hypothesis. Moreover, Riviere and colleagues have reported that patients with milder disabilities in the previous phase III trials had a slower rate of progression if prescribed riluzole (Riviere et al., 1998). Consistently, a more recent retrospective cohort study conducted in the Irish ALS population has demonstrated that this drug prolongs survival even in patients with suspected and possible forms of ALS (Traynor et al., 2003a). All these reports seem to support the use of riluzole in the early stages of the disease before significant degeneration of spinal neurons has occurred.

However, several key issues concerning treatment with riluzole remain unresolved, *i.e.*, whether it is more effective in certain clinical forms of ALS or what is the appropriate duration of treatment (previous clinical trials followed subjects for only 18 months and studies beyond this timeframe have been confined to the safety profile of the drug).

The effect of riluzole on ALS progression reported in the two reported clinical trials has strengthened belief in the glutamate hypothesis and prompted excitotoxicity studies; at the same time it has paved the way for further testing of drugs potentially interfering with this mechanism.

Branched-Chain Amino Acids (BCAAs)

The branched-chain amino acids L-leucine and, to a lesser extent, L-isoleucine and L-valine, have proved to activate *in vitro* glutamate dehydrogenase (GD), the enzyme that interconverts glutamate and α-ketoglutarate. In the first 12 months of a double-blind trial (Plaitakis et al., 1988), BCAAs seemed to slow the rate of decline of some spinal scores compared with placebo, but these data were not confirmed by subsequent studies. In 1993, The Italian Subgroup of The European Study Group (1993) reported a possible increase in the risk of death in the treated group, based on a double-blind, placebo–controlled trial.

Gabapentin

Gabapentin is a BCAA homolog stereosimilar to L-leucine. Its mechanism of action is unknown, although experimental evidence seems to suggest that it could decrease the synthesis of glutamate (Taylor, 1994). Gabapentin was first tested in a double-blind, phase II placebo-controlled trial (Miller et al., 1996) in 152 patients at doses ranging from 800 mg/day to 2000-2400 mg/day (adjusted on the basis of adverse reactions), for six months. The primary end-point, *i.e.*, the mean arm megascore slope of the intention-to-treat population, was not achieved. No treatment effect was observed on secondary end-point results (rates of decline of forced vital capacity, FVC, and of arm megascore slope of the subjects completing the study).

A phase III longer (nine months), larger (204 patients), higher dose (3600 mg/day) study with gabapentin performed in North America failed to confirm the encouraging preliminary findings provided by the previous phase II trial. It showed no significant differences between patients treated with gabapentin respect to placebo in the mean rate of decline of arm strength (primary outcome) or in the other secondary outcome measures (Miller et al., 2001).

Dextromethorphan (DMP)

This is a non-competitive antagonist of NMDA glutamate receptors. The results of four trials using DMP at dosages ranging from 100 to 150 mg/day gave no significant results. Phase II and III trials, at higher dosages (about 7 mg/Kg/day), shown to be tolerable in phase I safety and pharmacokinetic studies (Hollander et al., 1994), are under way.

Topiramate

This drug displays antiexcitotoxic properties through its ability to diminish glutamate release from neurons and antagonize kainate activation of the AMPA receptors (Skradski and White, 2000). Topiramate protects motor neurons in an *in vitro* model of chronic glutamate toxicity but has no effect on survival in an ALS mouse model (Maragakis et al., 2003).

In a US double-blind multicenter clinical trial, 296 ALS patients were randomised to receive topiramate (maximum tolerated dose up to 800 mg/day) or placebo for 12 months. This study (Cudkowicz et al., 2003) has demonstrated a more rapid strength decline in treated patients, as measured by MVIC (maximum voluntary isometric contraction), the primary outcome measure. There was no impact on the rate of decline of FVC, ALS functional rating scale (ALSFRS), and tracheostomy-free survival. Since an increased risk for several side effects was observed, the more rapid strength decline in treated patients may have been related to a reduced tolerability. Further trials are warranted in order to determine whether topiramate may be neuroprotective and safer at lower doses.

COX-2 Inhibitors

Recent evidences indicate that COX-2 may play an important role in ALS pathogenesis by producing prostaglandins (particularly PGE2) that trigger astrocytic glutamate release and by inducing free radical formation (Almer et al., 2002). Celecoxib, a highly lipid soluble COX-2 inhibitor, was found to delay disease onset and prolong survival of treated ALS mice with a significant preservation of both large and small neurons in the spinal cord (Drachman et al., 2002). A multi-center double-blind placebo controlled study with celecoxib is currently ongoing in ALS patients.

Selective Inhibitors of Glutamate Carboxypeptidase II (GCPII)

Since GCPII converts NAAG (N-Actyl-Aspartyl-Glutamate), a peptide produced in the brain, into glutamate, its inhibition may represent a new approach to block the release of excess excitatory amino acids. Recently, selective inhibitors of glutamate carboxypeptidase II (GCPII) have been shown to protect motor neurons in both *in vitro* and animal models of FALS (Ghadge et al., 2003). However, no testing in humans has been performed yet.

Tamoxifen

A dose-ranging study of tamoxifen for ALS patients began enrollment in 2002 at the University of Wisconsin-Madison. On completion of the one-year trial, all patients would receive the drug on an "open label" program at the most effective dose. A possible disease mechanism being investigated in this clinical trial is that tamoxifen is a protein kinase C inhibitor that could produce an antiglutamate effect, as theorized also for riluzole.

Oxidative Stress

Although free radical-mediated damage to cellular function may not be the primary event initiating ALS, accumulating evidence indicates that this mechanism is involved in the pathogenetic cascade of the disorder. Indeed, increased free radical-mediated damage relates closely to the hypotheses of reduced energy metabolism, trace element toxicity, and excitotoxicity in neurodegeneration.

Oxidative stress occurs when cells are damaged by exposure to highly reactive free radicals that irreversibly damage cellular components (Benzie, 1996; Onorato et al., 1998; Keller and Mattson, 1998; Cookson and Shaw, 1999; Torreilles et al., 1999). A free radical is defined as any atom or molecule with an unpaired electron in its outer shell. Multiple radicals exist, but the most common are formed from the reduction of molecular oxygen to water, and are typically referred to as reactive oxygen species (ROS): superoxide anion (O_2^-), a free radical that participates in cellular signalling but does not appear to be reactive with DNA or lipids, hydroxyl radical (·OH), the most reactive oxygen radical capable of oxidizing lipids, carbohydrates, proteins, and DNA.

Nitric oxide (NO·) is another free radical synthesized by the enzymatic oxidation of L-arginine to form citrulline through the action of calcium-activated, calmodulin-dependent nitric oxide synthases (NOS). Nitric oxide is produced in excitotoxicity, and can react with O_2^- to produce peroxynitrite ($ONOO^-$), a powerful oxidant capable of damaging lipids, proteins, and DNA. It can also form ·OH and the nitrogen dioxide radical (NO_2·).

In order to defend the cells against free radicals and maintain homeostasis, extensive antioxidant systems and repair enzymes remove and repair oxidized molecules. Antioxidants have multiple mechanisms of action, including preventing initiation of oxidation by radical scavenging, binding or removing catalyzing metal ions, limiting the propagation of the oxidative reaction, and decomposing peroxide. Important enzymatic antioxidants present in the brain include copper-zinc (Cu/Zn) superoxide dismutase (SOD), manganese (Mn)-SOD, glutathione peroxidase (GSH-Px), and glutathione reductase (GSSH-R). The brain also contains a small amount of catalase (CAT) together with numerous other non-enzymatic antioxidants and more complex forms of protection represented by systems for metal transport and buffering, such as glutathione, ascorbic acid, ceruloplasmin, uric acid, bilirubin, melatonin.

Although antioxidant defense mechanisms can be upregulated in response to increased free radical production (Sen et al., 2003), they may only confer a partial protection, without completely prevent oxidative damage.

Noteworthy, different tissues display different susceptibility to oxidative stress. The CNS is particularly sensitive to this kind of damage for its anatomical and physiological characteristics. For example, CNS high O_2 consumption – in fact, in humans the brain processes 20% of basal oxygen consumption – produces, via mitochondria, ATP needed to maintain transmembrane gradients of various ionic species (high intracellular K^+, low Na^+, very low "free" Ca^{2+}). The respiratory chain of mitochondria is responsible for most of the reactive oxygen species (ROS), especially superoxide anion (O_2^-). As a matter of fact, in physiological conditions, 1-2% of the O_2 consumed by neurons is converted to ROS.

Moreover, nitric oxide (NO) behaves as a reactive nitrogen species (RNS). This gaseous free radical is an important biological messenger, highly diffusible, that plays a prominent role in CNS physiology (Yun et al., 1996). Three enzymatic isoforms account for NO production and include neuronal NO synthase (nNOS), indicible NO synthase (iNOS) which is present in very large amounts in activated microglia, and endothelial NO synthase (eNOS). In the CNS, nNOS, whose expression is regulated by both physiological and pathophysiological stimuli (Shimizu et al., 2003), accounts for most NO activity. Interestingly, NO reacts rapidly with O_2^- to form peroxynitrite ($ONOO^-$) which is the most reactive RNS (Dawson and Dawson, 1996).

Classically oxidative stress is described as an imbalance between generation and elimination of ROS and RNS, that can react with lipids, proteins and DNA, often causing irreparable damage leading to cell death (Simpson et al., 2003). These reactive species were originally considered to be exclusively detrimental to cells. It is now recognized that redox regulation involving ROS is the key of the modulation of critical cellular functions, such as mitogene-activated protein (MAP) kinase cascade activation, ion transport, calcium mobilization, and apoptosis program activation, both in neurons, astrocytes, and microglia (Hidelman et al., 2003).

Mutant SOD1 and Familial ALS

Mutations of the gene for the cytosolic form of the SOD1 have been found in a subgroup of patients affected by a familial form of ALS (Rosen et al., 1993). Interestingly, to date, more than 100 different mutations (see the ALS online database for mutations in ALS related genes, www.alsod.org) have been detected in the enzyme in about 20% of patients with familial ALS (Andersen, 2001). Mutations are distributed in all five exons of the gene and result in amino acid substitutions scattered throughout the SOD structure: while some mutations affect the active site, others are positioned at the dimmer interface, or inside beta-strands or connecting loops.

Epidemiological studies have also shown SOD1 mutations in 3-7% of patients with apparently sporadic ALS, although some of these latter patients may be misdiagnosed familial forms, possibly due to low penetrance (Andersen, 2001).

SOD1 is a well-characterized homodimeric enzyme, abundant in the cytoplasm and present in the intermembrane space of mitochondria (Higgins et al., 2002), with each subunit binding a catalitically essential copper ion and a stabilising zinc ion, and protects against oxidative damage by catalyzing the disproportion of superoxide radicals to dioxygen and hydrogen peroxide, according to the following formulae:

$$M^{3+} + O_2^- \rightarrow M^{2+} + O_2$$
$$M^{2+} + O_2^- + 2H^+ \rightarrow M^{3+} + H_2O_2$$

However, many of the mutations observed in familial ALS neither abolish nor decrease this dismutase activity and their deleterious consequences are thought to be due to a "gain-of-function" rather than a loss-of-function. Strong evidence for the causal role of SOD mutations in ALS is derived from experiments in which transgenic mice overexpressing specific ALS mutations were shown to develop progressive paralysis caused by the death of motor neurons (Gurney et al., 1994). Interestingly, because the complete knockout of the endogenous gene encoding SOD in mouse does not produce motor neuron disease, toxicity cannot be solely caused by the loss of superoxide scavenging activity (Reaume et al., 1996). However, the recent report of a slow decline in motor units with aging in SOD1 knock-out mice seems to partially challenge the latter affirmation (Shefner et al., 1999).

Moreover, recent evidence from transgenic mice has established that mutant SODs may selectively activate apoptosis in motor neurons (Pasinelli et al., 1998; Li et al., 2000; Kostic et al., 1997).

The apparent gain of function conferred by the SOD mutations in ALS remains elusive. It was originally proposed that the SOD mutants might be more likely to catalyze tyrosine nitration by peroxynitrite (Beckman et al., 1993), but this theory posits that toxicity is independent of oxidative stress and is caused by protein aggregation (Cleveland and Liu, 2000). The basis for this hypothesis lies in the observation that the toxicity of SODs in ALS appears to be independent of the capacity of the cell to scavenge superoxide, since disease progression in transgenic mice is independent of the presence of SOD. However, aggregates of SOD protein *per se* have not been demonstrated to be toxic (Johnston et al., 2000). Metal-deficient apoSODs are nontoxic to motor neurons even though they are considerably more prone to aggregation (Estevez et al., 1999). Furthermore, mice carrying the A4V SOD mutation do not develop motor neuron disease (though, paradoxically, this mutation causes the most rapid progression of ALS in humans; Gurney et al., 1994). The level of A4V SOD expression in mice is similar to that of the G93A mutant and produces large aggregates in motor neurons without cell death (Gurney et al., 1994). Aggregation of neurofilaments and other proteins is certainly a hallmark of ALS, but aggregation of SOD protein *per se* might not be the primary cause of toxicity. Indeed, nitrative stress, generated by SOD and peroxynitrite could promote the aggregation of structural proteins.

However, the mutant SODs do have more problems binding metals (Goto et al., 2000). The ALS mutants have diminished zinc affinity and often accumulate in Zn-deficient states when expressed *in vitro* (Crow et al., 1997). The reduced affinity for Zn appears to be an indirect consequence of the ALS mutations structurally weakening the backbone of the SOD protein (Deng et al., 1993). Because Zn is held about 7000-fold less tightly than Cu even in wild-type SOD, structural defects cause Zn to be lost before Cu (Crow et al., 1997). The loss of Zn profoundly alters the redox properties of SOD and makes SOD toxic to motor neurons (Estevez et al., 1999). Rather than acting as a scavenger of superoxide, Zn-deficient SOD can steal electrons to oxygen to produce superoxide. This slow production of superoxide by Zn-deficient SOD is not toxic by itself because remaining Cu-Zn SOD present in a cell recaptures superoxide. However, nitric oxide reacts so rapidly with superoxide to produce peroxynitrite that can effectively compete with SOD for superoxide.

Since Zn-deficient wild-type SOD has been demonstrated to be just as toxic as the mutant SODs, by inducing tyrosine nitration and motor neuron apoptosis, it is proposed that the mutations to SOD do not directly confer a gain of function, rather they increase the susceptibility to lose Zn. Thus, wild-type SOD can participate in sporadic ALS pathogenesis in conditions of Zn deficiency.

Copper is essential for the toxicity of Zn-deficient SOD, and it has been reported that apoSOD (SOD lacking in Cu and Zn) is not toxic to the motor neurons (Estevez et al., 1999). Recently, considerable attention has focused on the Cu chaperone protein for SOD (CCS). In knockout mice that lack CCS, the activity of endogenous SOD is decreased by about 70-80% (Wong et al., 2000). Although CCS is the major source of Cu *in vivo*, SOD can apparently acquire Cu from other sources in cells as 20-30% of activity remains in the knockout mice. Moreover, Cu is absolutely required for SOD to scavenge superoxide (McCord and Fridovich, 1969). A probable source for SOD to acquire Cu is the mitochondria, where a separate transport system provides substantial amounts of Cu for cytochrome C oxidase. These alternative sources of Cu might explain why deletion of the gene encoding CCS has little effect on the development of motor neuron disease in ALS mutant SOD mice (Cleveland and Liu, 2000). Other studies have shown that CCS selectively inserts Cu into Zn-containing SOD (Rae et al., 2001), which will produce Cu-Zn SOD. When replete with Zn, even SODs that are mutated in ALS are protective. In the absence of the CCS protein, the mutant SODs might acquire Cu without Zn from other sources (*e.g.*, the mitochondria) contributing to the formation of Zn-deficient SOD. This could explain why mitochondrial damage is the earliest marker of injury in ALS-SOD mutant mice (Kong and Xu, 1998).

From Familial to Sporadic ALS: Evidence for Oxidative Damage

Although there is no evidence that SOD1 function is altered in the majority of patients with ALS, the similarity of the familial and sporadic forms in terms of clinical symptoms and disease course suggests that oxidative damage might be important in all patients affected by the disorder. In line with this, evidence for oxidative damage has been found both in sporadic and familial ALS patients, with or without mutations in SOD1, and in several model systems as well.

Staining for 8-hydroxy-2'-deoxyguanosine, an index of oxidation-induced modification of nucleic acids, has been found to be increased in spinal motor neurons of SOD1-associated and non-SOD1-associated FALS patients (Ferrante et al., 1997). Oxidative damage to membrane lipids has been suggested because of increased immunocytochemical staining of malondialdehyde-modified proteins in motor neurons of FALS patients (Ferrante et al., 1997). Moreover, increased free nitrotyrosine staining has been reported in spinal motor neurons of SALS patients (Abe et al., 1995; Beal et al., 1997; Chou et al., 1996). Consistently, an increased level of carbonyl peptides has been found in motor cortex or spinal cord of SALS patients (Bowling et al., 1993; Ferrante et al., 1997; Shaw et al., 1995b), and similarly to what has been observed in FALS, increased staining for 8-hydroxy-2'-deoxyguanosine and malondialdehyde-modified protein has been reported in SALS spinal cord (Ferrante et al., 1997). 4-Hydroxynonenal, a lipid peroxidation product of fatty acids, was found to be increased in CSF of SALS patients (Smith et al., 1996). Moreover, the content of protein modified by 4-hydroxynonenal was found to be increased in the spinal cord of SALS patients, by immunohistochemistry and immunoblotting (Pedersen et al., 1998). Noteworthy, immunoprecipitation studies have suggested that one of the targets of this oxidation may be the glial glutamate transporter EAAT2 (Pedersen et al., 1998).

Consistently with a systemic rather than selective involvement in ALS, primary fibroblast cultures from both patients with SOD1-associated FALS (SOD1 $^{L38F, D90A, G93C}$) and sporadic ALS (SALS) were found to be more sensitive than controls to 3-morpholinosydnonimine hydrochloride (SIN-1), but not to serum withdrawal (Aguirre et al., 1998). Moreover, in the same study, fibroblasts from SOD1 FALS patients were demonstrated to be more sensitive to oxidative stress induced by H_2O_2 than SALS fibroblasts and controls. On the other hand, SALS fibroblasts were more sensitive to SIN-1 exposure with respect to SOD1 FALS cells (Aguirre et al., 1998).

Our group reported that the expression of mutant G93A SOD1 specifically causes a decrease in MTT reduction rate and ATP levels and an increase in both cytosolic and mitochondrial ROS production in a human neuroblastoma SH-SY5Y cell line. Indeed, exposure to the antioxidant N-acetylcysteine lowers ROS production and returns mitochondrial function assays to control levels. We did not detect large aggregates of human SOD1 under basal growth conditions in any of the investigated cell lines; however, following proteasome activity inhibition, we demonstrated SOD1 aggregates exclusively in G93A

SOD1 cells. These findings indicate that mitochondrial homeostasis is affected by mutant SOD1-generated ROS independently from the formation of aggregates and that this alteration is reversed by antioxidants (Beretta et al., 2003d). Moreover, V_{max} of glutamate uptake was reduced in mutant cells, with no change in K_m (Ferrarese et al., 2001a) No difference in EAAT1, EAAT2 and EAAT3 glutamate transporter mRNAs and immuno-reactive proteins was found, suggesting that one and/or more transporters are functionally inactivated, possibly due to increased oxidative stress induced by the G93A mutation. Mutant cells showed a marked sensitivity to oxidants, resulting in a higher reduction of glutamate uptake. No rescue of impaired glutamate uptake was demonstrated in G93A cells after short-term antioxidant treatment, suggesting that such a treatment, while offering partial protection against exogenous oxidative insults, is unable to act effectively on damaged transporters (G.S. et al., submitted manuscript).

Interactions Between Excitotoxicity and Oxidative Stress in ALS

The excitotoxic and oxidative stress theories of ALS are not mutually exclusive. Free radical-mediated damage could sensitize neurons to glutamate-mediated excitotoxic mechanisms and, conversely, the increase in intracellular calcium concentrations that accompanies excitotoxicity can increase free radical production (Gurney, 2000; Atlante et al., 2001; Doble, 1999; Gurney, 1997).

Evidence suggesting a link between free radical formation and glutamate transporter dysfunction comes from a Xenopus oocyte model, where it has been shown that co-expression of the A4V or I113T mutant forms of human copper/zinc superoxide dismutase (SOD1) protein with GLT1/EAAT2 caused selective inactivation of the glutamate transporter molecules via oxidative reactions triggered by hydrogen peroxide (Trotti et al., 1999). Moreover, 4-hydroxynonenal, a product of membrane lipid peroxidation, oxidizes EAAT2 protein in the lumbar spinal cord of sporadic ALS patients (Pedersen et al, 1998). These evidences suggest that EAAT2 might be vulnerable to oxidant stress, which could lead to impaired glutamate clearance at the synaptic cleft and resultant motor neuron injury.

The redox modulation of EAAT2 provides an other important link between oxidative stress and excitotoxicity pathways. Rao and colleagues recently demonstrated that ROS generated within motor neurons in response to glutamate can disrupt the glutamate transport function of neighboring astrocytes (Rao et al., 2003). ROS-induced decrease in glutamate transport would cause additional rises in extracellular glutamate, which, in turn, would lead to further excitotoxic activation of neurons. Similarly, this cycle could be initiated by ROS arising in microglial cells with following involvement of both neurons, and astrocytes (Rao and Weiss, 2004).

With the recent cloning and characterization of the promoter for EAAT2 (Su et al., 2003), further insights may soon be made into other mechanisms by which human astrocytes can regulate EAAT2 expression. For example, through effects on transcription regulatory motifs upstream of the EAAT2 promoter, the growth factors epidermal growth factor (EGF) and transforming growth factor-α (TGF- α) have been shown to stimulate EAAT2 mRNA expression, whereas tumor necrosis factor- α (TNF-α) decreases EAAT2 expression

(Simpson et al., 2003). Therefore, soluble signals from neighboring neurons and microglial cells may exert a regulatory influence on astrocytic glutamate transporter expression, hence further emphasizing the importance of intracellular crosstalk.

Mitochondrial Dysfunction in ALS

The mitochondrial respiratory chain is one of the major sites for intracellular generation of free radicals, and, as previously described, this might be expected to cause cell damage and increase cellular vulnerability to secondary excitotoxicity.

Both human $SOD1^{G93A}$ and $SOD1^{G37R}$ mice show mitochondrial vacuolization and swelling (Gurney et al., 1994; Wong et al., 1995), and, consequently, it has been suggested that massive mitochondrial degeneration is an early event in the development of the disease in these animals (Kong and Xu, 1998).

Interestingly, morphological changes in mitochondria have been reported in the spinal motor neurons of ALS patients, together with a decrease in cytochrome C oxidase activity in ventral horn and individual spinal motor neurons (Borthwick et al., 1999; Beal, 1998; Browne et al., 1998; Swerdlow et al., 1998; Wiedemann et al., 1998; Dhaliwal and Grewal, 2000; Menzies et al., 2002).

Our group recently demonstrated the presence of mitochondrial dysfunction due to mutant $SOD1^{G93A}$ in a cell model of familial ALS, and that this alteration can be reversed by N-acetylcysteine treatment (Beretta et al., 2003d), suggesting that the use of antioxidants in the therapy of ALS should be further examined with the specific aim to protect mitochondrial homeostasis.

Antioxidant Agents for ALS Therapy

N-Acetylcysteine

N-acetylcysteine (NAC) is a free-radical scavenger that promotes hydrogen peroxide and hydroxyl radicals removal and also acts as a precursor of the intracellular antioxidant glutathione. It has shown benefits in a cell-culture model of ALS and in SOD1 transgenic mice (Rothstein et al., 1994; Andreassen et al., 2000).

A double-blind, placebo-controlled trial with acetylcysteine sc 50 mg/kg/day for 12 months was conducted in 111 patients (Louwerse et al., 1995). The primary end-point, *i.e.*, one year-survival, was not achieved. No differences in the rate of progression of the various parameters measured (muscle strength, pulmonary function, disability, and bulbar function) were observed.

Selegiline

Selegiline, a selective monoamine oxidase B inhibitor, was tested in a 6-month, double-blind, placebo-controlled trial involving 133 patients. The results were not significant (Lange et al., 1998). Analogously, an earlier open-randomized clinical trial failed to report any effect (Mazzini et al., 1994). In another trial, Jossan and colleagues performed a double-blind, crossover trial with 10 patients, with negative results (Jossan et al., 1994).

Vitamin E

This lipophilic antioxidant agent diffuses into cell membranes and protects fatty acids against damage caused by lipid peroxidation. Studies in cell cultures and in SOD1 animals have pointed out a role for α-tocopherol in ALS (Pioro, 2000). However, uncontrolled clinical trials with large doses of vitamin E and a recent large, controlled study in European patients have failed to show benefit in ALS patients (Desnuelle et al., 2001).

Chelating Agents

Another proposed strategy for preventing oxidative damage is to chelate metal ions required for the intracellular reactions that produce hydroxyl radicals and lipid peroxidation. Increasing evidences indicate the importance of aberrant copper/zinc-mediated chemistry in toxicity linked to SOD1 mutation in the mouse model (Azzouz et al., 2000). Actually several chelating agents, such as ethylenediaminetetraacetic acid (EDTA) or the copper chelator tetraethylenepentamine (TEPA), have been tested in cell cultures occasionally with some benefit. D-penicillamine delays disease onset and improves survival in SOD1 mice (Hottinger et al., 1997), as does vitamin C combined with the copper chelator trientine (Nagano et al., 1999), a drug currently used in Wilson's disease treatment. Some reports have been published two decades ago including small numbers of ALS patients treated with D-penicillamine with no benefit, but there are not more recent studies.

Mitochondria as Targets for ALS Therapy

Various agents that improve mitochondrial function have been tested in ALS patients and in animal models of the disease.

Creatine is one of such compounds and is believed to act by increasing glutamate uptake into synaptic vesicles and by stabilizing the mitochondrial energy transfer complex through inhibiting the mitochondrial permeability transition pore opening. Klivenyi and colleagues showed that creatine oral supplementation induces significant neuroprotection in SOD1 mice, by reducing markers of oxidative damage in the spinal cord and increasing survival by 26 days, twice the effect of riluzole in the same model (Klivenyi et al., 1999). A small, non-placebo controlled study recently reported a temporary increase in muscle strength in ALS patients treated with oral creatine (Mazzini et al., 2001).

More recently, a double-blind placebo-controlled sequential clinical trial has demonstrated the lack of effect of oral supplementation with 10 mg daily creatine monohydrate on survival and disease progression in 175 patients with ALS (Groeneveld et al., 2003). Rate of decline of the secondary outcome measures (isometric arm muscle strength, FVC, functional status as assessed by ALSFRS and quality of life) were unaffected.

Coenzyme Q_{10} (CoQ_{10}) is an essential cofactor of the electron transport chain, as well as an important antioxidant, which is particularly effective within mitochondria. A number of prior studies have shown that it can be effective in the treatment of patients with known mitochondrial disorders. CoQ_{10} significantly extended survival in a transgenic mouse model of ALS (Beal, 2002) and, recently, an open label trial on 16 ALS patients has reported a positive trend in ALSFRS scores, motor unit number estimate and slowing of vital capacity reduction. Moreover, CoQ_{10} was well tolerated and demonstrated no adverse effects on any major organ system.

Ex Vivo Peripheral Cells to Model Neuronal Dysfunction in ALS

Since the first El Escorial consensus criteria (Brooks, 1994) the evaluation of the disease progression represents one of the core points to allow the diagnosis of ALS. The possible drawback of applying such restrictive diagnostic criteria is represented by the delay by which a therapeutic strategy can be defined. As a matter of fact, it is reasonable to propose that early therapeutic intervention in ALS patients would lead to better results both in term of disease progression, and disability control. One possible strategy to increase the sensibility of the diagnosis, even from the first sub-clinical phases, is represented by the use of biological parameters reflecting for example glutamate homeostasis dysfunction, or oxidative stress associated to ALS. Such bio-markers would be extremely valuable tools both for a better diagnostic evaluation, and for studying the impact of therapeutic interventions on the disease course.

A special category of such biomarkers is represented by peripheral cells obtained directly from patients (*ex vivo*). The assumption underlying the use of these models consists in postulating a systemic involvement rather than a neuronal specific one, an assumption that is, at least in part, in line with the revision of the concept of the selectivity of motor neuron involvement in ALS. In this paragraph we will focus on two classes of cells that have been successfully used in ALS studies: blood cells and fibroblasts.

Blood Cells

Human platelets have been repeatedly considered as potentially useful tools for modeling CNS dysfunction in neurological patients (Da Prada et al., 1988; Di Luca et al., 2000), because they store, release, and uptake several neurotransmitters, such as serotonin, glutamate, GABA, and dopamine, and also frequently express the relative functional receptor molecules (Yang et al., 1996; Mangano and Schwarcz, 1981b; Sherif, 1994; Altamura et al., 1993). Interestingly, platelets represent an extremely suitable model to study the glutamatergic system dysfunction in ALS, as well as in other neuropsychiatric disorders (Ferrarese et al., 2001b; Ferrarese et al., 2001c; Ferrarese et al., 1999; Ferrarese et al., 2000; Mangano and Schwarcz, 1981a). In fact, platelets display all the components of a functional glutamatergic system, although its role is not completely cleared. For example, NMDA receptors have been repeatedly shown both in platelets and megakaryocytes (Genever et al., 1999; Skerry and Genever, 2001; Reilmann et al., 1997), and a role for glutamate in platelet activation and/or aggregation has already been proposed (Franconi et al., 1996; Franconi et al., 1998; Franconi et al., 2000). Moreover, we recently demonstrated in human platelets (Zoia et al., 2004) the presence of the three major glutamate transporters, namely EAAT1, EAAT2, and EAAT3, while a functional high-affinity sodium-dependent glutamate re-uptake system have been successfully described more than twenty years ago (Mangano and Schwarcz, 1981b). The possible significance of this finding still need to be definitively addressed, although it is conceivable that glutamate uptake in platelets, a major source of the amino acid removal from blood, may represent a suitable window for studying CNS glutamate uptake alterations (Begni et al., 2005). As a matter of fact, we recently reported in platelets obtained from ALS patients (Ferrarese et al., 2001b) a decrease in the maximal velocity of high-affinity sodium-dependent glutamate uptake (without changes in affinity), of the same order of magnitude observed in CNS (Rothstein et al., 1992), with respect to both healthy controls, and subjects affected by other neurological, non-neurodegenerative disorders. This data apparently indicate a more widespread involvement than previously believed in ALS patients. As a matter of fact, oxidative stress, endogenously generated or derived from xenobiotic exposure, may directly impair energy-dependent glutamate uptake and also can lead to the generation of lipid peroxydation products and free radicals, which in turn may damage glutamate transporters. A role for inflammatory mechanisms may also be proposed to explain the observed ALS-associated impairment of glutamate uptake, both in periphery, and CNS. For example, several cytokines have been reported to affect glutamate uptake (Fine et al., 1996) in neuronal and peripheral cell models, and plasma levels of some of these inflammatory mediators have been found increased in ALS patients (Houi et al., 2002). An alternative hypothesis may be indicated in the existence of a genetic trait predisposing to the development of motor neuron disease, possibly reducing the neuronal threshold to ROS- or other agents- mediated injury. In line with the latter hypothesis, preliminary data indicate that platelet uptake values are stable over time in individual ALS patients, thus suggesting that decreased transport is a disease trait rather than disease state marker. Although our data indicate a systemic involvement in ALS, other groups failed to report in platelets (Gluck et al., 2000) and leukocytes (Lanius et al., 1995) obtained from ALS patients a reduction of the activity of the enzymes cytochrome oxidase, glutamate dehydrogenase, glutaminase, and PKC histone H1 phosphotransferase, as described in motor neuron disease affected areas. It is reasonable to conclude that only some ALS-associated markers may be usefully studied in platelets, possibly due to the implicit phenotypic differences among different cell types.

Interestingly, our more recent observations also indicate that platelets release glutamate upon aggregation (Aliprandi et al., 2005), possibly allowing future studies addressing the role of excessive glutamate release in the pathogenesis of ALS.

Also lymphocytes have been proposed as model for studying oxidative metabolism and calcium homeostasis. While no difference was found in lymphocytes from ALS patients in basal oxygen consumption rate (QO_2), cytochrome c oxidase activity, catalase activity, and lactate production, a decrease in QO_2, induced by an uncoupler of oxidative phosphorylation, FCCP, was observed (Curti et al., 1996). Moreover, the basal (resting) level of free cytosolic calcium was higher in lymphocytes from sporadic ALS patients. Further increase in free intracellular calcium challenged by a K^+ channel blocker or by FCCP was similar in ALS and control lymphocytes (Curti et al., 1996).

Fibroblasts

Another model we are currently investigating is represented by fibroblasts, obtained through a very small skin biopsy with almost no nuisance for the patients and propagated by simple cell-culture procedures (Connolly, 1998). Fibroblasts, with respect to platelets, offer the advantage of being able to survive in culture and of displaying a nuclear structure, allowing a better approximation of what is the complex neuronal situation.

An early study indicated that fibroblasts from 5 patients with non-SOD1 familial ALS did not display signs of abnormal oxidative stress, based on the assay of ROS metabolism and of thiobarbituric-acid-reactive species (TBARS), a marker of lipid peroxidation (Jansen et al., 1996). On the other hand, other authors demonstrated an increased sensitivity to oxidative stress of fibroblasts from patients with sporadic and SOD1-associated familial ALS following treatment with free radical-generating agents (Aguirre et al., 1998).

Because fibroblasts possess a sodium-dependent high affinity uptake of L-glutamate mediated by a transport system similar to that observed in brain tissue (Balcar et al., 1994) and express at least moderate levels of glutamate transporters (Cooper et al., 1998), we are using fibroblasts from sporadic ALS patients in order to verify whether these peripheral cells can be used to model the alterations of the glutamate uptake system already demonstrated in the CNS of ALS patients.

Preliminary kinetic analyses of sodium-dependent glutamate uptake, determined as [^{3}H]-glutamate influx, showed that only a subgroup of ALS patient fibroblasts displays a reduced glutamate reuptake. Currently we are also measuring in this model EAAT2 glutamate transporter subtype both mRNA, and immunoreactive peptide. No significant change in whole-cell ROS amount, after exposure to the oxidative sensitive dye 2',7'-dichlorofluorescein diacetate, was demonstrated in ALS versus control fibroblasts (G.S. et al., unpublished observations). Collectively, our data support a possible use of fibroblasts as useful model for exploring the role of excitotoxicity and oxidative stress in the pathogenesis of ALS, allowing new anti-oxidant or anti-glutamate compounds, or combination therapies to be tested, as well as agents able to increase the expression of EAAT2 and/or other putative protective genes.

Conclusions: Are We Closer to a Therapy?

Although in the recent years several pieces of evidence have been accumulating about both ALS pathogenesis, motor neuronal selectivity, extra-neural involvement, and new possible therapeutic strategies, still we lack of a really effective pharmacological option. As previously suggested (Kriz et al., 2003; Zhang et al., 2003), a combined approach targeting different pathogenic mechanisms may prove to be an optimal strategy for preventing motor neuronal death in ALS. Excitotoxicity and oxidative stress, reciprocally sustaining each other in a complex pathogenic interplay, may represent two major mechanisms to address, especially in light of their repeatedly demonstrated role in ALS pathogenesis.

May We Prevent Excitotoxicity in ALS by Targeting EAAT2 Downregulation?

The recent report of the EAAT2 promoter sequence (Su et al., 2003) allows to think to future studies aimed at addressing the issue of the modulation of the expression of this transporter. This task appears to be extremely appealing, in light of the putative role played by EAAT2 in ALS pathogenesis, as discussed above. In fact, the possibility of a pharmacological intervention correcting EAAT2 (or other candidate genes, for example VEGF) downregulation may eventually prove to be a good strategy for arresting and/or preventing motor neuronal death in ALS.

Along this line, an interesting novel target of pharmacological intervention may be represented by epigenetic modifications (Beck and Olek, 2003), *i.e.*, chromatin rearrangements consequent to DNA or histones covalent changes (such as methylation or acetylation), resulting in gene expression rate mutations. For example, valproate, an old anti-epileptic drug that is widely used by neurologists, has been recently shown to display histone deacetylase (HDAC) inhibitor activity (Phiel et al., 2001), increasing acetylated histone immunoreactive content in mouse brain, following systemic administration (Tremolizzo et al., 2002). Noteworthy, in the same study, valproate chronic exposure was able to increase reelin and GAD_{67} expression in an animal model expressing schizophrenia-related endophenotypes (Tremolizzo et al., 2002). Similarly, valproate has been recently used to increase SMN expression rate in fibroblasts from patients affected by spinal muscular atrophy (Sumner et al., 2003), resulting in a partial compensation of the SMN1 loss at the nuclear level. This latter report appears to be especially interesting in light of the discussed role of the SMN gene as a protective factor in ALS (Veldnik et al., 2001; Corcia et al., 2002; Gamez et al., 2002).

Also EAAT2 may represent a suitable target for an epigenetic strategy of pharmacological intervention, especially in light of the presence in its promoter region of a CpG island, *i.e.*, a cytosine-guanidine dynucleotide rich region (Gardiner-Garden and Frommer, 1987), that represents a structural presuppose for epigenetic regulation of the expression of the gene through DNA methylation (analysis preformed on the sequence deposited by Su et al., 2003).

Considering these evidences, and in light of the low-toxicity profile and the high permeability through the blood-brain barrier, valproate might be indicated as the prototype of a new class of drugs (the HDAC inhibitors), able to target gene expression downregulation in neurological disorders, by inducing chromatin relaxation. However, before being able to prevent excitotoxicity in ALS by upregulating EAAT2 expression, one should address the issues of the target specificity, regarding both cell types, and genes modulated by the drugs. In fact, the list of genes that may be regulated through this mechanism may be very long, including "bad" genes as well "good" ones (for example, inflammatory genes may be upregulated by valproate, Koyama et al., 2002). Moreover, although EAAT2 upregulation has already been reported in the hippocampus of rats treated for 90 days with valproate (Hassel et al., 2001), several issues still need to be clarified, regarding the mechanisms involved in this putative overexpression, time- and dose-dependency, effective function of the upregulated proteins, and most important of all, human applicability.

In conclusion, given the complex interactions among oxidative stress, excitotoxicity, as well as other pathways implicated in ALS pathogenesis, it is unlikely that a single therapeutic modality will arrest the disease progression. Ideally, as new information is uncovered about these intertwined pathways, more effective cocktail treatments will emerge (Morrison, 2002).

Moreover, peripheral cells obtained from ALS patients will surely prove to be suitable models for studying multi-targeted therapeutic options, combining drugs acting synergistically. Discerning patients who "biologically" respond to the treatment might also serve to plan and optimize future more targeted trials. In fact, this is a critical issue, especially if we consider that trials of neuroprotective drugs in neurodegenerative diseases as ALS are extremely expensive, time-consuming and, last but not least, generating great expectations in patients and their care-givers.

References

Abe K, Pan LH, Watanabe M, Kato T, Itoyama Y (1995) Induction of nitrotyrosine-like immunoreactivity in the lower motor neuron of amyotrophic lateral sclerosis. *Neurosci Lett. 199*:152-154.

Aguirre T, Van Den Bosch L, Goetschalckx K, Tilkin P, Mathijs G, Cassiman JJ, Robberecht W (1998) Increased sensitivity of fibroblasts from amyotrophic lateral sclerosis patients to oxidative stress. *Ann Neurol. 43*:452-457.

Aliprandi A, Longoni M, Stanzani L, Tremolizzo L, Vaccaro M, Begni B, Galimberti G, Garofolo R, Ferrarese C (2005) Increased plasma glutamate in stroke patients may be linked to altered platelet release and uptake. *J Cereb Blood Flow Metab. 25*:513-519.

Almer G, Teismann P, Stevic Z, Halaschek-Wiener J, Deecke L, Kostic V, Przedborski S (2002) Increased levels of the pro-inflammatory prostaglandin PGE2 in CSF from ALS patients. *Neurology. 58*:1277-1279.

Altamura CA, Mauri MC, Ferrara A, Moro AR, D'Andrea G and Zamberlan F (1993) Plasma and platelet excitatory amino acids in psychiatric disorders. *Am J Psychiatry 150*:1731-1733.

Amara SG, Fontana AC (2002) Excitatory amino acid transporters: keeping up with glutamate. *Neurochem Int. 41*:313-318.

Andersen PM (2001) Genetics of sporadic ALS. *Amyotroph Lateral Scler Other Motor Neuron Disord.* 2 Suppl.*1*:S37-S41.

Andreassen OA, Dedeoglu A, Klivenyi P, Beal MF, Bush AI (2000) N-acetyl-L-cysteine improves survival and preserves motor performance in an animal model of familial amyotrophic lateral sclerosis. *Neuroreport. 11*:2491-2493.

Aoki M, Lin CL, Rothstein JD, Geller BA, Hosler BA, Munsat TL, Horvitz HR, Brown RH Jr (1998) Mutations in the glutamate transporter EAAT2 gene do not cause abnormal EAAT2 transcripts in amyotrophic lateral sclerosis. *Ann Neurol. 43*:645-653.

Atlante A, Calissano P, Bobba A, Giannattasio S, Marra E, Passarella S (2001) Glutamate neurotoxicity, oxidative stress and mitochondria. *FEBS Lett. 497*:1-5.

Azzouz M, Poindron P, Guettier S, Leclerc N, Andres C, Warter JM, Borg J (2000) Prevention of mutant SOD1 motoneuron degeneration by copper chelators in vitro. *J Neurobiol. 42*:49-55.

Baker DA, Shen H, Kalivas PW (2002) Cystine/glutamate exchange serves as the source for extracellular glutamate: modifications by repeated cocaine administration. *Amino Acids. 23*:161-162.

Balcar VJ, Shen J, Bao S, King NJ (1994) Na(+)-dependent high affinity uptake of L-glutamate in primary cultures of human fibroblasts isolated from three different types of tissue. *FEBS Lett. 339(1-2)*:50-54.

Banack SA, Cox PA (2003) Biomagnification of cycad neurotoxins in flying foxes: implications for ALS-PDC in Guam. *Neurology. 61*:387-389.

Bannai S (1986) Exchange of cystine and glutamate across plasma membrane of human fibroblasts. *J Biol Chem. 261*:2256-2263.

Beal MF (1992a) Does impairment of energy metabolism result in excitotoxic neuronal death in neurodegenerative illnesses? *Ann Neurol. 31*:119-130.

Beal MF (1992b) Mechanisms of excitotoxicity in neurologic diseases. *FASEB J. 6*:3338-3344.

Beal MF (1998) Mitochondrial dysfunction in neurodegenerative diseases. *Biochim Biophys Acta. 1366*:211-223.

Beal MF (2002) Coenzyme Q10 as a possible treatment for neurodegenerative diseases. *Free Radic Res. 36*:455-460.

Beal MF, Ferrante RJ, Browne SE, Matthews RT, Kowall NW, Brown RH Jr (1997) Increased 3-nitrotyrosine in both sporadic and familial amyotrophic lateral sclerosis. *Ann Neurol. 42*:644-654.

Beck S, Olek A, editors (2003) The epigenome. Molecular hide and seek. Weinheim: Wiley-VCH.

Beckman JS, Carson M, Smith CD, Koppenol WH (1993) ALS, SOD and peroxynitrite. *Nature. 364*:584.

Begni B, Tremolizzo L, D'Orlando C, Bono MS, Garofolo R, Longoni M, Ferrarese C (2005) Substrate modulation of glutamate uptake in human platelets. *Br J Pharmacol.* advance online publication, 09 May, 2005; doi: 10.1038/sj.bjp.0706242.

Bensimon G, Lacomblez L, Meininger V and the ALS/Riluzole Study Group (1994) A controlled trial of riluzole in amyotrophic lateral sclerosis. *N Engl J Med. 330*:585-591.

Benzie IF (1996) Lipid peroxidation: a review of causes, consequences, measurement and dietary influences. *Int J Food Sci Nutr. 47*:233-261.

Beretta S, Aliprandi A, Ferrarese C (2003a) Markers of excitotoxicity in patients: tool for diagnosis and therapy? In: Ferrarese C and Beal MF, editors (2003) Excitotoxicity in Neurological Diseases: New Therapeutic Challenge. Kluwer Academic Publishers.

Beretta S, Begni B, Ferrarese C (2003b) Pharmacological manipulation of glutamate transport. *Drug News Perspect. 16*:435-445.

Beretta S, Carri MT, Beghi E, Chio A, Ferrarese C (2003c) The sinister side of Italian soccer. *Lancet Neurol. 2*:656-657.

Beretta S, Sala G, Mattavelli L, Ceresa C, Casciati A, Ferri A, Carri MT, Ferrarese C (2003d) Mitochondrial dysfunction due to mutant copper/zinc superoxide dismutase associated with amyotrophic lateral sclerosis is reversed by N-acetylcysteine. *Neurobiol Dis.* 13:213-221.

Borthwick GM, Johnson MA, Ince PG, Shaw PJ, Turnbull DM (1999) Mitochondrial enzyme activity in amyotrophic lateral sclerosis: implications for the role of mitochondria in neuronal cell death. *Ann Neurol. 46*:787-790.

Bowling AC, Schulz JB, Brown RH Jr, Beal MF (1993) Superoxide dismutase activity, oxidative damage, and mitochondrial energy metabolism in familial and sporadic amyotrophic lateral sclerosis. *J Neurochem. 61*:2322-2325.

Bredt DS, Nicoll RA (2003) AMPA receptor trafficking at excitatory synapses. *Neuron. 40*:361-379.

Brighina L, Sala G, Ceresa C, Tremolizzo L, Ferrarese C. (2001) Recent advances in the therapy of amyotrophic lateral sclerosis: focus on excitotoxicity. *Funct Neurol.* 16(4Suppl.):*189*-202.

Bristol LA, Rothstein JD (1996) Glutamate transporter gene expression in amyotrophic lateral sclerosis motor cortex. *Ann Neurol. 39*:676-679.

Broer S, Brookes N (2001) Transfer of glutamine between astrocytes and neurons. *J Neurochem. 77*:705-719.

Brooks BR (1994) El Escorial World Federation of Neurology criteria for the diagnosis of amyotrophic lateral sclerosis. Subcommittee on Motor Neuron Diseases/Amyotrophic Lateral Sclerosis of the World Federation of Neurology Research Group on Neuromuscular Diseases and the El Escorial "Clinical limits of amyotrophic lateral sclerosis" workshop contributors. *J Neurol Sci. 124 Suppl.*:96-107.

Browne SE, Bowling AC, Baik MJ, Gurney M, Brown RH Jr, Beal MF (1998) Metabolic dysfunction in familial, but not sporadic, amyotrophic lateral sclerosis. *J Neurochem. 71*:281-287.

Camu W, Billiard M, Baldy-Moulinier M (1993) Fasting plasma and CSF amino acid levels in amyotrophic lateral sclerosis: a subtype analysis. *Acta Neurol Scand. 88*:51-55.

Chen W, Aoki C, Mahadomrongkul V, Gruber CE, Wang GJ, Blitzblau R, Irwin N, Rosenberg PA (2002) Expression of a variant form of the glutamate transporter GLT1 in neuronal cultures and in neurons and astrocytes in the rat brain. *J Neurosci. 22*:2142-2152.

Choi DW (1988) Glutamate neurotoxicity and diseases of the nervous system. *Neuron. 1*:623-634.

Chou SM, Wang HS, Komai K (1996) Colocalization of NOS and SOD1 in neurofilament accumulation within motor neurons of amyotrophic lateral sclerosis: an immunohistochemical study. *J Chem Neuroanat. 10:*249-258.

Cleveland DW, Liu J (2000) Oxidation versus aggregation - how do SOD1 mutants cause ALS? *Nat Med. 6*:1320-1321.

Connolly GP (1998) Fibroblast models of neurological disorders: fluorescence measurement studies. *Trends Pharmacol Sci. 19*:171-177.

Conti F, DeBiasi S, Minelli A, Rothstein JD, Melone M (1998) EAAC1, a high-affinity glutamate tranporter, is localized to astrocytes and gabaergic neurons besides pyramidal cells in the rat cerebral cortex. *Cereb Cortex. 8*:108-116.

Cookson MR, Shaw PJ (1999) Oxidative stress and motor neurone disease. *Brain Pathol. 9:*165-186.

Cooper B, Chebib M, Shen J, King NJ, Darvey IG, Kuchel PW, Rothstein JD, Balcar VJ (1998) Structural selectivity and molecular nature of L-glutamate transport in cultured human fibroblasts. *Arch Biochem Biophys. 353*:356-364.

Corcia P, Mayeux-Portas V, Khoris J, de Toffol B, Autret A, Muh JP, Camu W, Andres C; French ALS Research Group. Amyotrophic Lateral Sclerosis (2002) Abnormal SMN1 gene copy number is a susceptibility factor for amyotrophic lateral sclerosis. *Ann Neurol. 51*:243-246.

Cotman CW, Monaghan DT, Ganong AH (1988) Excitatory amino acid neurotransmission: NMDA receptors and Hebb-type synaptic plasticity. *Annu Rev Neurosci. 11*:61-80.

Cox PA, Banack SA, Murch SJ (2003) Biomagnification of cyanobacterial neurotoxins and neurodegenerative disease among the Chamorro people of Guam. *Proc Natl Acad Sci U S A. 100*:13380-13383.

Cox PA, Sacks OW (2002) Cycad neurotoxins, consumption of flying foxes, and ALS-PDC disease in Guam. *Neurology. 58*:956-959.

Crow JP, Sampson JB, Zhuang Y, Thompson JA, Beckman JS (1997) Decreased zinc affinity of amyotrophic lateral sclerosis-associated superoxide dismutase mutants leads to enhanced catalysis of tyrosine nitration by peroxynitrite. *J Neurochem. 69*:1936-1944.

Cudkowicz ME, Shefner JM, Schoenfeld DA, Brown RH Jr, Johnson H, Qureshi M, Jacobs M, Rothstein JD, Appel SH, Pascuzzi RM, Heiman-Patterson TD, Donofrio PD, David WS, Russell JA, Tandan R, Pioro EP, Felice KJ, Rosenfeld J, Mandler RN, Sachs GM, Bradley WG, Raynor EM, Baquis GD, Belsh JM, Novella S, Goldstein J, Hulihan J; Northeast ALS Consortium (2003) A randomized, placebo-controlled trial of topiramate in amyotrophic lateral sclerosis. *Neurology. 61*:456-464.

Curti D, Malaspina A, Facchetti G, Camana C, Mazzini L, Tosca P, Zerbi F, Ceroni M (1996) Amyotrophic lateral sclerosis: oxidative energy metabolism and calcium homeostasis in peripheral blood lymphocytes. *Neurology. 47*:1060-1064.

Curtis DR, Phillis JW, Watkins JC (1959) Chemical excitation of spinal neurones. *Nature. 183*:611-612.

Curtis DR, Watkins JC (1960) The excitation and depression of spinal neurones by structurally related amino acids. *J Neurochem. 6*:117-141.

Da Prada M, Cesura AM, Launay JM, Richards JG (1988) Platelets as a model for neurones? *Experientia 44*:115-126.

Danbolt NC (2001) Glutamate uptake. *Prog Neurobiol. 65:*1-105.

Danbolt NC; Holmseth, S, Skar, A, Lehre KP, Furness DN (2003) Glutamate uptake transporters. In: Ferrarese C and Beal MF, editors (2003) Excitotoxicity in Neurological Diseases: New Therapeutic Challenge. Kluwer Academic Publishers.

Daw NW, Stein PS, Fox K (1993) The role of NMDA receptors in information processing. *Annu Rev Neurosci. 16*:207-222.

Dawson VL, Dawson TM (1996) Nitric oxide neurotoxicity. *J Chem Neuroanat.* 10:179-190.

Dehnes Y, Chaudhry FA, Ullensvang K, Lehre KP, Storm-Mathisen J, Danbolt NC (1998) The glutamate transporter EAAT4 in rat cerebellar Purkinje cells: a glutamate-gated chloride channel concentrated near the synapse in parts of the dendritic membrane facing astroglia. *J Neurosci. 18*:3606-3619.

del Aguila MA, Longstreth WT Jr, McGuire V, Koepsell TD, van Belle G (2003) Prognosis in amyotrophic lateral sclerosis: a population-based study. *Neurology. 60:*813-819.

Deng HX, Hentati A, Tainer JA, Iqbal Z, Cayabyab A, Hung WY, Getzoff ED, Hu P, Herzfeldt B, Roos RP, et al. (1993) Amyotrophic lateral sclerosis and structural defects in Cu,Zn superoxide dismutase. *Science. 261*:1047-1051.

Desnuelle C, Dib M, Garrel C, Favier A (2001) A double-blind, placebo-controlled randomized clinical trial of alpha-tocopherol (vitamin E) in the treatment of amyotrophic lateral sclerosis. ALS riluzole-tocopherol Study Group. *Amyotroph Lateral Scler Other Motor Neuron Disord. 2*:9-18.

Dhaliwal GK, Grewal RP (2000) Mitochondrial DNA deletion mutation levels are elevated in ALS brains. *Neuroreport. 11*:2507-2509.

Di Luca M, Colciaghi F, Pastorino L, Borroni B, Padovani A, Cattabeni F (2000) Platelets as a peripheral district where to study pathogenetic mechanism of Alzheimer disease: the case of amyloid precursor protein. *Eur J Pharmacol 405*:277-283.

Doble A (1999) The role of excitotoxicity in neurodegenerative disease: implications for therapy. *Pharmacol Ther.* 8*1*:163-221.

Drachman DB, Frank K, Dykes-Hoberg M, Teismann P, Almer G, Przedborski S, Rothstein JD (2002) Cyclooxygenase 2 inhibition protects motor neurons and prolongs survival in a transgenic mouse model of ALS. *Ann Neurol. 52*:771-778.

Duan S, Anderson CM, Stein BA, Swanson RA (1999) Glutamate induces rapid upregulation of astrocyte glutamate transport and cell-surface expression of GLAST. *J Neurosci. 19*:10193-10200.

Estevez AG, Crow JP, Sampson JB, Reiter C, Zhuang Y, Richardson GJ, Tarpey MM, Barbeito L, Beckman JS (1999) Induction of nitric oxide-dependent apoptosis in motor neurons by zinc-deficient superoxide dismutase. *Science. 286*:2498-2500.

Ferrante RJ, Browne SE, Shinobu LA, Bowling AC, Baik MJ, MacGarvey U, Kowall NW, Brown RH Jr, Beal MF (1997) Evidence of increased oxidative damage in both sporadic and familial amyotrophic lateral sclerosis. *J Neurochem. 69:*2064-2074.

Ferrarese C and Beal MF, editors (2003) Excitotoxicity in Neurological Diseases: New Therapeutic Challenge. Kluwer Academic Publishers.

Ferrarese C, Begni B, Canevari C, Zoia C, Piolti R, Frigo M, Appollonio I, Frattola L (2000) Glutamate uptake is decreased in platelets from Alzheimer's disease patients. *Ann Neurol. 47*:641-643.

Ferrarese C, Pecora N, Frigo M, Appollonio I, Frattola L (1993) Assessment of reliability and biological significance of glutamate levels in cerebrospinal fluid. *Ann Neurol. 33*:316-319.

Ferrarese C, Sala G, Ceresa C, Tremolizzo L, Ferri A, Carrì MT (2001a) Interactions between oxidative stress and excitotoxicity in a cellular model of familial amyotrophic lateral sclerosis. *Amyotroph Lateral Scler Other Motor Neuron Disord. 2(Suppl.2):*146-147.

Ferrarese C, Sala G, Riva R, Begni B, Zoia C, Tremolizzo L, Galimberti G, Millul A, Bastone A, Mennini T, Balzarini C, Frattola L, Beghi E; Italian ALS Study Group (2001b) Decreased platelet glutamate uptake in patients with amyotrophic lateral sclerosis. *Neurology. 56:*270-272.

Ferrarese C, Tremolizzo L, Rigoldi M, Sala G, Begni B, Brighina L, Ricci G, Albizzati MG, Piolti R, Crosti F, Dalpra L, Frattola L (2001c) Decreased platelet glutamate uptake and genetic risk factors in patients with Parkinson's disease. *Neurol Sci. 22*:65-66.

Ferrarese C, Zoia C, Pecora N, Piolti R, Frigo M, Bianchi G, Sala G, Begni B, Riva R, Frattola L (1999) Reduced platelet glutamate uptake in Parkinson's disease. *J Neural Transm 106*:685-692.

Fiermonte G, Palmieri L, Todisco S, Agrimi G, Palmieri F, Walker JE (2002) Identification of the mitochondrial glutamate transporter. Bacterial expression, reconstitution, functional characterization, and tissue distribution of two human isoforms. *J Biol Chem. 277*:19289-19294.

Fine SM, Angel RA, Perry SW, Epstein LG, Rothstein JD, Dewhurst S, Gelbard HA (1996) Tumor necrosis factor alpha inhibits glutamate uptake by primary human astrocytes. Implications for pathogenesis of HIV-1 dementia. *J Biol Chem. 271*:15303-15306.

Flowers JM, Powell JF, Leigh PN, Andersen P, Shaw CE (2001) Intron 7 retention and exon 9 skipping EAAT2 mRNA variants are not associated with amyotrophic lateral sclerosis. *Ann Neurol. 49*:643-649.

Flynn J, McBean GJ (2000) Kinetic and pharmacological analysis of L-[35S]cystine transport into rat brain synaptosomes. *Neurochem Int. 36*:513-521.

Franconi F, Micele M, De Montis MG, Crisafi EL, Bennardini F, Tagliamonte A (1996) NMDA receptors play an anti-aggreganting role in human palatelets. *Thromb Haemost 76*:84-87.

Franconi F, Miceli M, Alberti L, Seghieri G, De Montis MG, Tagliamonte A (1998) Futher insights into the anti-aggregating activity of NMDA in human platelets. *Br J Pharmacol 124*:35-40.

Franconi F, Miceli M, De Montis MG, Lupis Crisafi E, Bennardini F, Tagliamonte A (2000): NMDA receptors play an antiaggregating role in human platelets. *Thromb Haemost 76*:84-87.

Fray AE, Ince PG, Banner SJ, Milton ID, Usher PA, Cookson MR, Shaw PJ (1998) The expression of the glial glutamate transporter protein EAAT2 in motor neuron disease: an immunohistochemical study. *Eur J Neurosci. 10*:2481-2489.

Gardiner-Garden M, Frommer M (1987) CpG islands in vertebrate genomes. *J Mol Biol. 196*:261-282.

Garthwaite J, Garthwaite G, Palmer RM, Moncada S (1989) NMDA receptor activation induces nitric oxide synthesis from arginine in rat brain slices. *Eur J Pharmacol. 172*:413-416.

Genever PG, Wilkinson DJP, Patton AJ, Peet NM, Hong Y, Mathur A, Erusalimsky JD, Skerry TM (1999) Expression of a functional N-methyl-D-aspartate-type glutamate receptor by bone marrow megakaryocytes. *Blood 23*:2876-2883.

Ghadge GD, Slusher BS, Bodner A, Canto MD, Wozniak K, Thomas AG, Rojas C, Tsukamoto T, Majer P, Miller RJ, Monti AL, Roos RP (2003) Glutamate carboxypeptidase II inhibition protects motor neurons from death in familial amyotrophic lateral sclerosis models. *Proc Natl Acad Sci U S A. 100*:9554-9559.

Gluck MR, Thomas RG, Sivak MA (2000) Unaltered cytochrome oxidase, glutamate dehydrogenase and glutaminase activities in platelets from patients with sporadic amyotrophic lateral sclerosis--a study of potential pathogenetic mechanisms in neurodegenerative diseases. *J Neural Transm. 107*:1437-1447.

Gamez J, Barcelo MJ, Munoz X, Carmona F, Cusco I, Baiget M, Cervera C, Tizzano EF (2002) Survival and respiratory decline are not related to homozygous SMN2 deletions in ALS patients. *Neurology. 59*:1456-1460.

Goto JJ, Zhu H, Sanchez RJ, Nersissian A, Gralla EB, Valentine JS, Cabelli DE (2000) Loss of in vitro metal ion binding specificity in mutant copper-zinc superoxide dismutases associated with familial amyotrophic lateral sclerosis. *J Biol Chem. 275*:1007-1014.

Groeneveld GJ, Veldink JH, van der Tweel I, Kalmijn S, Beijer C, de Visser M, Wokke JH, Franssen H, van den Berg LH (2003) A randomized sequential trial of creatine in amyotrophic lateral sclerosis. *Ann Neurol. 53:*437-445.

Gurney ME (1997) Transgenic animal models of familial amyotrophic lateral sclerosis. *J Neurol. 244 Suppl.2*:S15-S20.

Gurney ME (2000) Transgenic mouse model for familial amyotrophic lateral sclerosis. In: Brown Jr RH, Meininger V, Swash M, editors (2000) Amyotrophic lateral sclerosis. London: Martin Dunitz.

Gurney ME, Cutting FB, Zhai P et al. (1996) Benefit of vitamin E, riluzole and gabapentin in a transgenic model of familial amyotrophic lateral sclerosis. *Ann Neurol. 39*:147-157.

Gurney ME, Pu H, Chiu AY, Dal Canto MC, Polchow CY, Alexander DD, Caliendo J, Hentati A, Kwon YW, Deng HX, et al. (1994) Motor neuron degeneration in mice that express a human Cu,Zn superoxide dismutase mutation. *Science. 264*:1772-1775.

Hassel B, Iversen EG, Gjerstad L, Tauboll E (2001) Up-regulation of hippocampal glutamate transport during chronic treatment with sodium valproate. *J Neurochem. 77*:1285-1292.

Heath PR, Shaw PJ (2002) Update on the glutamatergic neurotransmitter system and the role of excitotoxicity in amyotrophic lateral sclerosis. *Muscle Nerve. 26*:438-458.

Heath PR, Tomkins J, Ince PG, Shaw PJ (2002) Quantitative assessment of AMPA receptor mRNA in human spinal motor neurons isolated by laser capture microdissection. *Neuroreport. 13*:1753-1757.

Henneberry RC, Novelli A, Cox JA, Lysko PG (1989) Neurotoxicity at the N-methyl-D-aspartate receptor in energy-compromised neurons. An hypothesis for cell death in aging and disease. *Ann N Y Acad Sci. 568*:225-233.

Hildeman DA, Mitchell T, Aronow B, Wojciechowski S, Kappler J, Marrack P (2003) Control of Bcl-2 expression by reactive oxygen species. *Proc Natl Acad Sci U S A. 100*:15035-15040.

Higgins CM, Jung C, Ding H, Xu Z (2002) Mutant Cu, Zn superoxide dismutase that causes motoneuron degeneration is present in mitochondria in the CNS. *J Neurosci.* 22:RC215.

Hinoi E, Takarada T, Ueshima T, Tsuchihashi Y, Yoneda Y (2004) Glutamate signaling in peripheral tissues. *Eur J Biochem. 271*:1-13.

Hisano S (2003) Vesicular glutamate transporters in the brain. *Anat Sci Int. 78*:191-204.

Hollander D, Pradas J, Kaplan R, McLeod HL, Evans WE, Munsat TL (1994) High dose dextromethorphan in amyotrophic lateral sclerosis: phase 1 safety and pharmacokinetic studies. *Ann Neurol. 36:*920-924.

Honig LS, Chambliss DD, Bigio EH, Carroll SL, Elliott JL (2000) Glutamate transporter EAAT2 splice variants occur not only in ALS, but also in AD and controls. *Neurology. 55*:1082-1088.

Hottinger AF, Fine EG, Gurney ME, Zurn AD, Aebischer P (1997) The copper chelator d-penicillamine delays onset of disease and extends survival in a transgenic mouse model of familial amyotrophic lateral sclerosis. *Eur J Neurosci. 9*:1548-1551.

Houi K, Kobayashi T, Kato S, Mochio S, Inoue K (2002) Increased plasma TGF-beta1 in patients with amyotrophic lateral sclerosis. *Acta Neurol Scand. 106*:299-301.

Huettner JE (2003) Kainate receptors and synaptic transmission. *Prog Neurobiol. 70:*387-407.

Ince PG, Eggett CJ, Shaw PJ (1997) The role of excitotoxicity in neurological disease. *Rev Contemp Pharmacother 8:*195-212.

Ince PG, Lowe J, Shaw PJ (1998) Amyotrophic lateral sclerosis: current issues in classification, pathogenesis and molecular pathology. *Neuropathol Appl Neurobiol. 24*:104-117.

Ince P, Stout N, Shaw P, Slade J, Hunziker W, Heizmann CW, Baimbridge KG (1993) Parvalbumin and calbindin D-28k in the human motor system and in motor neuron disease. *Neuropathol Appl Neurobiol. 19*:291-299.

Jackson M, Song W, Liu MY, Jin L, Dykes-Hoberg M, Lin CI, Bowers WJ, Federoff HJ, Sternweis PC, Rothstein JD (2001) Modulation of the neuronal glutamate transporter EAAT4 by two interacting proteins. *Nature. 410*:89-93.

Jansen GA, Wanders RJ, Jobsis GJ, Bolhuis PA, de Jong JM (1996) Evidence against increased oxidative stress in fibroblasts from patients with non-superoxide-dismutase-1 mutant familial amyotrophic lateral sclerosis. *J Neurol Sci. 139 Suppl.:*91-94.

Johnston JA, Dalton MJ, Gurney ME, Kopito RR (2000) Formation of high molecular weight complexes of mutant Cu, Zn-superoxide dismutase in a mouse model for familial amyotrophic lateral sclerosis. *Proc Natl Acad Sci U S A. 97*:12571-12576.

Jossan SS, Ekblom J, Gudjonsson O, Hagbarth KE, Aquilonius SM (1994) Double blind cross over trial with deprenyl in amyotrophic lateral sclerosis. *J Neural Transm Suppl. 41*:237-241.

Keller JN, Mark RJ, Bruce AJ, Blanc E, Rothstein JD, Uchida K, Waeg G, Mattson MP (1997) 4-hydroxynonenal, an aldehydic product of membrane lipid peroxidation, impairs glutamate transport and mitochondrial function in synaptosomes. *Neuroscience. 80*:685-696.

Keller JN, Mattson MP (1998) Roles of lipid peroxidation in modulation of cellular signaling pathways, cell dysfunction, and death in the nervous system. *Rev Neurosci. 9*:105-116.

Klivenyi P, Ferrante RJ, Matthews RT, Bogdanov MB, Klein AM, Andreassen OA, Mueller G, Wermer M, Kaddurah-Daouk R, Beal MF (1999) Neuroprotective effects of creatine in a transgenic animal model of amyotrophic lateral sclerosis. *Nat Med. 5*:347-350.

Kong J, Xu Z (1998) Massive mitochondrial degeneration in motor neurons triggers the onset of amyotrophic lateral sclerosis in mice expressing a mutant SOD1. *J Neurosci. 18*:3241-3250.

Kostic V, Jackson-Lewis V, de Bilbao F, Dubois-Dauphin M, Przedborski S (1997) Bcl-2: prolonging life in a transgenic mouse model of familial amyotrophic lateral sclerosis. *Science. 277*:559-562.

Koyama N, Koschmieder S, Tyagi S, Nurnberger H, Wagner S, Bocker U, Hoelzer D, Gerhard Ottmann O, Kalina U (2002) Differential effects of histone deacetylase inhibitors on interleukin-18 gene expression in myeloid cells. *Biochem Biophys Res Commun. 292*:937-943.

Kriz J, Gowing G, Julien JP (2003) Efficient three-drug cocktail for disease induced by mutant superoxide dismutase. *Ann Neurol. 53*:429-436.

Lacomblez L, Bensimon G, Leigh PN, Guillet P, Meininger V (1996) A dose-ranging study of riluzole in amyotrophic lateral sclerosis. *Lancet. 347*:1425-1431.

Lange DJ, Murphy PL, Diamond B, Appel V, Lai EC, Younger DS, Appel SH (1998) Selegiline is ineffective in a collaborative double-blind, placebo-controlled trial for treatment of amyotrophic lateral sclerosis. *Arch Neurol. 55*:93-96.

Lanius RA, Paddon HB, Mezei M, Wagey R, Krieger C, Pelech SL, Shaw CA (1995) A role for amplified protein kinase C activity in the pathogenesis of amyotrophic lateral sclerosis. *J Neurochem. 65*:927-930.

Lazarewicz JW, Wroblewski JT, Palmer ME, Costa E (1988) Activation of N-methyl-D-aspartate-sensitive glutamate receptors stimulates arachidonic acid release in primary cultures of cerebellar granule cells. *Neuropharmacology. 27*:765-769.

Lehre KP, Danbolt NC (1998) The number of glutamate transporter subtype molecules at glutamatergic synapses: chemical and stereological quantification in young adult rat brain. *J Neurosci. 18*:8751-8757.

Li M, Ona VO, Guegan C, Chen M, Jackson-Lewis V, Andrews LJ, Olszewski AJ, Stieg PE, Lee JP, Przedborski S, Friedlander RM (2000) Functional role of caspase-1 and caspase-3 in an ALS transgenic mouse model. *Science. 288*:335-339.

Li YV, Hough CJ, Sarvey JM (2003) Do we need zinc to think? *Sci STKE.* 2003(182):pe19.

Lin CI, Orlov I, Ruggiero AM, Dykes-Hoberg M, Lee A, Jackson M, Rothstein JD (2001) Modulation of the neuronal glutamate transporter EAAC1 by the interacting protein GTRAP3-18. *Nature. 410*:84-88.

Lin CL, Bristol LA, Jin L, Dykes-Hoberg M, Crawford T, Clawson L, Rothstein JD (1998) Aberrant RNA processing in a neurodegenerative disease: the cause for absent EAAT2, a glutamate transporter, in amyotrophic lateral sclerosis. *Neuron. 20*:589-602.

Lipton SA, Singel DJ, Stamler JS (1994) Nitric oxide in the central nervous system. *Prog Brain Res. 103:*359-364.

Louwerse ES, Weverling GJ, Bossuyt PM, Meyjes FE, de Jong JM (1995) Randomized, double-blind, controlled trial of acetylcysteine in amyotrophic lateral sclerosis. *Arch Neurol. 52*:559-564.

Lucas DR, Newhouse JP (1957) The toxic effect of sodium L-glutamate on the inner layers of the retina. *Ama Arch Opthalmol. 58*:193-201.

Ludolph AC, Riepe M, Ullrich K (1993) Excitotoxicity, energy metabolism and neurodegeneration. *J Inherit Metab Dis. 16*:716-723.

Mangano RM, Schwarcz R (1981a) Platelet glutamate and aspartate uptake in Huntington's disease. *J Neurochem. 37:*1072-1074.

Mangano RM, Schwarcz R (1981b) The human platelet as a model for the glutamatergic neuron: platelet uptake of L-Glutamate. *J Neurochem 36*:1067-1076.

Maragakis NJ, Jackson M, Ganel R, Rothstein JD (2003) Topiramate protects against motor neuron degeneration in organotypic spinal cord cultures but not in G93A SOD1 transgenic mice. *Neurosci Lett. 338*:107-110.

Marie H, Billups D, Bedford FK, Dumoulin A, Goyal RK, Longmore GD, Moss SJ, Attwell D (2002) The amino terminus of the glial glutamate transporter GLT-1 interacts with the LIM protein Ajuba. *Mol Cell Neurosci. 19*:152-164.

Massieu L, Garcia O (1998) The role of excitotoxicity and metabolic failure in the pathogenesis of neurological disorders. *Neurobiology. 6:*99-108.

Mattson MP (2003a) Excitotoxic and excitoprotective mechanisms: abundant targets for the prevention and treatment of neurodegenerative disorders. *Neuromolecular Med. 3*:65-94.

Mattson MP (2003b) Mechanisms of excitotoxicity and excitoprotection. In: Ferrarese C and Beal MF, editors (2003) Excitotoxicity in Neurological Diseases: New Therapeutic Challenge. Kluwer Academic Publishers.

Mazzini L, Balzarini C, Colombo R, Mora G, Pastore I, De Ambrogio R, Caligari M (2001) Effects of creatine supplementation on exercise performance and muscular strength in amyotrophic lateral sclerosis: preliminary results. *J Neurol Sci. 191*:139-144.

Mazzini L, Testa D, Balzarini C, Mora G (1994) An open-randomized clinical trial of selegiline in amyotrophic lateral sclerosis. *J Neurol. 241*:223-227.

McCord JM, Fridovich I (1969) Superoxide dismutase. An enzymic function for erythrocuprein (hemocuprein). *J Biol Chem. 244*:6049-6055.

Melcher T, Maas S, Herb A, Sprengel R, Seeburg PH, Higuchi M (1996) A mammalian RNA editing enzyme. *Nature. 379*:460-464.

Mennini T, Bendotti C (2003) Excitotoxicity in amyotrophic lateral sclerosis: selective vulnerability of motor neurons. In: Ferrarese C and Beal MF, editors (2003) Excitotoxicity in Neurological Diseases: New Therapeutic Challenge. Kluwer Academic Publishers.

Menzies FM, Ince PG, Shaw PJ (2002) Mitochondrial involvement in amyotrophic lateral sclerosis. *Neurochem Int. 40*:543-551.

Meyer T, Fromm A, Munch C, Schwalenstocker B, Fray AE, Ince PG, Stamm S, Gron G, Ludolph AC, Shaw PJ (1999) The RNA of the glutamate transporter EAAT2 is variably spliced in amyotrophic lateral sclerosis and normal individuals. *J Neurol Sci. 170*:45-50.

Miller RG, Moore D, Young LA, Armon C, Barohn RJ, Bromberg MB, Bryan WW, Gelinas DF, Mendoza MC, Neville HE, Parry GJ, Petajan JH, Ravits JM, Ringel SP, Ross MA (1996) A placebo-controlled trial of gabapentin in amyotrophic lateral sclerosis. *Neurology. 47*:1383-1388.

Miller RG, Moore DH 2nd, Gelinas DF, Dronsky V, Mendoza M, Barohn RJ, Bryan W, Ravits J, Yuen E, Neville H, Ringel S, Bromberg M, Petajan J, Amato AA, Jackson C, Johnson W, Mandler R, Bosch P, Smith B, Graves M, Ross M, Sorenson EJ, Kelkar P, Parry G, Olney R; Western ALS Study Group (2001) Phase III randomized trial of gabapentin in patients with amyotrophic lateral sclerosis. *Neurology. 56*:843-848.

Miller RJ, Murphy SN, Glaum SR (1989) Neuronal Ca2+ channels and their regulation by excitatory amino acids. *Ann N Y Acad Sci. 568*:149-158.

Mody I, MacDonald JF (1995) NMDA receptor-dependent excitotoxicity: the role of intracellular Ca2+ release. *Trends Pharmacol Sci. 16*:356-359.

Mori H, Mishina M (2003) Roles of diverse glutamate receptors in brain functions elucidated by subunit-specific and region-specific gene targeting. *Life Sci. 74*:329-336.

Morrison KE (2002) Therapies in amyotrophic lateral sclerosis–beyond riluzole. *Curr Opin Pharmacol 2*:302-309.

Munir M, Correale DM, Robinson MB (2000) Substrate-induced up-regulation of Na(+)-dependent glutamate transport activity. *Neurochem Int. 37*:147-162.

Nagai M, Abe K, Okamoto K, Itoyama Y (1998) Identification of alternative splicing forms of GLT-1 mRNA in the spinal cord of amyotrophic lateral sclerosis patients. *Neurosci Lett. 244*:165-168.

Nagano S, Ogawa Y, Yanagihara T, Sakoda S (1999) Benefit of a combined treatment with trientine and ascorbate in familial amyotrophic lateral sclerosis model mice. *Neurosci Lett. 265*:159-162.

Northington FJ, Traystman RJ, Koehler RC, Martin LJ (1999) GLT1, glial glutamate transporter, is transiently expressed in neurons and develops astrocyte specificity only after midgestation in the ovine fetal brain. *J Neurobiol. 39*:515-526.

Olney JW (1969) Brain lesions, obesity and other disturbances in mice treated with monosodium glutamate. *Science. 164*:719-721.

Olney JW (1989) Excitatory amino acids and neuropsychiatric disorders. *Biol Psychiatry. 26*:505-525.

Onorato JM, Thorpe SR, Baynes JW (1998) Immunohistochemical and ELISA assays for biomarkers of oxidative stress in aging and disease. *Ann N Y Acad Sci. 20*:277-290.

O'Shea RD (2002) Roles and regulation of glutamate transporters in the central nervous system. *Clin Exp Pharmacol Physiol.* 29:1018-1023.

Pasinelli P, Borchelt DR, Houseweart MK, Cleveland DW, Brown RH Jr (1998) Caspase-1 is activated in neural cells and tissue with amyotrophic lateral sclerosis-associated mutations in copper-zinc superoxide dismutase. *Proc Natl Acad Sci U S A. 95*:15763-15768.

Pedersen WA, Fu W, Keller JN, Markesbery WR, Appel S, Smith RG, Kasarskis E, Mattson MP (1998) Protein modification by the lipid peroxidation product 4-hydroxynonenal in the spinal cords of amyotrophic lateral sclerosis patients. *Ann Neurol. 44*:819-824.

Peghini P, Janzen J, Stoffel W (1997) Glutamate transporter EAAC-1-deficient mice develop dicarboxylic aminoaciduria and behavioral abnormalities but no neurodegeneration. *EMBO J. 16*:3822-3832.

Perry TL, Krieger C, Hansen S, Eisen A (1990) Amyotrophic lateral sclerosis: amino acid levels in plasma and cerebrospinal fluid. *Ann Neurol. 28*:12-17.

Phiel CJ, Zhang F, Huang EY, Guenther MG, Lazar MA, Klein PS (2001) Histone deacetylase is a direct target of valproic acid, a potent anticonvulsant, mood stabilizer, and teratogen. *J Biol Chem. 276:*36734-36741.

Pioro EP (2000) Antioxidant therapy in ALS. *Amyotroph Lateral Scler Other Motor Neuron Disord. 1(Suppl.4):*5-12.

Plaitakis A, Caroscio JT (1987) Abnormal glutamate metabolism in amyotrophic lateral sclerosis. *Ann Neurol. 22*:575-579.

Plaitakis A, Smith J, Mandeli J, Yahr MD (1988) Pilot trial of branched-chain aminoacids in amyotrophic lateral sclerosis. *Lancet. 1*:1015-1018.

Rae TD, Torres AS, Pufahl RA, O'Halloran TV (2001) Mechanism of Cu,Zn-superoxide dismutase activation by the human metallochaperone hCCS. J Biol Chem. *276*:5166-5176.

Rao SD, Weiss JH (2004) Excitotoxic and oxidative cross-talk between motor neurons and glia in ALS pathogenesis. *Trends Neurosci. 27*:17-23.

Rao SD, Yin HZ, Weiss JH (2003) Disruption of glial glutamate transport by reactive oxygen species produced in motor neurons. *J Neurosci. 23*:2627-2633.

Rauen T, Fischer F, Wiessner M (1999) Glia-neuron interaction by high-affinity glutamate transporters in neurotransmission. *Adv Exp Med Biol. 468*:81-95.

Reaume AG, Elliott JL, Hoffman EK, Kowall NW, Ferrante RJ, Siwek DF, Wilcox HM, Flood DG, Beal MF, Brown RH Jr, Scott RW, Snider WD (1996) Motor neurons in Cu/Zn superoxide dismutase-deficient mice develop normally but exhibit enhanced cell death after axonal injury. *Nat Genet. 13*:43-47.

Reilmann R, Rolf LH, Lange HW (1997) Huntington's disease: N-methyl-D-aspartate receptor coagonist glycine is increased in platelets. *Exp Neurol. 144*:416-419.

Riviere M, Meininger V, Zeisser P, Munsat T (1998) An analysis of extended survival in patients with amyotrophic lateral sclerosis treated with riluzole. *Arch Neurol.* 55:526-528.

Rosen DR, Siddique T, Patterson D, Figlewicz DA, Sapp P, Hentati A, Donaldson D, Goto J, O'Regan JP, Deng HX, et al. (1993) Mutations in Cu/Zn superoxide dismutase gene are associated with familial amyotrophic lateral sclerosis. *Nature. 362*:59-62.

Rothstein JD, Bristol LA, Hosler B, Brown RH Jr, Kuncl RW (1994) Chronic inhibition of superoxide dismutase produces apoptotic death of spinal neurons. *Proc Natl Acad Sci U S A. 91*:4155-4159.

Rothstein JD, Martin LJ, Kuncl RW (1992) Decreased glutamate transport by the brain and spinal cord in amyotrophic lateral sclerosis. *N Engl J Med. 326*:1464-1468.

Rothstein JD, Tsai G, Kuncl RW, Clawson L, Cornblath DR, Drachman DB, Pestronk A, Stauch BL, Coyle JT (1990) Abnormal excitatory amino acid metabolism in amyotrophic lateral sclerosis. *Ann Neurol. 28*:18-25.

Rothstein JD, Van Kammen M, Levey AI, Martin LJ, Kuncl RW (1995) Selective loss of glial glutamate transporter GLT-1 in amyotrophic lateral sclerosis. *Ann Neurol. 38*:73-84.

Sato H, Tamba M, Ishii T, Bannai S (1999) Cloning and expression of a plasma membrane cystine/glutamate exchange transporter composed of two distinct proteins. *J Biol Chem. 274:*11455-11458.

Schmitt A, Asan E, Lesch KP, Kugler P (2002) A splice variant of glutamate transporter GLT1/EAAT2 expressed in neurons: cloning and localization in rat nervous system. *Neuroscience. 109*:45-61.

Sen P, Mukherjee S, Bhaumik G, Das P, Ganguly S, Choudhury N, Raha S (2003) Enhancement of catalase activity by repetitive low-grade H2O2 exposures protects fibroblasts from subsequent stress-induced apoptosis. *Mutat Res. 529*:87-94.

Shaw PJ, Chinnery RM, Ince PG (1994) [3H]D-aspartate binding sites in the normal human spinal cord and changes in motor neuron disease: a quantitative autoradiographic study. *Brain Res. 655*:195-201.

Shaw PJ, Eggett CJ (2000) Molecular factors underlying selective vulnerability of motor neurons to neurodegeneration in amyotrophic lateral sclerosis. *J Neurol.* 247(Suppl.1):I17-I27.

Shaw PJ, Forrest V, Ince PG, Richardson JP, Wastell HJ (1995a) CSF and plasma amino acid levels in motor neuron disease: elevation of CSF glutamate in a subset of patients. *Neurodegeneration. 4:*209-216.

Shaw PJ, Ince PG, Falkous G, Mantle D (1995b) Oxidative damage to protein in sporadic motor neuron disease spinal cord. *Ann Neurol. 38*:691-695.

Shaw PJ, Kuncl RW (2002) Current concepts in the pathogenesis of ALS. In: Kuncl RW, editor (2002) Motor Neuron Disease. W.B. Saunders.

Shaw PJ, Williams TL, Slade JY, Eggett CJ, Ince PG (1999) Low expression of GluR2 AMPA receptor subunit protein by human motor neurons. *Neuroreport. 10*:261-265.

Shefner JM, Reaume AG, Flood DG, Scott RW, Kowall NW, Ferrante RJ, Siwek DF, Upton-Rice M, Brown RH Jr (1999) Mice lacking cytosolic copper/zinc superoxide dismutase display a distinctive motor axonopathy. *Neurology. 53*:1239-1246.

Sherif FM (1994) GABA-transaminase in brain and blood platelets: basic and clinical aspects. *Prog Neuropsycopharmacol Biol Psychiatry. 18:*1219-1233.

Shibata N (2001) Transgenic mouse model for familial amyotrophic lateral sclerosis with superoxide dismutase-1 mutation. *Neuropathology. 21*:82-92.

Shimizu S, Shiota K, Yamamoto S, Miyasaka Y, Ishii M, Watabe T, Nishida M, Mori Y, Yamamoto T, Kiuchi Y (2003) Hydrogen peroxide stimulates tetrahydrobiopterin synthesis through the induction of GTP-cyclohydrolase I and increases nitric oxide synthase activity in vascular endothelial cells. *Free Radic Biol Med. 34*:1343-1352.

Simpson EP, Yen AA, Appel SH (2003) Oxidative Stress: a common denominator in the pathogenesis of amyotrophic lateral sclerosis. *Curr Opin Rheumatol. 15*:730-736.

Skerry TM, Genever PG (2001) Glutamate signalling in non-neuronal tissues. *Trends Pharmacol Sci. 22*:174-181.

Skradski S, White HS (2000) Topiramate blocks kainate-evoked cobalt influx into cultured neurons. *Epilepsia. 41(Suppl.1):*S45-S47.

Smith MA, Sayre LM, Monnier VM, Perry G (1996) Oxidative posttranslational modifications in Alzheimer disease. A possible pathogenic role in the formation of senile plaques and neurofibrillary tangles. *Mol Chem Neuropathol. 28*:41-48.

Spencer PS (1987) Guam ALS/parkinsonism-dementia: a long-latency neurotoxic disorder caused by "slow toxin(s)" in food? *Can J Neurol Sci. (3Suppl.):*347-357.

Spencer PS, Kisby GE, Ludolph AC (1991) Slow toxins, biologic markers, and long-latency neurodegenerative disease in the western Pacific region. *Neurology. 41(5Suppl.2):*62-66.

Spencer PS, Schaumburg HH (1983) Lathyrism: a neurotoxic disease. *Neurobehav Toxicol Teratol. 5*:625-629.

Springer JE, Azbill RD, Mark RJ, Begley JG, Waeg G, Mattson MP (1997) 4-hydroxynonenal, a lipid peroxidation product, rapidly accumulates following traumatic spinal cord injury and inhibits glutamate uptake. *J Neurochem. 68*:2469-2476.

Strong M, Rosenfeld J (2003) Amyotrophic lateral sclerosis: a review of current concepts. *Amyotroph Lateral Scler Other Motor Neuron Disord. 4*:136-143.

Su ZZ, Leszczyniecka M, Kang DC, Sarkar D, Chao W, Volsky DJ, Fisher PB (2003) Insights into glutamate transport regulation in human astrocytes: cloning of the promoter for excitatory amino acid transporter 2 (EAAT2). *Proc Natl Acad Sci U S A. 100*:1955-1960.

Sumner CJ, Huynh TN, Markowitz JA, Perhac JS, Hill B, Coovert DD, Schussler K, Chen X, Jarecki J, Burghes AHM, Taylor JP, Fischbeck KH (2003) Valproic acid increases SMN levels in spinal muscular atrophy patient cells. *Ann Neurol. 54*:647–654.

Swerdlow RH, Parks JK, Cassarino DS, Trimmer PA, Miller SW, Maguire DJ, Sheehan JP, Maguire RS, Pattee G, Juel VC, Phillips LH, Tuttle JB, Bennett JP Jr, Davis RE, Parker WD Jr (1998) Mitochondria in sporadic amyotrophic lateral sclerosis. *Exp Neurol. 153*:135-142.

Tanaka K, Watase K, Manabe T, Yamada K, Watanabe M, Takahashi K, Iwama H, Nishikawa T, Ichihara N, Kikuchi T, Okuyama S, Kawashima N, Hori S, Takimoto M, Wada K (1997) Epilepsy and exacerbation of brain injury in mice lacking the glutamate transporter GLT-1. *Science. 276*:1699-1702.

Taylor CP (1994) Emerging perspectives on the mechanism of action of gabapentin. Neurology. *44(6Suppl.5):*S10-S16.

The Italian ALS Study Group (1993) Branched-chain amino acids and amyotrophic lateral sclerosis: a treatment failure? *Neurology.* 43:2466-2470.

Torgner I, Kvamme E (1990) Synthesis of transmitter glutamate and the glial-neuron interrelationship. *Mol Chem Neuropathol. 12*:11-17.

Torreilles F, Salman-Tabcheh S, Guerin M, Torreilles J (1999) Neurodegenerative disorders: the role of peroxynitrite. *Brain Res Brain Res Rev. 30*:153-163.

Traynor BJ, Alexander M, Corr B, Frost E, Hardiman O (2003a) An outcome study of riluzole in amyotrophic lateral sclerosis--a population-based study in Ireland, 1996-2000. *J Neurol. 250*:473-479.

Traynor BJ, Alexander M, Corr B, Frost E, Hardiman O (2003b) Effect of a multidisciplinary amyotrophic lateral sclerosis (ALS) clinic on ALS survival: a population based study, 1996-2000. *J Neurol Neurosurg Psychiatry. 74*:1258-1261.

Tremolizzo L, Carboni G, Ruzicka WB, Mitchell CP, Sugaya I, Tueting P, Sharma R, Grayson DR, Costa E, Guidotti A (2002) An epigenetic mouse model for molecular and behavioral neuropathologies related to schizophrenia vulnerability. *Proc Natl Acad Sci U S A. 99*:17095-17100.

Trotti D, Aoki M, Pasinelli P, Berger UV, Danbolt NC, Brown RH Jr, Hediger MA (2001) Amyotrophic lateral sclerosis-linked glutamate transporter mutant has impaired glutamate clearance capacity. *J Biol Chem. 276*:576-582.

Trotti D, Rolfs A, Danbolt NC, Brown RH Jr, Hediger MA (1999) SOD1 mutants linked to amyotrophic lateral sclerosis selectively inactivate a glial glutamate transporter. *Nat Neurosci. 2*:427-433.

Trotti D, Rossi D, Gjesdal O, Levy LM, Racagni G, Danbolt NC, Volterra A (1996) Peroxynitrite inhibits glutamate transporter subtypes. *J Biol Chem. 271*:5976-5979.

Trotti D, Volterra A, Lehre KP, Rossi D, Gjesdal O, Racagni G, Danbolt NC (1995) Arachidonic acid inhibits a purified and reconstituted glutamate transporter directly from the water phase and not via the phospholipid membrane. *J Biol Chem. 270:*9890-9895.

Veldink JH, van den Berg LH, Cobben JM, Stulp RP, De Jong JM, Vogels OJ, Baas F, Wokke JH, Scheffer H (2001) Homozygous deletion of the survival motor neuron 2 gene is a prognostic factor in sporadic ALS. *Neurology. 56*:749-752.

Vielhaber S, Winkler K, Kirches E, Kunz D, Buchner M, Feistner H, Elger CE, Ludolph AC, Riepe MW, Kunz WS (1999) Visualization of defective mitochondrial function in skeletal muscle fibers of patients with sporadic amyotrophic lateral sclerosis. *J Neurol Sci. 169*:133-139.

Volterra A, Trotti D, Cassutti P, Tromba C, Galimberti R, Lecchi P, Racagni G (1992) A role for the arachidonic acid cascade in fast synaptic modulation: ion channels and transmitter uptake systems as target proteins. *Adv Exp Med Biol. 318*:147-158.

Volterra A, Trotti D, Floridi S, Racagni G (1994) Reactive oxygen species inhibit high-affinity glutamate uptake: molecular mechanism and neuropathological implications. *Ann N Y Acad Sci. 738*:153-162.

Wiedemann FR, Winkler K, Kuznetsov AV, Bartels C, Vielhaber S, Feistner H, Kunz WS (1998) Impairment of mitochondrial function in skeletal muscle of patients with amyotrophic lateral sclerosis. *J Neurol Sci. 156*:65-72.

Williams K (1997) Interactions of polyamines with ion channels. *Biochem J. 325*:289-297.

Williams TL, Day NC, Ince PG, Kamboj RK, Shaw PJ (1997) Calcium-permeable alpha-amino-3-hydroxy-5-methyl-4-isoxazole propionic acid receptors: a molecular determinant of selective vulnerability in amyotrophic lateral sclerosis. *Ann Neurol. 42*:200-207.

Wong PC, Pardo CA, Borchelt DR, Lee MK, Copeland NG, Jenkins NA, Sisodia SS, Cleveland DW, Price DL (1995) An adverse property of a familial ALS-linked SOD1 mutation causes motor neuron disease characterized by vacuolar degeneration of mitochondria. *Neuron. 14*:1105-1116.

Wong PC, Waggoner D, Subramaniam JR, Tessarollo L, Bartnikas TB, Culotta VC, Price DL, Rothstein J, Gitlin JD (2000) Copper chaperone for superoxide dismutase is essential to activate mammalian Cu/Zn superoxide dismutase. *Proc Natl Acad Sci U S A*. 97:2886-2891.

Yang M, Srikiatkhachorn A, Anthony M, Chong BH (1996) Serotonin stimulates megakaryocytopoiesis via the 5-HT2 receptor. *Blood Coagul Fibrinolysis* 7:127-133.

Yun HY, Dawson VL, Dawson TM (1996) Neurobiology of nitric oxide. *Crit Rev Neurobiol. 10*:291-316.

Zhang W, Narayanan M, Friedlander RM (2003) Additive neuroprotective effects of minocycline with creatine in a mouse model of ALS. *Ann Neurol. 53*:267-270.

Zoia C, Cogliati T, Tagliabue E, Cavaletti G, Sala G, Galimberti G, Rivolta I, Rossi V, Frattola L, Ferrarese C (2004) Glutamate transporters in platelets: EAAT1 decrease in aging and in Alzheimer's disease. *Neurobiol Aging. 25*:149-157.

In: Amyotrophic Lateral Sclerosis: New Research
Editor: Christine A. Murray, pp. 111-134
ISBN 1-59454-179-5

Chapter IV

Mitochondrial Alterations in a Murine Model of Amyotrophic Lateral Sclerosis

C. Bendotti[1*] and S. De Biasi[2]

[1]Lab. Molecular Neurobiology, Dept Neuroscience, Istituto Ricerche Farmacologiche "Mario Negri," Milan, Italy

[2]Dept Biomolecular Sciences and Biotechnologies, University of Milan, Milan, Italy

Abstract

Accumulating evidence indicates that alterations of the mithochondrial pool in motor neurons are implicated in the pathogenesis of Amyotrophic Lateral Sclerosis (ALS) and therefore mitochondrial damage has become an important area of the investigation in the causes of this pathology. Ultrastructural investigations have shown that morphological abnormalities of mitochondria in spinal motor neurons are a very early sign in the disease progression in murine models of familial ALS represented by transgenic mice carrying a mutated form of the gene coding for human Cu, Zn superoxide dismutase (SOD1). In particular, in a transgenic line of mice expressing human SOD1 with a glycine to alanine mutation in position 93 (Tg SOD1G93A mice) we have detected swollen mitochondria with dilated and disorganized cristae in spinal motor neurons as early as two weeks after birth, when the animals are completely asymptomatic. Similar mitochondrial abnormalities were detected also in motor neurons of the hypoglossal and trigeminal motor nuclei of young Tg SOD1G93A mice and do not seem to depend on the number of transgene copies expressed as they are present even in low expressor mice with a late onset of the pathology.

The mechanisms that can lead to mitochondrial damage, which include excitotoxicity, oxidation of mitochondrial components and accumulation of protein aggregates are discussed in light of possible therapeutic interventions.

---

* Correspondence concerning this article should be addressed to Dr. Caterina Bendotti, Lab. Molecular Neurobiology, Dept Neuroscience, Istituto Ricerche Farmacologiche "Mario Negri", via Eritrea 62, 20157 Milan, Italy; e-mail: bendotti@irfmn.mnegri.it

Keywords: motor neurons, mutant superoxide dismutase-1, transgenic mice, mitochondrial permeability transition pore, excitotoxicity

Background

Mitochondria are cytoplasmic organelles that play a crucial role in the life of the cells, not only as major producers of the ATP necessary to support all cellular functions, but also for their ability to generate free radicals and to remove calcium from the cytosol when its concentration rises at toxic levels. Mitochondrial damage or dysfunction inevitably leads to cellular alterations and death, which may follow a physiological programmed cell death process mediated by the activation of proteases and endonucleases (apoptosis) or may be accidental (necrosis), with a severe ATP loss accompanied by mitochondrial and cytoplasmic swelling (reviewed in [46, 56]). It is therefore not surprising that accumulating evidence suggests a pivotal role of mitochondrial dysfunction in the mechanisms underlying the development of several types of neurodegenerative pathologies and that mitochondrial abnormalities have been identified in a large proportion of neurodegenerative diseases, including amyotrophic lateral sclerosis (ALS) [45, 66].

Abnormal mitochondrial function in central nervous system (CNS) tissues of ALS patients was first demonstrated by Bowling and collaborators [10] who showed an increase in mitochondrial complex I activity in the frontal cortex of patients with mutations in the gene encoding Cu, Zn superoxide dismutase (SOD1) which was absent in other cases of ALS. Similar changes were confirmed later in motor and parietal cortex of patients with familial ALS (fALS) linked to SOD1 mutations [11], whereas mitochondrial complex II and III activities were found to be increased in motor cortex and cerebellum in fALS not linked to SOD1 mutations, but not in sporadic ALS (sALS). On the other hand, different studies on spinal cord tissue or skeletal muscle homogenates from sALS patients demonstrated a decrease in mitochondrial complex IV (cytochrome oxidase) activities [9, 19, 25, 77]. In some cases such deficiency was associated with mutations in the mitochondrial DNA [19, 77]. Controversial evidences have been presented regarding changes in the Mn superoxide dismutase (SOD2), which is responsible for the removal of superoxide in mitochondria. An increased labeling for this enzyme was found in motor neurons and astrocytes of brainstem and spinal cord from ALS patients using immunohistochemical techniques [49, 67], whereas the analysis of total protein levels and activities of SOD2 from motor cortex homogenates showed no changes [63]. A major problem in the study of ALS, as well as of other neurodegenerative diseases affecting humans, is related to the possibility of analyzing only post-mortem tissues whose results are confounded by the variability in the post-mortem interval, pre-terminal hypoxia, tissues treatment procedures and other factors. Moreover, they generally represent a very late stage of the pathology. This makes it difficult to interpret the relevance of the observed abnormalities with respect to the initial development of the disorders. Therefore, it is still debated whether the mitochondrial alterations are a primary cause of the disease or whether they represent a consequence of the disease processes.

Attempts to circumvent this problem have been made by looking at muscle biopsies or at peripheral cells, such as lymphocytes or fibroblasts, obtained from patients at different time points during the progression of the disease. Taking advantage of the fact that spinal motor neurons have axons that exit the CNS to innervate muscle fibers, Siklos and collaborators examined axonal terminals in bioptic muscle specimens from patients with early diagnosed sporadic ALS [69]. Using electron microscopy they demonstrated an increased mitochondrial volume associated with elevated intra-mitochondrial calcium levels in neuromuscular terminals from ALS patients with respect to control samples. Mitochondrial changes in muscle biopsies from ALS patients have also been demonstrated by Atsumi [3], who showed a decrease in the number of mitochondria in intramuscular nerves, and by Vielhaber and collaborators [77], who found differences in the activity of cytochrome oxidase (mitochondrial complex IV) in saponin-permeabilized muscle fibers from patients with sALS with respect to control subjects. Nevertheless, these results are at variance with a recent study showing no changes of mitochondrial function in skeletal muscle of patients with early stage sALS [22], leaving uncertain whether systemic abnormalities of mitochondria may precede the effects in the CNS. However, mitochondrial alterations were also found in body districts not strictly related to the ALS vulnerable regions. For example, a curious description of "bizarre giant mitochondria" was given by Nakano in liver biopsies from sALS patients [55], while a functional mitochondial impairment with respect to calcium homeostasis and complex I activity was present in lymphocytes from sALS patients [20]. Using the technique of the cytoplasmic hybrid cell (cybrids) obtained by fusing platelets, which are devoid of nucleus, from sporadic ALS patients, with rho° cells depleted of mitochondria, Swerdlow and collaborators showed several defects, including altered mitochondrial ultrastructure, decreased mitochondrial complex I activity, increase in free radical scavenging enzymes and perturbations in calcium homeostasis [72].

Altogether these evidences suggest that mitochondria are susceptible of alterations in ALS, but the causes and the consequences of these alterations remain elusive. The use of appropriate experimental models is mandatory to settle this issue. A major breakthrough in this direction came with the discovery that about 20% of fALS cases and 2-3% of sALS cases possess a mutation in the gene encoding the antioxidant enzyme Cu, Zn superoxide dismutase (SOD1) [64]. This metalloenzyme is abundantly expressed in all vertebrate tissues and is responsible for the conversion of superoxide anion to hydrogen peroxide, thus playing a major role in the cell defense against oxygen free radicals. So far more than 100 mutations of this enzyme have been associated with ALS and several lines of evidence indicate that the neurotoxicity of the mutant enzyme is not due to a loss of its function, but instead to the gain of a toxic function [18]. The most straightforward evidence for this derives from the development of cellular and animal models of motor neuron degeneration expressing SOD1 mutants. In particular, transgenic rodents (mice and rats) expressing mutant human SOD1 develop progressive skeletal muscle atrophy, paralysis and death associated with selective motor neuron loss, similar to those observed in human ALS cases [32, 67]. These transgenic rodent models provide therefore a unique opportunity to investigate in detail the mechanisms that trigger the cascade of events leading to motor neuron death.

Transgenic Rodent Models Expressing Mutant Human SOD1

Several lines of transgenic mice carrying different human SOD1 mutants have been produced and examined [67]. So far the most extensively studied SOD1 transgenic mice are those carrying the G93A mutation (Tg SOD1 G93A mice) [28] that are commercially available (The Jackson Laboratories, Bar Harbor, ME). In general, transgenic mice expressing a high number of copies of the mutated SOD1 gene develop an early-onset disease with respect to transgenic mice expressing a low number of copies of the mutated SOD1 gene. However, the duration of the disease does not correlate with the time of onset or with the number of transgene copies [67]. Accordingly, we have found that Tg SOD1 G93A mice, maintained on homogenous C57BL/6 genetic background expressing 20-25 copies of the transgene, develop the first neuromuscular deficits (tremor in legs and loss of extension reflex of the hind paw) at about 12±1 weeks of age and die at 22±1.5 weeks, whereas those with about one third of transgene copy number, probably due to a cross over event leading to a loss of transgene copies, show the first motor dysfunction symptoms at 32±3.1 weeks and die at 36.4±3.3 weeks [17].

Almost all of the SOD1 transgenic rodent models overexpress the mutant human SOD1 while maintaining their normal murine SOD1 activity, thus demonstrating that mutant human SOD1 kills motor neurons by gaining a toxic function. Several hypotheses have been postulated to explain the toxic mechanism of mutant human SOD1. Among these are: 1) oxidative damage induced by enhancement of pro-oxidant activities of the mutant enzyme, including peroxidation and generation of hydroxyl radicals [81]; 2) decrease affinity of the mutant enzyme for zinc that would increase its reaction with nitric oxide to induce nitration of protein tyrosine residues by peroxynitrite [5]; 3) enhanced propensity of the mutant SOD1 to form intracellular protein aggregates, which in turn can induce cellular toxicity in analogy to what occurs in other neurodegenerative diseases [35]. Interestingly, increased expression of markers of oxidative stress, such as nitrotyrosine and oxidized proteins, and accumulation of SOD1-containing aggregates are also found in some cases of sALS [68], thus suggesting that common pathophysiological mechanisms may contribute to the different form of ALS. In the light of this, studies conducted in transgenic mice expressing mutant human SOD1 at different stages of the disease provide useful informations underlying the sequence of pathological events correlated with the clinical progression of the disease that may be also relevant to clarify the pathogenesis of sALS.

The most prominent alterations found in transgenic mice at times preceeding any behavioral symptoms of motor neuron dysfunction are: i) mitochondrial swelling and cytoplasmic vacuolization [6, 43]; ii) fragmentation of the Golgi apparatus [26]; iii) accumulation of phosphorylated neurofilaments and intracellular kinases [73]. Electron microscopy analysis showed that the earliest alteration observed in spinal motor neurons of both Tg SOD1 G93A mice [6, 43] and of mice carrying the SOD1 G37R mutation [82] was a massive mitochondrial vacuolization and swelling. These morphological changes precede motor neuron loss and decrease at the end stage of the pathology [43]. This might explain why these abnormalities are hardly found in motor neurons of autoptic samples from ALS patients that are obtained at a final stage of the disease.

It has been suggested that mitochondrial pathology may be related to the presence of a high number of mutant SOD1 gene copies, and that therefore mitochondrial alterations may not be evident in transgenic low expressor mice or in fALS patients with low levels of mutant SOD1 [70]. In this study we examined more extensively the ultrastructure of motor neurons from spinal cord and brainstem motor nuclei of high expressor Tg SOD1G93A mice in comparison with low expressor Tg SOD1G93A mice that develop the disease much later and which more closely mimic the human SOD1 levels. The results will be examined and discussed in the context of the accumulating evidence suggesting a role of abnormal mitochondrial function in the development of motor neuron disease.

Methods

Animals

Female C57BL/6 and transgenic mice were maintained at a temperature of 21 ± 1°C with relative humidity 55 ± 10% and 12 hours of light. Food (standard pellets) and water were supplied ad libitum. Transgenic mice originally obtained from The Jackson Laboratories (Bar Harbor, ME, USA) and expressing either a high copy number (20-25 copies, high expressor mice) or a low copy number (7-10 copies, low expressor mice) of mutant human SOD1 with a Gly 93 Ala substitution (Tg SOD1 G93A) were bred and maintained on a C57BL/6 mice strain at the Consorzio Mario Negri Sud, Santa Maria Imbaro (CH), Italy. Transgenic mice were identified by polymerase chain reaction (PCR) [64]. The high expressor mice become symptomatic at around 11 weeks and die at about 21-22 weeks of age, and about 50 % motor neuron loss is found in the oldest mice compared to age-matched controls [53]. Female high expressor mice were killed at the following ages: a) 2, 4, 6 and 8 weeks, corresponding to a presymptomatic stage; b) 12 weeks, corresponding to an early symptomatic stage; c) 14 and 15 weeks, corresponding to a symptomatic stage; and d) 18, 19, 21 weeks corresponding to an end stage of disease. The low expressor mice become symptomatic at around 30-32 weeks and die at about 36-40 weeks of age. Female low expressor mice were killed at 20 weeks of age, corresponding to a presymptomatic stage of disease. Non transgenic litttermates were used as controls.

Tissue Processing

Transgenic and non transgenic mice were fixed by intracardiac perfusion with 2.5% glutaraldehyde and 0.5% paraformaldehyde (for electron microscopy) or with 4% paraformaldehyde (for light microscopy immunocytochemistry). Their brains and lumbar spinal cords were then coronally cut with a Vibratome at 50 microns and the sections serially collected in cell wells in PBS. Brain areas were identified according to the atlas of mouse brain [60].

Procedures involving animals and their care were conducted in conformity with the institutional guidelines that are in compliance with national (D.L. no. 116, G.U. suppl. 40,

Feb. 18, 1992, Circolare No. 8, G.U., 14 luglio 1994) and international laws and policies (EEC Council Directive 86/609, OJ L 358, 1 DEC.12, 1987; NIH Guide for the Care and use of Laboratory Animals, U.S. National Research Council, 1996). All efforts were made to minimize the number of animals used and their suffering.

Electron Microscopy

Vibratome sections of the lumbar spinal cord and of the brainstem at the level of the motor trigeminal and of the hypoglossal nuclei were osmicated, dehydrated and flat-embedded in Epon-Spurr resin. Areas of interest were trimmed out under a dissection microscope and glued to blank resin blocks for ultramicrotomy. Semithin (1 micron-thick) sections were stained with toluidine blue and examined with a light microscope, whereas thin sections collected on copper grids were counterstained with uranyl acetate and lead citrate and then observed and photographed with a Jeol T8 electron microscope.

Immunocytochemistry

Vibratome sections of lumbar spinal cord were immersed in 0.05M NH4Cl in phosphate buffered saline (PBS) to remove unbound aldehydes from the tissue, blocked for 1 h in 1% bovine serum albumine (BSA) in PBS containing 0.2% Triton-X100 and then incubated overnight in the primary antiserum (mouse monoclonal anti-cytochrome oxidase subunit I, clone 1D6, Molecular Probes, a mitochondrial marker) diluted 1:200 in PBS containing 0.1% BSA and 0.2% Triton-X100. The immunoreaction was then visualized using a secondary horse-anti mouse antibody conjugated with red-X. Controls were carried out by omitting either the primary or the secondary antibody.

The sections were then observed with a TCS NT confocal laser scan microscope equipped with a 75-mW krypton/argon mixed gas laser (Leica Lasertecknik GmbH, Heidelberg, Germany).

Results

To detect the first signs of morphological alterations we performed detailed electron microscopy analyses on thin sections of lumbar spinal cord, trigeminal and hypoglossal motor nuclei obtained from a) Tg SOD1G93A high expressor mice starting at 2 weeks of age and proceeding up to the end stage of disease, b) Tg SOD1G93A low expressor mice at 20 weeks of age and c) age-matched non transgenic mice.

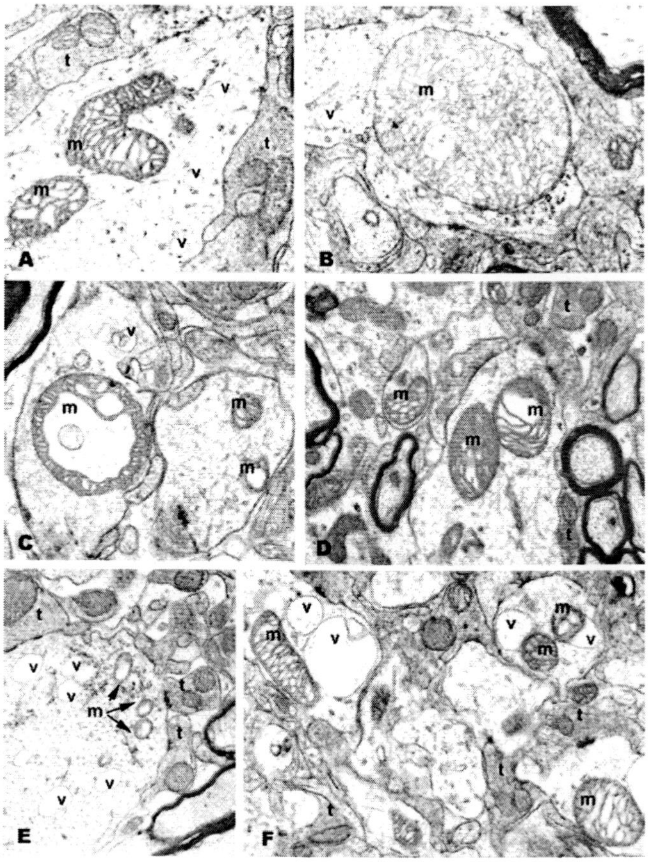

Figure 1. Electron micrographs showing alterations of mitochondria (m) and presence of vacuoles (v) in dendrites located in the ventral horn (A-D), motor trigeminal nuclei (E), hypoglossal nuclei (F) of both high expressor (A-C,E,F) and low expressor (D) Tg SOD1 G93A mice at early presymptomatic stages of disease. Note that in adjacent synaptic terminals (t) mitochondria have a normal morphology. A, B: ventral horn of high expressors at 2 weeks of age. Original magnifications 20,000x. C: ventral horn of a high expressor at 5 weeks of age. Original magnification 20,000x. D: ventral horn of a low expressor 20 weeks of age. Original magnification 16,000x. E: motor trigeminal nucleus of a high expressor at 4 weeks of age. Original magnification 16,000x. F: hypoglossal nucleus of a high expressor at 4 weeks of age. Original magnification 16,000x

Presymptomatic Mice

In all high expressor transgenic mice examined, mitochondrial abnormalities can be easily observed already in the presymptomatic stages of disease progression (2-6 weeks) both in the lumbar spinal cord and in the brainstem hypoglossal and motor trigeminal nuclei, with no significant differences among the three areas investigated (Figs. 1A-F, 2B). At these ages, mitochondria in dendrites (Fig. 1 A-F) and in motor neuron cell bodies (Fig.2B) appear swollen, with disorganized or indistinct cristae, and are often located close to clear vacuoles of variable sizes (Figs. 1A-C, 1E-F, 2B). In general, during the first postnatal week, mitochondrial abnormalities tend to affect predominantly the dendrites with respect to the cell bodies and they also tend to increase in frequency and severity with the age of the animal. Moreover, neuronal mitochondria also show alterations in size, as a significant number of enlarged mitochondria are present in trangenic mice (Fig. 1A-C, 2B) with respect to controls (Fig. 2A). These giant mitochondria are often located close to each other and they seem to form clusters (Fig. 2B), thus giving rise to an uneven distribution in motor neuron perikarya. The presence of abnormally large mitochondria in motor neurons of transgenic mice is also confirmed by immunocytochemical experiments in which the subunit I of the enzymatic complex cytochrome oxidase (cox), which is located in the inner mitochondrial membrane and is considered a reliable marker of mitochondria, is visualized with fluorescent light microscopy in thick vibratome sections (Fig. 3). In control mice, in fact, the large perikarya in lamina IX of the the ventral horn, identifiable for their size and location as motor neurons, display a homogeneous distribution of several cox-labeled puncta with a regular size (Fig. 3A), whereas in transgenic mice the cell bodies of motor neurons contain cox-labeled puncta unevenly distributed and sometimes of very large size (Fig. 3B). Large, cox-labeled puncta are also found dispersed in the neuropil of transgenic mice and they likely represent enlarged mitochondria present in dendrites (Fig. 3B).

Mitochondrial alterations similar to those described in young Tg SOD1G93A high expressor mice were also observed in low expressor transgenic mice at the age of 20 weeks, which in these animals corresponds to an early presymptomatic stage, both in the lumbar spinal cord (Fig.1D) and in the two brainstem nuclei investigated.

Finally, another typical morphological alteration observed in all Tg SOD1 G93A mice since the early presymptomatic stages is the presence of clear vacuoles located in both dendrites and neuronal cell bodies. The vacuoles are initially small (Figs. 1A-C, 1E, 2B) and then increase in size and number with the progression of the disease (Fig. 2B, 4).

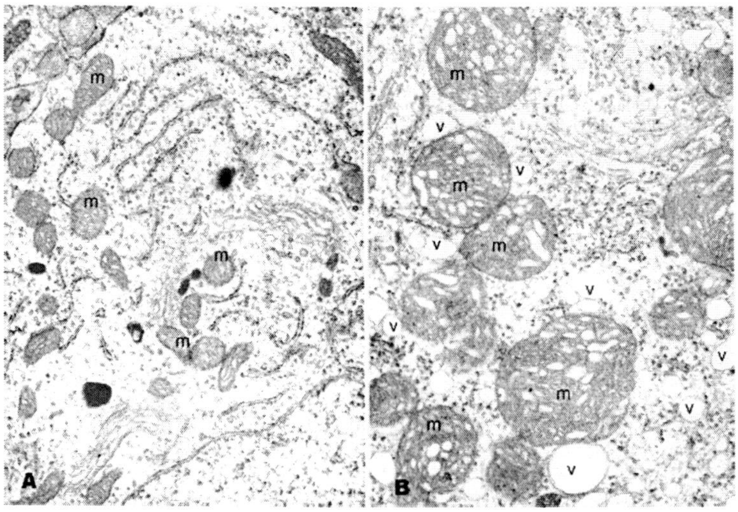

Figure 2. Electron micrographs showing early alterations and enlargement of somatic mitochondria (m) and presence of small vacuoles in ventral horn motor neurons of Tg SOD1 G93A mice at 4 weeks of age (B) compared to an age-matched non transgenic mice (A). Original magnifications: 16,000x.

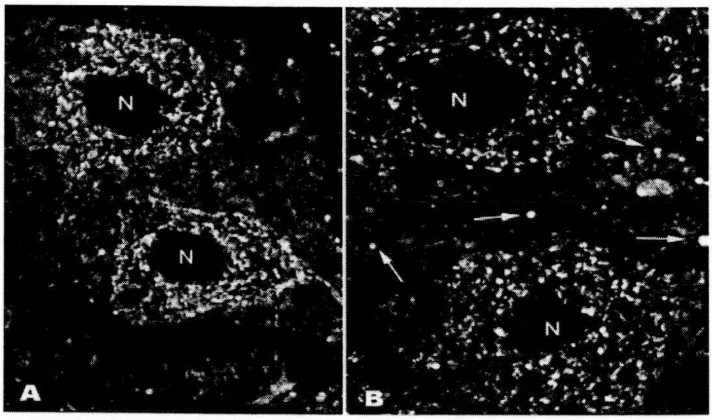

Figure 3. Confocal images of immunolabeling with an antiserum against the subunit I of cytochrome oxidase in two ventral horn motor neurons of a non transgenic (A) and a Tg SOD1 G93A (B) mouse at 4 weeks of age. Fluorescent dots labeled by the antiserum indicate mitochondria. In the non transgenic mice (A) motor neurons have several mitochondria of regular size homogenously distributed in their perikarya, whereas in TgSOD1G93A mice (B) some of the mitochondria in motor neuron perikarya and in the neuropil (arrows) appear enlarged. N, unlabeled nuclei. Original magnifications: 2,200x

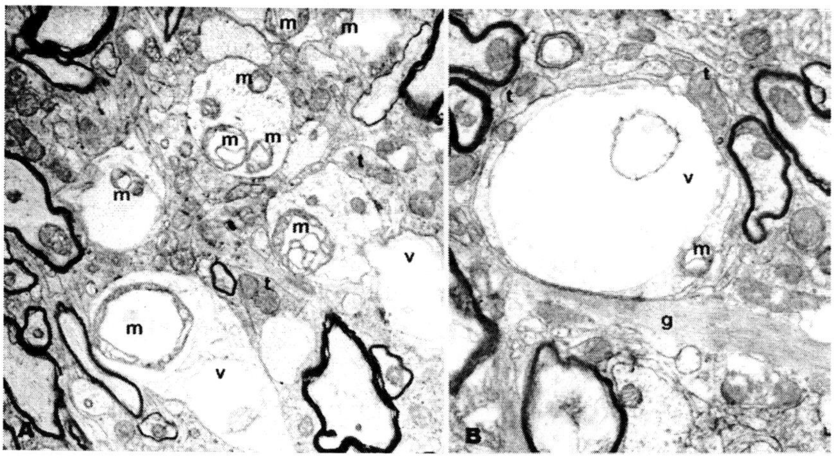

Figure 4. Electron micrographs showing alterations of mitochondria (m) and presence of vacuoles (v) in dendrites located in the ventral horn of high expressor Tg SOD1 G93A mice at symptomatic (A) and final (B) stages of disease. Note that in adjacent synaptic terminals (t) mitochondria have a normal morphology. In B the presence of a large bundle of gliofilaments (g) indicates a prominent astrocytosis. A: 12 weeks of age. Original magnification 10,000x. B: 19 weeks of age. Original magnification 16,000x

Symptomatic Mice

As the disease proceeds, mitochondrial alterations become more severe in both ventral horn and brainstem nuclei of all the high expressor Tg SOD1 G93A mice, and in symptomatic stages (12-15 week) several mitochondria appear completely swollen, with a marked or total disruption of their cristae (Fig. 4A). Morover, numerous clear vacuoles of variable size and shape are found in dendrites (Fig. 4A) and cell bodies at these ages.

End Stage Mice

The surviving motor neurons of transgenic high expressor mice in the final stage of the disease (18-21 weeks) mostly show accumulations of filamentous or granular material in their perikarya and dendrites. However, swollen mitochondria and clear vacuoles of variable size are still present in these samples, although with a minor frequency with respect to the earlier stages (Fig. 4B).

It is important to mention that in all the transgenic mice examined the mitochondrial abnormalities found in spinal cord are characteristically confined to the ventral horn and never detected in the dorsal horn, thus indicating that they are not due to technical artifacts. Moreover, both in the ventral horn and in the brainstem nuclei, mitochondria are always found to be normal in synaptic terminals adjacent to dendrites or cell bodies containing altered mitochondria, again emphasizing the specificity of the phenotype observed (Fig. 1A, 1D-F, 4).

Controls

The control, non transgenic, mice at all ages examined do not show mitochondrial alterations or cytoplasmic vacuoles in the spinal cord or in the brainstem hypoglossal and trigeminal motor nuclei.

Discussion

Overall, our ultrastructural examination of samples from lumbar spinal cord and from brainstem hypoglossal and trigeminal motor nuclei of Tg SOD1 G93A mice shows that mitochondrial swelling occurs always very early, in a presymptomatic stage of the disease, both in high expressor and in low expressor mice, and is accompanied by the presence of cytoplasmic clear vacuoles that are absent in controls. Interestingly, at these stages mitochondrial alterations tend to affect predominantly the dendrites and only later become conspicuous also in the perikarya and axons of motor neurons, and this process is accompanied by an increase in size of cytoplasmic vacuoles that often include altered mitochondria. The origin of the vacuoles is not yet clearly defined but it has been recently shown that the specific mitochondrial outer membrane markers TOM40 and TOM20 are localised in the vacuolar membrane [31]. Thus, vacuole formation may be a consequence of mitochondrial swelling due to the increase of intermembrane space, in concomitance with the expansion and likely the fusion of the outer membranes from different swollen mitochondria with a possible contribution of peroxisomes [31]. We have previously shown that in the ventral spinal horn of Tg SOD1 G93A mice the thin rim of cytoplasm surrounding large vacuoles is intensely labeled with an antiserum directed against human SOD1 [6]. Later, Higgins and collaborators also demonstrated that vacuoles are surrounded by SOD1 colocalized with outer membrane markers and that they contain many small SOD1 aggregates

[31]. Different mechanisms have been hypothesized by which mutant human SOD1 can induce mitochondrial alterations; they are discussed below.

Mutant SOD1 Could Directly Damage Mitochondria

Although SOD1 is generally considered cytosolic, there is increasing evidence demonstrating that this enzyme, both in wild type and in mutant form, is localized in the intermembrane space of mitochondria in yeast and in many mammalian cells [30, 51, 57, 71]. Recently, it has also been demonstrated that the partially or wholly demetallated SOD1, but not the holo enzyme, is taken up by mitochondria [57]. Therefore, mutant SOD1 molecules that have an altered metal binding affinity may acquire copper in the intermitochondrial space and generate aberrant reactions with peroxynitrite or hydrogen peroxide, that in turn may produce toxicity inside the mitochondria. In fact, a significant proportion of enzymatically active SOD1 was localized in the intermembrane space of mitochondria in SOD1 mutant mice [51]. Accumulation of SOD1 was also found in neuronal mitochondria of transgenic mice expressing wild type human SOD1 [34]. These mice develop a very mild and late mitochondrial vacuolization compared to transgenic mice expressing mutant human SOD1, thus suggesting that a mitochondrial-related toxicity may also exist in the presence of high levels of wild type human protein, although at a much lower extent compared to the mutant SOD1 [34].

Mitochondrial damage by mutant SOD1 may also depend on the propensity of the mutant enzyme to aggregate. SOD1 aggregates have been in fact observed associated with vacuolar membranes in motor neurons of transgenic mice expressing mutant human SOD1 [31]. Interestingly, interactions between membranes and toxic proteins were shown to produce a dual effect, consisting in promoting protein aggregation and membrane damage [52]. Thus, by interacting with mitochondria the aggregates of mutant SOD1 might damage the outer mitochondrial membrane and favor its expansion and/or fusion with other damaged membranes to form vacuoles. On the other hand, it is known that the formation of abnormal protein aggregates can be initiated by an impairment of mitochondrial function [47]. Thus, the damage of mitochondria, that appears very early in motor neurons of transgenic mice expressing mutant human SOD1, could induce the formation of protein aggregates which in turn may cause a further damage of mitochondrial membranes, giving rise in this way to a self-amplifying process that could underlie the progression of neurodegeneration.

However, it should be noted that vacuolization and mitochondrial damage are not common features of all fALS transgenic mouse models. In fact mice expressing the G85R [12] or the H46R/H48Q [78] variants of human SOD1 show a propensity to form aberrant aggregates but lack the vacuolar pathology in the degenerating motor neurons. The discrepancy with respect to the mouse models carrying the G93A and G37R human SOD1 variants might be due to the higher affinity for copper of the latter two variants compared to the G85R and H46R/H48Q variants. This may result in an abnormal reactivity of the G93A and G37R SOD1 variants with hydrogen peroxide and peroxynitrite, leading to a massive ROS production in motor neurons. In light of this, oxidative stress may therefore play a major role in the mitochondrial degeneration in motor neurons.

Alteration of the Mitochondrial Permeability Transition Pore

A possible explanation for the swelling of mitochondria is the change in the permeability of this organelle due to a dysfunction in the mitochondrial permeability transition pore (MPTP). The MPTP is a voltage-gated, cation-permeable proteinaceous channel whose opening may trigger two pathways of death. One of these pathways initiates with the release of cytochrome c, which activates a cascade of caspases leading to apoptotic death, whereas the other pathway implies the dissipation of the inner membrane potential $\Delta\psi_m$ with consequent alterations of redox potentials, ATP comsumption and depletion, and an energetic catastrophe followed by necrotic cell death (see [46] for review). The opening of the MPTP is favored by several factors including depolarisation, intramatrix calcium accumulation and oxidising agents like reactive oxygen species (ROS) [54]. All these factors can be altered in motor neurons by the presence of mutant human SOD1. For example, G93A mutant human SOD1 transfected in a neuroblastoma cell line induced a significant loss of mitochondrial membrane potential and increased the depolarisation of mitochondrial membranes, the cytosolic levels of Ca^{2+} and both the mitochondrial and cytosolic ROS [8,14]. Excitotoxic stimuli also play an important role in the MPTP activation that may lead to mitochondrial degeneration (see below). MPTP is made by different components, including the adenine nucleotide translocator, the voltage-dependent anion channel, cyclophilin D, the antiapoptotic protein Bcl2 and creatine kinase, a key enzyme that uses creatine as substrate for the energy supply of the cell through ATP production. Interestingly, a series of agents or strategies which are able to interact with the different components of the MPTP and to inhibit its activation, were shown to produce a delay in disease onset and/or an increase in survival when applied to mice transgenic for mutant SOD1, thus suggesting that alterations of these proteins may play a relevant role in the pathogenesis of the disease (see Table 1).

Functional Alterations in Mouse Models of Motor Neuron Degeneration

SOD1 mutant mice exhibit not only morphological but also functional alterations of mitochondria during the course of disease progression. For example, Jung and collaborators [36], using three different methods to measure the activities of the mitochondrial electron transport chain complex, found a decrease in complexes I, II and IV in the ventral horn of lumbar spinal cord prior to the disease onset, and this effect increased with the disease progression. Moreover, mitochondrial respiration, electron transfer chain and ATP synthesis were severely defective in Tg SOD1 G93A mice at the time of disease onset [51]. The same group also found evidence of oxidative damage to mitochondrial proteins and lipids. The possibility that an enhanced production of oxygen free radicals in the mitochondria of SOD1 mutant mice is associated with the onset of the disease is also supported by the observed increase in the immunoreactivity for Mn SOD, that represents the main superoxide scavenger of mitochondria, in motor neurons of Tg SOD1G93A mice at presymptomatic and symptomatic stages of the disease [16].

In line with the hypothesis of a pathogenic role of ROS production in mitochondria of SOD1 mutant mice, it has been found that transgenic SOD1 mutant mice with a deficiency in

MnSOD show an exacerbation of the disease progression and a significant reduction in survival compared with mice with mutant SOD1 alone [2]. On the other hand, the overexpression of Mn SOD protects neuroblastoma cell lines by the toxicity of mutant human SOD1 G37R [24], a mutation that was reported to produce mitochondrial vacuolization in transgenic mice [82].

Table 1. Effect of agents acting on mitochondria in transgenic SOD1 mutant mice

Agent	Effect on mitochondria	Therapeutic effect	Reference
Coenzyme Q10	essential cofactor in ETC	- onset ND - extens life span	[50]
Creatine	-Stabilizes mitochondrial creatine kinase -inhibits MPTP	-retards onset -extends life span	[41] [42]a
Cyclosporin A	-binds cyclophylin D and inhibits MPTP	- onset ND -extends life span	[39] [40]b
Bcl- 2 overexpression	- inhibits ROS induced MPTP	-retards onset -extends life span	[44]
Bcl-2 r-AAV		- retards onset - survival unchanged	[4]
Minocyclin	-inhibits MPTP and cytochrome c release	- retards onset - extends life span	[85] [84]c
Gingko biloba	- stimulates complexes I and III	- extends life span	[23]d
MnSOD deficiency	-reduces ROS scavenging	- exhacerbates disease	[2]

ND not determined, [a] additive effect of creatine in association with cyclooxygenase 2 inhibitor; [b] cyclosporine A was administerd to transgenic SOD1G93A mice with a permeable blood-brain barrier, the beneficial effect was significant only in males; [c] additive beneficial effect of creatine with mimocycline; [d] the effect was significant only in male transgenic SOD1G93A mice. ETC: electron transport chain; MPTP: mitochondrial permeability transition pore; ROS: reactive oxygen species

Evidence that mitochondrial dysfunction may play a role in the pathogenesis of motor neuron degeneration has been also found in wobbler mice, a spontaneous mouse mutant exhibiting motor neuron pathology [62]. A significant decrease in mitochondrial state 3 and 4 respiration rates has been in fact reported in the wobbler mice spinal cord at an early age, and this effect was accompanied by impairment of complex I activity in mitochondria isolated from spinal cord [21]. Therefore, the possible implication of mitochondria in motor neuron degeneration does not seem to be limited to mice expressing mutant human SOD1 and this finding further suggests that mitochondrial damage may indeed be an initial step in the cascade of events leading to motor neuron death. Another example of abnormal mitochondria associated with cytoplasmic vacuolization of motor neurons was also reported in mice with a specific deletion of the hypoxia responsive element of the promoter of vascular endothelial growth factor, which have been recently proposed as a new model of motor neuron degeneration [58]. This finding further suggests that mitochondrial alterations represent a hallmark of progressive motor neuron degeneration, independently of the trigger stimuli.

Interplay Between Excitotoxicity and Mitochondrial Dysfunction

A pathogenetic hypothesis for ALS that can be applied to the different forms of this disease is the glutamate-induced excitotoxicity. Glutamate levels and metabolism were shown to be altered in ALS and this is likely to be the direct consequence of a decreased reuptake of the amino acid caused by a pronounced loss of the astroglial glutamate transporter protein EAAT2/GLT1, detected in the affected regions of ALS patients [65] as well as in rodent models of motor neuron degeneration [7, 12, 32]. This effect was found only in presence of the reactive astrocytosis and of the motor neuron loss that occur in advanced stages of the disease, thus suggesting that it could be a consequence rather than a primary cause of the neuronal death. However, a reduced function of the astroglial glutamate transporter may occur before its loss as a consequence of its oxidation due to mutant SOD1 [74], and this may be sufficient to induce an early increase in the extracellular levels of glutamate.

The neurotoxic activity of glutamate occurs through the overactivation of its receptors. Although motor neurons possess all three different types of glutamate receptors, i.e. the ionotropic (NMDA and AMPA) and the metabotropic receptors, in vitro studies have demonstrated that they are particularly sensitive to glutamate excitotoxicity exerted through the AMPA receptors [15]. In particular, the selective vulnerability of motor neurons in ALS has been explained by a higher calcium permeability of these cells compared to other neurons, which in turn is likely due to a specific subunit composition of AMPA receptors expressed on their membranes. In fact, large rises in intracellular calcium levels induced by brief periods of AMPA-kainate channel activation were shown to cause a particularly rapid mitochondrial calcium overload and a strong mithochondrial ROS generation in motor neurons, thus suggesting a direct effect of glutamate excitotoxicity on mitochondrial function in these cells [15].

AMPA receptors are heteromers consisting of four subunits (GluR1-4) of which the GluR2 subunit specifically confers calcium impermeability [80], and therefore a lack of this subunit increases the permeability of neurons to calcium [61]. Cultured spinal motor neurons were shown to contain both GluR2-immunopositive and GluR2-immunonegative AMPA receptor clusters, the latter predominating in dendrites, where their activation might greatly amplify the local calcium signal [76]. Interestingly, in samples of ventral spinal cord, motor trigeminal and hypoglossal nuclei from Tg SOD1G93A mice we observed that mitochondrial alterations tend to appear first and to be more severe in dendrites than in perikarya of motor neurons. The earlier vulnerability of this neuronal compartment in transgenic mice might thus depend on the higher sentitivity of dendritic mitochondria to excitotoxicity. In turn, dendritic alterations may possibly be further exacerbated by increased mitochondrial production of

ROS due to the presence of mutant human SOD1. Thus, the relative low percentage of GluR2 subunits in functional AMPA glutamate receptors may be a major determinant of the selective vulnerability of motor neurons to excitotoxicity. In line with this, a relatively low adundance of GluR2 mRNA was found in human spinal motor neurons with respect to other neurons from spinal cord and brain [29, 38]. In addition, a defect in GluR2 mRNA editing at the Q/R site, that gives rise to glutamate receptors which are highly permeable to calcium influx [61], was found in spinal motor neurons from ALS patients [37]. A role of AMPA receptors in the pathogenesis of transgenic SOD1 mutant mice has also been postulated, since treatments with AMPA receptors antagonists were able to slow down the disease progression and to prolong the survival of these mice [13, 75]. The complex of these data therefore indicates that the increase of calcium influx through glutamate receptors, in particular the AMPA receptors, can be considered a trigger stimulus inducing mitochondrial damage; in turn, mitochondrial dysfunctions are themselves known to sensitize neurons to glutamate toxicity. Hence, we suggest that the synergic action exerted by the presence of mutant human SOD1 and by glutamatergic stimuli in motor neurons may be an initial step in the cascade of events leading to disease progression in transgenic mutant SOD1 mice.

Mitochondrial Dysfunction and Mechanisms of Cell Death

As reported before, mitochondrial dysfunction is at the base of the initiation of a programmed cell death pathway. Changes in the permeability of mitochondria, with consequent release of cytochrome c, are in fact thought to be a key event in initiating the cascade of reactions that culminates in apoptotic cell death through the activation of caspases [46]. However, in every specimen from Tg SOD1 G93A mice that we examined, the spinal cord and brainstem motor neurons displaying mitochondrial swelling and vacuolization always exhibited clearly euchromatic nuclei that did not stain with TUNEL, a common cytochemical procedure designed to reveal apoptotic nuclei [6,53], thus suggesting that an alternative mechanism is involved in the motor neuron death of these mice. Other researchers [27, 83] also reported that dying neurons in transgenic SOD1 mutant mice exhibit a non-apoptotic morphology, although some molecular components of the programmed cell death process, such as caspases, are activated and inhibition of the caspases pathway seems to be beneficial to mice survival [27, 33, 44, 48, 59]. In this context the paradox is that, unlike necrosis, apoptosis is an ATP-requiring process and ATP production is likely to be reduced in ALS as a consequence of mitochondrial functional damage.

Taken together, all these considerations suggest that a mechanism alternative to the "classic" apoptotic process is involved in motor neuron death affecting SOD1 mutant mice and perhaps also ALS patients. Deficiency of a vital energy source such as ATP may affect several different cellular mechanisms that are relevant for the survival of motor neurons. For example, ATP depletion may determine an impairment of ionic pumps function, thus reducing the ability of the cell to remove the excess of intracellular calcium with a consequent calcium overload due to the activation of glutamate receptors. In addition, the ubiquitin-proteasome system (UPP), which keeps the intracellular environment clean from misfolded proteins by rapidly destroying them, also requires ATP. The possibility that the

UPP is disrupted in ALS has been suggested by several recent in vitro studies[1, 35]. Therefore a failure of the UPP may be one of the mechanisms underlying the formation of the ubiquitinated inclusions that are the most consistent neuropathological features of both sporadic and familial ALS and also of transgenic mice expressing different types of mutant human SOD1 [79].

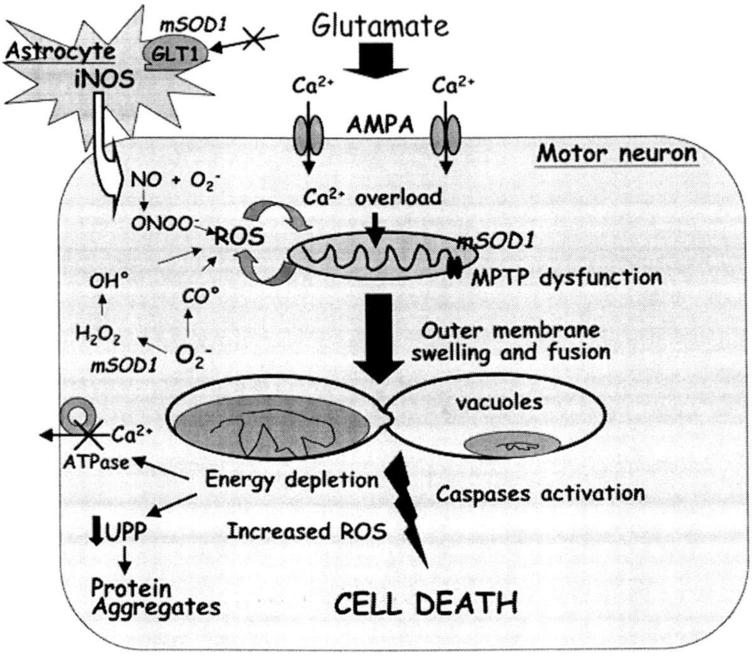

Figure 5. Potential role of mitochondrial dysfunction in the motor neurons death triggered by mutant SOD1.

In addition, as mitochondria are also a major source of oxidative free radicals in cells, their damage may provide aberrant substrates for the mutant SOD1 that in turn can generate a massive oxidation of cellular protein, lipid and DNA leading to irreversible damage of neurons.

Mitochondrial swelling and dysfunction may be triggered by different stimuli: 1) Direct action by mutant SOD1 (mSOD1) which is taken up by mitochondria and might interact and damage mitochondrial membranes through the formation of aggregates and/or the oxidation of proteins and lipids due to the increased production of reactive oxygen species (ROS). 2) Overproduction of cytosolic free radicals, such as peroxinitrite ($ONOO^-$) and the highly reactive OH° radical, which is one of the main toxic effects of mutant SOD1 in the cells. 3) Overactivation of glutamate receptors, in particular the AMPA subtype, that may induce a massive increase in calcium influx which in turn is known to cause toxicity through the mitochondria. This may be the consequence of an increased level of extracellular glutamate due to an inhibition of its uptake from astrocytes (reduced function and levels of astrocytic glutamate transporter GLT1) induced by mutant SOD1. 4) Calcium accumulation, increased ROS and the direct action of mutant SOD1 may activate the mitochondrial permeability transition pore (MPTP) thus inducing swelling and rupture of the outer mitochondrial membrane. The alterations of mitochondria may then reduce the production of energy (ATP) with a consequent inhibition of different ATP-dependent cellular processes. One of these processes is the ubiquitin-proteasome pathway (UPP) necessary for degradation and elimination of aberrant or misfolded cellular proteins, such as mutant SOD1. The failure of the UPP can give raise to intracellular aggregates followed by the formation of proteinaceous inclusions that may damage the motor neuron. In addition, energy deficiency may impair the activity of cellular ionic pumps, producing a further increase of intracellular Ca^{2+} which activates a vicious circle that eventually leads to cell death. The damage of mitochondria also induces the release of cytochrome c, which in turn activates a caspases cascade. Although this pathway is known to preceed the apoptotic cell death, motor neurons do not exhibit alterations in the nuclei, thus suggesting that an alternative "non-classic" mechanism of death is the result of such complex scenario.

Conclusions and Perspectives

The involvement of mitochondria in motor neuron degeneration seems to be clearly established in animal models of ALS represented by trangenic mice expressing a mutated form of human SOD1. Moreover, morphological abnormalities and functional deficiencies of mitochondria are early events also in cases of motor neuron degeneration that are not related to the toxicity induced by mutant SOD1. The scenario of the mechanisms leading to mitochondrial damage is likely to be multifactorial, based on interplay between excitotoxicity, oxidation of mitochondrial components and accumulation of protein aggregates. At the same time, mitochondrial dysfunction may itself exacerbate all these mechanisms, thus activating a vicious cycle that leads to motor neuron death (Fig. 5À). As shown in Table 1, strategies aimed to interfere with mitochondrial dysfunction have been shown to delay the onset of the disease and to improve motor behavior in mouse models of ALS. This suggests that indeed mytochondrial abnormalities may play a key role in the initial steps of the disease development and may also contribute to the pathology progression, together with other primary insults. A better comprehension of these interactive mechanisms might eventually help to identify more effective therapeutic strategies for ALS.

Acknowledgments

CB is supported by grants from Fondazione Monzino, Fondazione Cariplo, the Italian Ministry for Health, the Italian Ministry for University and Research (MIUR) and Telethon, Italy; SDB is supported by grants from MIUR (COFIN), FIRST and Telethon.

References

[1] Allen S, Heath P R, Kirby J, Wharton S B, Cookson M R, Menzies F M, Banks R E Shaw P J. Analysis of the cytosolic proteome in a cell culture model of familial amyotrophic lateral sclerosis reveals alterations to the proteasome, antioxidant defenses, and nitric oxide synthetic pathways. *J Biol Chem.* 2003; 278: 6371-83.

[2] Andreassen O A, Ferrante R J, Klivenyi P, Klein A M, Shinobu L A, Epstein C J Beal M F. Partial deficiency of manganese superoxide dismutase exacerbates a transgenic mouse model of amyotrophic lateral sclerosis. *Ann Neurol.* 2000; 47: 447-55.

[3] Atsumi T. The ultrastructure of intramuscular nerves in amyotrophic lateral sclerosis. *Acta Neuropathol (Berl).* 1981; 55: 193-8.

[4] Azzouz M, Hottinger A, Paterna J C, Zurn A D, Aebischer P Bueler H. Increased motoneuron survival and improved neuromuscular function in transgenic ALS mice after intraspinal injection of an adeno-associated virus encoding Bcl-2. *Hum Mol Genet.* 2000; 9: 803-11.

[5] Beckman J S, Estevez A G, Crow J P Barbeito L. Superoxide dismutase and the death of motoneurons in ALS. *Trends Neurosci.* 2001; 24: S15-20.

[6] Bendotti C, Calvaresi N, Chiveri L, Prelle A, Moggio M, Braga M, Silani V De Biasi S. Early vacuolization and mitochondrial damage in motor neurons of FALS mice are not associated with apoptosis or with changes in cytochrome oxidase histochemical reactivity. *J Neurol Sci.* 2001; 191: 25-33.

[7] Bendotti C, Tortarolo M, Suchak S K, Calvaresi N, Carvelli L, Bastone A, Rizzi M, Rattray M Mennini T. Transgenic SOD1 G93A mice develop reduced GLT-1 in spinal cord without alterations in cerebrospinal fluid glutamate levels. *J Neurochem.* 2001; 79: 737-46.

[8] Beretta S, Sala G, Mattavelli L, Ceresa C, Casciati A, Ferri A, Carri M T Ferrarese C. Mitochondrial dysfunction due to mutant copper/zinc superoxide dismutase associated with amyotrophic lateral sclerosis is reversed by N-acetylcysteine. *Neurobiol Dis.* 2003; 13: 213-21.

[9] Borthwick G M, Johnson M A, Ince P G, Shaw P J Turnbull D M. Mitochondrial enzyme activity in amyotrophic lateral sclerosis: implications for the role of mitochondria in neuronal cell death. *Ann Neurol.* 1999; 46: 787-90.

[10] Bowling A C, Schulz J B, Brown R H, Jr. Beal M F. Superoxide dismutase activity, oxidative damage, and mitochondrial energy metabolism in familial and sporadic amyotrophic lateral sclerosis. *J Neurochem.* 1993; 61: 2322-5.

[11] Browne S E, Bowling A C, Baik M J, Gurney M, Brown R H, Jr. Beal M F. Metabolic dysfunction in familial, but not sporadic, amyotrophic lateral sclerosis. *J Neurochem.* 1998; 71: 281-7.

[12] Bruijn L I, Becher M W, Lee M K, Anderson K L, Jenkins N A, Copeland N G, Sisodia S S, Rothstein J D, Borchelt D R, Price D L Cleveland D W. ALS-linked SOD1 mutant G85R mediates damage to astrocytes and promotes rapidly progressive disease with SOD1-containing inclusions. *Neuron.* 1997; 18: 327-38.

[13] Canton T, Bohme G A, Boireau A, Bordier F, Mignani S, Jimonet P, Jahn G, Alavijeh M, Stygall J, Roberts S, Brealey C, Vuilhorgne M, Debono M W, Le Guern S, Laville

M, Briet D, Roux M, Stutzmann J M Pratt J. RPR 119990, a novel alpha-amino-3-hydroxy-5-methyl-4-isoxazolepropionic acid antagonist: synthesis, pharmacological properties, and activity in an animal model of amyotrophic lateral sclerosis. *J Pharmacol Exp Ther*. 2001; 299: 314-22.

[14] Carri M T, Ferri A, Battistoni A, Famhy L, Gabbianelli R, Poccia F Rotilio G. Expression of a Cu,Zn superoxide dismutase typical of familial amyotrophic lateral sclerosis induces mitochondrial alteration and increase of cytosolic Ca2+ concentration in transfected neuroblastoma SH-SY5Y cells. *FEBS Lett*. 1997; 414: 365-8.

[15] Carriedo S G, Sensi S L, Yin H Z Weiss J H. AMPA exposures induce mitochondrial Ca(2+) overload and ROS generation in spinal motor neurons in vitro. *J Neurosci*. 2000; 20: 240-50.

[16] Chung Y H, Joo K M, Lee Y J Cha C I. Immunohistochemical study on the distribution of MnSOD in the central nervous system of the transgenic mice expressing a human Cu/Zn SOD mutation. *Brain Res*. 2003; 990: 215-20.

[17] Ciavarro G L, Calvaresi N, Botturi A, Bendotti C, Andreoni G Pedotti A. The densitometric physical fractionator for counting neuronal populations: application to a mouse model of familial amyotrophic lateral sclerosis. *J Neurosci Methods*. 2003; 129: 61-71.

[18] Cleveland D W. From Charcot to SOD1: mechanisms of selective motor neuron death in ALS. *Neuron*. 1999; 24: 515-20.

[19] Comi G P, Bordoni A, Salani S, Franceschina L, Sciacco M, Prelle A, Fortunato F, Zeviani M, Napoli L, Bresolin N, Moggio M, Ausenda C D, Taanman J W Scarlato G. Cytochrome c oxidase subunit I microdeletion in a patient with motor neuron disease. *Ann Neurol*. 1998; 43: 110-6.

[20] Curti D, Malaspina A, Facchetti G, Camana C, Mazzini L, Tosca P, Zerbi F Ceroni M. Amyotrophic lateral sclerosis: oxidative energy metabolism and calcium homeostasis in peripheral blood lymphocytes. *Neurology*. 1996; 47: 1060-4.

[21] Dave K R, Bradley W G Perez-Pinzon M A. Early mitochondrial dysfunction occurs in motor cortex and spinal cord at the onset of disease in the Wobbler mouse. *Exp Neurol*. 2003; 182: 412-20.

[22] Echaniz-Laguna A, Zoll J, Ribera F, Tranchant C, Warter J M, Lonsdorfer J Lampert E. Mitochondrial respiratory chain function in skeletal muscle of ALS patients. *Ann Neurol*. 2002; 52: 623-7.

[23] Ferrante R J, Klein A M, Dedeoglu A Beal M F. Therapeutic efficacy of EGb761 (Gingko biloba extract) in a transgenic mouse model of amyotrophic lateral sclerosis. *J Mol Neurosci*. 2001; 17: 89-96.

[24] Flanagan S W, Anderson R D, Ross M A Oberley L W. Overexpression of manganese superoxide dismutase attenuates neuronal death in human cells expressing mutant (G37R) Cu/Zn-superoxide dismutase. *J Neurochem*. 2002; 81: 170-7.

[25] Fujita K, Yamauchi M, Shibayama K, Ando M, Honda M Nagata Y. Decreased cytochrome c oxidase activity but unchanged superoxide dismutase and glutathione peroxidase activities in the spinal cords of patients with amyotrophic lateral sclerosis. *J Neurosci Res*. 1996; 45: 276-81.

[26] Gonatas N K, Stieber A, Mourelatos Z, Chen Y, Gonatas J O, Appel S H, Hays A P, Hickey W F Hauw J J. Fragmentation of the Golgi apparatus of motor neurons in amyotrophic lateral sclerosis. *Am J Pathol.* 1992; 140: 731-7.

[27] Guegan C Przedborski S. Programmed cell death in amyotrophic lateral sclerosis. *J Clin Invest.* 2003; 111: 153-61.

[28] Gurney M E, Pu H, Chiu A Y, Dal Canto M C, Polchow C Y, Alexander D D, Caliendo J, Hentati A, Kwon Y W, Deng H X et al. Motor neuron degeneration in mice that express a human Cu,Zn superoxide dismutase mutation. *Science.* 1994; 264: 1772-5.

[29] Heath P R, Tomkins J, Ince P G Shaw P J. Quantitative assessment of AMPA receptor mRNA in human spinal motor neurons isolated by laser capture microdissection. *Neuroreport.* 2002; 13: 1753-7.

[30] Higgins C M, Jung C, Ding H Xu Z. Mutant Cu, Zn superoxide dismutase that causes motoneuron degeneration is present in mitochondria in the CNS. *J Neurosci.* 2002; 22: RC215.

[31] Higgins C M, Jung C Xu Z. ALS-associated mutant SOD1G93A causes mitochondrial vacuolation by expansion of the intermembrane space and by involvement of SOD1 aggregation and peroxisomes. *BMC Neurosci.* 2003; 4: 16.

[32] Howland D S, Liu J, She Y, Goad B, Maragakis N J, Kim B, Erickson J, Kulik J, DeVito L, Psaltis G, DeGennaro L J, Cleveland D W Rothstein J D. Focal loss of the glutamate transporter EAAT2 in a transgenic rat model of SOD1 mutant-mediated amyotrophic lateral sclerosis (ALS). *Proc Natl Acad Sci U S A.* 2002; 99: 1604-9.

[33] Inoue H, Tsukita K, Iwasato T, Suzuki Y, Tomioka M, Tateno M, Nagao M, Kawata A, Saido T C, Miura M, Misawa H, Itohara S Takahashi R. The crucial role of caspase-9 in the disease progression of a transgenic ALS mouse model. *Embo J.* 2003; 22: 6665-74.

[34] Jaarsma D, Haasdijk E D, Grashorn J A, Hawkins R, van Duijn W, Verspaget H W, London J Holstege J C. Human Cu/Zn superoxide dismutase (SOD1) overexpression in mice causes mitochondrial vacuolization, axonal degeneration, and premature motoneuron death and accelerates motoneuron disease in mice expressing a familial amyotrophic lateral sclerosis mutant SOD1. *Neurobiol Dis.* 2000; 7: 623-43.

[35] Johnston J A, Dalton M J, Gurney M E Kopito R R. Formation of high molecular weight complexes of mutant Cu, Zn-superoxide dismutase in a mouse model for familial amyotrophic lateral sclerosis. *Proc Natl Acad Sci U S A.* 2000; 97: 12571-6.

[36] Jung C, Higgins C M Xu Z. Mitochondrial electron transport chain complex dysfunction in a transgenic mouse model for amyotrophic lateral sclerosis. *J Neurochem.* 2002; 83: 535-45.

[37] Kawahara Y, Ito K, Sun H, Aizawa H, Kanazawa I Kwak S. Glutamate receptors: RNA editing and death of motor neurons. *Nature.* 2004; 427: 801.

[38] Kawahara Y, Kwak S, Sun H, Ito K, Hashida H, Aizawa H, Jeong S Y Kanazawa I. Human spinal motoneurons express low relative abundance of GluR2 mRNA: an implication for excitotoxicity in ALS. *J Neurochem.* 2003; 85: 680-9.

[39] Keep M, Elmer E, Fong K S Csiszar K. Intrathecal cyclosporin prolongs survival of late-stage ALS mice. *Brain Res.* 2001; 894: 327-31.

[40] Kirkinezos I G, Hernandez D, Bradley W G Moraes C T. An ALS mouse model with a permeable blood-brain barrier benefits from systemic cyclosporine A treatment. *J Neurochem.* 2004; 88: 821-6.

[41] Klivenyi P, Ferrante R J, Matthews R T, Bogdanov M B, Klein A M, Andreassen O A, Mueller G, Wermer M, Kaddurah-Daouk R Beal M F. Neuroprotective effects of creatine in a transgenic animal model of amyotrophic lateral sclerosis. *Nat Med.* 1999; 5: 347-50.

[42] Klivenyi P, Kiaei M, Gardian G, Calingasan N Y Beal M F. Additive neuroprotective effects of creatine and cyclooxygenase 2 inhibitors in a transgenic mouse model of amyotrophic lateral sclerosis. *J Neurochem.* 2004; 88: 576-82.

[43] Kong J Xu Z. Massive mitochondrial degeneration in motor neurons triggers the onset of amyotrophic lateral sclerosis in mice expressing a mutant SOD1. *J Neurosci.* 1998; 18: 3241-50.

[44] Kostic V, Jackson-Lewis V, de Bilbao F, Dubois-Dauphin M Przedborski S. Bcl-2: prolonging life in a transgenic mouse model of familial amyotrophic lateral sclerosis. *Science.* 1997; 277: 559-62.

[45] Krieger C Duchen M R. Mitochondria, Ca(2+) and neurodegenerative disease. *Eur J Pharmacol.* 2002; 447: 177-88.

[46] Kroemer G, Dallaporta B Resche-Rigon M. The mitochondrial death/life regulator in apoptosis and necrosis. *Annu Rev Physiol.* 1998; 60: 619-42.

[47] Lee H J, Shin S Y, Choi C, Lee Y H Lee S J. Formation and removal of alpha-synuclein aggregates in cells exposed to mitochondrial inhibitors. *J Biol Chem.* 2002; 277: 5411-7.

[48] Li M, Ona V O, Guegan C, Chen M, Jackson-Lewis V, Andrews L J, Olszewski A J, Stieg P E, Lee J P, Przedborski S Friedlander R M. Functional role of caspase-1 and caspase-3 in an ALS transgenic mouse model. *Science.* 2000; 288: 335-9.

[49] Liu Y, Brooks B R, Taniguchi N Hartmann H A. CuZnSOD and MnSOD immunoreactivity in brain stem motor neurons from amyotrophic lateral sclerosis patients. *Acta Neuropathol* (Berl). 1998; 95: 63-70.

[50] Matthews R T, Yang L, Browne S, Baik M Beal M F. Coenzyme Q10 administration increases brain mitochondrial concentrations and exerts neuroprotective effects. *Proc Natl Acad Sci U S A.* 1998; 95: 8892-7.

[51] Mattiazzi M, D'Aurelio M, Gajewski C D, Martushova K, Kiaei M, Beal M F Manfredi G. Mutated human SOD1 causes dysfunction of oxidative phosphorylation in mitochondria of transgenic mice. *J Biol Chem.* 2002; 277: 29626-33.

[52] Michikawa M, Gong J S, Fan Q W, Sawamura N Yanagisawa K. A novel action of alzheimer's amyloid beta-protein (Abeta): oligomeric Abeta promotes lipid release. *J Neurosci.* 2001; 21: 7226-35.

[53] Migheli A, Atzori C, Piva R, Tortarolo M, Girelli M, Schiffer D Bendotti C. Lack of apoptosis in mice with ALS. *Nat Med.* 1999; 5: 966-7.

[54] Miller R J. Mitochondria - the Kraken wakes! *Trends Neurosci.* 1998; 21: 95-7.

[55] Nakano Y, Hirayama K Terao K. Hepatic ultrastructural changes and liver dysfunction in amyotrophic lateral sclerosis. *Arch Neuro*l. 1987; 44: 103-6.

[56] Newmeyer D D Ferguson-Miller S. Mitochondria: releasing power for life and unleashing the machineries of death. *Cell.* 2003; 112: 481-90.

[57] Okado-Matsumoto A Fridovich I. Amyotrophic lateral sclerosis: a proposed mechanism. *Proc Natl Acad Sci U S A.* 2002; 99: 9010-4.

[58] Oosthuyse B, Moons L, Storkebaum E, Beck H, Nuyens D, Brusselmans K, Van Dorpe J, Hellings P, Gorselink M, Heymans S, Theilmeier G, Dewerchin M, Laudenbach V, Vermylen P, Raat H, Acker T, Vleminckx V, Van Den Bosch L, Cashman N, Fujisawa H, Drost M R, Sciot R, Bruyninckx F, Hicklin D J, Ince C, Gressens P, Lupu F, Plate K H, Robberecht W, Herbert J M, Collen D Carmeliet P. Deletion of the hypoxia-response element in the vascular endothelial growth factor promoter causes motor neuron degeneration. *Nat Genet.* 2001; 28: 131-8.

[59] Pasinelli P, Houseweart M K, Brown R H, Jr. Cleveland D W. Caspase-1 and -3 are sequentially activated in motor neuron death in Cu,Zn superoxide dismutase-mediated familial amyotrophic lateral sclerosis. *Proc Natl Acad Sci U S A.* 2000; 97: 13901-6.

[60] Paxinos G F K, The mouse brain in sterotaxic coordinates., Academic press, 2001.

[61] Pellegrini-Giampietro D E, Gorter J A, Bennett M V Zukin R S. The GluR2 (GluR-B) hypothesis: Ca(2+)-permeable AMPA receptors in neurological disorders. *Trends Neurosci.* 1997; 20: 464-70.

[62] Pioro E P Mitsumoto H. Animal models of ALS. *Clin Neurosci.* 1995; 3: 375-85.

[63] Radunovic A, Porto W G, Zeman S Leigh P N. Increased mitochondrial superoxide dismutase activity in Parkinson's disease but not amyotrophic lateral sclerosis motor cortex. *Neurosci Lett.* 1997; 239: 105-8.

[64] Rosen D R, Siddique T, Patterson D, Figlewicz D A, Sapp P, Hentati A, Donaldson D, Goto J, O'Regan J P, Deng H X et al. Mutations in Cu/Zn superoxide dismutase gene are associated with familial amyotrophic lateral sclerosis. *Nature.* 1993; 362: 59-62.

[65] Rothstein J D, Van Kammen M, Levey A I, Martin L J Kuncl R W. Selective loss of glial glutamate transporter GLT-1 in amyotrophic lateral sclerosis. *Ann Neurol.* 1995; 38: 73-84.

[66] Schon E A Manfredi G. Neuronal degeneration and mitochondrial dysfunction. *J Clin Invest.* 2003; 111: 303-12.

[67] Shibata N. Transgenic mouse model for familial amyotrophic lateral sclerosis with superoxide dismutase-1 mutation. *Neuropathology.* 2001; 21: 82-92.

[68] Shibata N, Asayama K, Hirano A Kobayashi M. Immunohistochemical study on superoxide dismutases in spinal cords from autopsied patients with amyotrophic lateral sclerosis. *Dev Neurosci.* 1996; 18: 492-8.

[69] Siklos L, Engelhardt J, Harati Y, Smith R G, Joo F Appel S H. Ultrastructural evidence for altered calcium in motor nerve terminals in amyotropic lateral sclerosis. *Ann Neurol.* 1996; 39: 203-16.

[70] Stieber A, Gonatas J O Gonatas N K. Aggregation of ubiquitin and a mutant ALS-linked SOD1 protein correlate with disease progression and fragmentation of the Golgi apparatus. *J Neurol Sci.* 2000; 173: 53-62.

[71] Sturtz L A, Diekert K, Jensen L T, Lill R Culotta V C. A fraction of yeast Cu,Zn-superoxide dismutase and its metallochaperone, CCS, localize to the intermembrane

space of mitochondria. A physiological role for SOD1 in guarding against mitochondrial oxidative damage. *J Biol Chem.* 2001; 276: 38084-9.

[72] Swerdlow R H, Parks J K, Cassarino D S, Trimmer P A, Miller S W, Maguire D J, Sheehan J P, Maguire R S, Pattee G, Juel V C, Phillips L H, Tuttle J B, Bennett J P, Jr., Davis R E Parker W D, Jr. Mitochondria in sporadic amyotrophic lateral sclerosis. *Exp Neurol.* 1998; 153: 135-42.

[73] Tortarolo M, Veglianese P, Calvaresi N, Botturi A, Rossi C, Giorgini A, Migheli A Bendotti C. Persistent activation of p38 mitogen-activated protein kinase in a mouse model of familial amyotrophic lateral sclerosis correlates with disease progression. *Mol Cell Neurosci.* 2003; 23: 180-92.

[74] Trotti D, Rolfs A, Danbolt N C, Brown R H, Jr. Hediger M A. SOD1 mutants linked to amyotrophic lateral sclerosis selectively inactivate a glial glutamate transporter. *Nat Neurosci.* 1999; 2: 848.

[75] Van Damme P, Leyssen M, Callewaert G, Robberecht W Van Den Bosch L. The AMPA receptor antagonist NBQX prolongs survival in a transgenic mouse model of amyotrophic lateral sclerosis. *Neurosci Lett.* 2003; 343: 81-4.

[76] Vandenberghe W, Bindokas V P, Miller R J, Robberecht W Brorson J R. Subcellular localization of calcium-permeable AMPA receptors in spinal motoneurons. *Eur J Neurosci.* 2001; 14: 305-14.

[77] Vielhaber S, Kunz D, Winkler K, Wiedemann F R, Kirches E, Feistner H, Heinze H J, Elger C E, Schubert W Kunz W S. Mitochondrial DNA abnormalities in skeletal muscle of patients with sporadic amyotrophic lateral sclerosis. *Brain.* 2000; 123 (Pt 7): 1339-48.

[78] Wang J, Xu G, Gonzales V, Coonfield M, Fromholt D, Copeland N G, Jenkins N A Borchelt D R. Fibrillar inclusions and motor neuron degeneration in transgenic mice expressing superoxide dismutase 1 with a disrupted copper-binding site. *Neurobiol Dis.* 2002; 10: 128-38.

[79] Watanabe M, Dykes-Hoberg M, Culotta V C, Price D L, Wong P C Rothstein J D. Histological evidence of protein aggregation in mutant SOD1 transgenic mice and in amyotrophic lateral sclerosis neural tissues. *Neurobiol Dis.* 2001; 8: 933-41.

[80] Weiss J H Sensi S L. Ca2+-Zn2+ permeable AMPA or kainate receptors: possible key factors in selective neurodegeneration. *Trends Neurosci.* 2000; 23: 365-71.

[81] Wiedau-Pazos M, Goto J J, Rabizadeh S, Gralla E B, Roe J A, Lee M K, Valentine J S Bredesen D E. Altered reactivity of superoxide dismutase in familial amyotrophic lateral sclerosis. *Science.* 1996; 271: 515-8.

[82] Wong P C, Pardo C A, Borchelt D R, Lee M K, Copeland N G, Jenkins N A, Sisodia S S, Cleveland D W Price D L. An adverse property of a familial ALS-linked SOD1 mutation causes motor neuron disease characterized by vacuolar degeneration of mitochondria. *Neuron.* 1995; 14: 1105-16.

[83] Xu Z. Mechanism and treatment of motoneuron degeneration in ALS: what have SOD1 mutants told us? Amyotroph Lateral Scler Other Motor Neuron Disord. 2000; 1: 225-34.

[84] Zhang W, Narayanan M Friedlander R M. Additive neuroprotective effects of minocycline with creatine in a mouse model of ALS. *Ann Neurol.* 2003; 53: 267-70.

[85] Zhu S, Stavrovskaya I G, Drozda M, Kim B Y, Ona V, Li M, Sarang S, Liu A S, Hartley D M, Wu du C, Gullans S, Ferrante R J, Przedborski S, Kristal B S Friedlander R M. Minocycline inhibits cytochrome c release and delays progression of amyotrophic lateral sclerosis in mice. *Nature.* 2002; 417: 74-8.

In: Amyotrophic Lateral Sclerosis: New Research
Editor: Christine A. Murray, pp. 135-153

ISBN 1-59454-179-5

Chapter V

Blood Oxidative Stress in Amyotrophic Lateral Sclerosis

***D. Bonnefont-Rousselot*[1,*] *and V. Meininger*[2]**

[1]Fédération de Biochimie; [2]Fédération de Neurologie Mazarin,
Groupe Hospitalier Pitié-Salpêtrière (AP-HP), 47 boulevard de l'Hôpital,
75651 Paris Cedex 13, France

Abstract

The majority of cases of amyotrophic lateral sclerosis (ALS) are sporadic (primary or idiopathic ALD), while about 5 to 10% are familial (familial ALS). In sporadic ALS, recent studies showed abnormalities of glutamate metabolism, which would be responsible for motor neuron degeneration via neuroexcitotoxic mechanisms. Part of the familial forms of ALS have been linked with mutations of Cu,Zn-superoxide dismutase (Cu,Zn-SOD), an enzyme which is involved in the defense against superoxide free radicals. It has been shown that these mutations lead to a gain of toxic function of the enzyme rather than a loss of activity. Expression of the mutant human Cu,Zn-SOD in transgenic mice causes motor neuron disease while expression of wild type human Cu,Zn-SOD does not. Various hypotheses on the toxicity of the mutant SOD have been proposed such as increased access of the substrate to the active site, leading to increased oxidation of the substrate; disruption of the active site of the enzyme, allowing access of peroxynitrite to copper and leading to increased nitration by peroxynitrite. Oxidative stress may also be related to impaired ability of mutant SOD to bind zinc.

Moreover, glutamate excitotoxicity would be associated with increased oxidative stress, which could constitute a linkage between sporadic and familial forms of ALS. In relation with this mechanism, riluzole (2-amino-6-trifluoromethoxybenzothiazole) demonstrated a therapeutic activity in ALS patients. We conducted a study aiming to evaluate the

---

* Correspondence concerning this article should be addressed to Dr. D. Bonnefont-Rousselot, Fédération de Biochimie; Groupe Hospitalier Pitié-Salpêtrière (AP-HP), 47 boulevard de l'Hôpital, 75651 Paris Cedex 13, France.

blood oxidative stress status in a large population of 167 definite or probable ALS patients (without detected SOD mutation), with or without treatment with riluzole, in comparison with age- and sex-matched healthy control subjects. Our data supported an imbalance of the oxidant/antioxidant systems in favor of an oxidative stress in ALS, in patients without treatment as well as in patients treated with riluzole, as compared with healthy age-matched controls. No correlation was found between the level of oxidative stress markers and the disease duration nor the riluzole treatment duration. Patients treated with riluzole exhibited an erythrocyte Cu,Zn-SOD activity intermediate between the elevated SOD activity of ALS patients without treatment and that of controls. This suggests a possible activity of the drug on the oxidative stress.
Therapeutic trials using classical antioxidants alone, such as vitamin E, showed no effect on the survival and motor function in ALS. However, when using the ALS Health State scale, patients receiving riluzole plus alpha-tocopherol remained longer in a better condition and they showed changes in biochemical markers of oxidative stress. Additional studies are in course which could provide more information.
These results suggest that oxidative processes may play a critical role in the pathogenic mechanisms of neurodegeneration in ALS and therapeutic interventions targeted against this mechanism appear promising.

Keywords: oxidative stress; amyotrophic lateral sclerosis; superoxide dismutase; glutathione.

Introduction

ALS is one of the most common neurodegenerative disorders (incidence of about 1/100,000). It occurs either sporadically or as a familial disorder (5 to 10% of patients). In both forms, clinical and pathological criteria are indistinguishable (Hand and Rouleau, 2002) suggesting that these forms share common pathogenetic mechanisms. Approximately 20% of the familial ALS have been linked to mutations of Cu,Zn-superoxide dismutase (Cu,Zn-SOD). In both forms, an increased oxidative stress has been shown, suggesting that in both familial and sporadic cases there is an imbalance between production of reactive oxygen species (ROS) and antioxidant defence systems (Halliwell and Gutteridge, 1999). Therefore, association between glutamate excitotoxicity and increased oxidative stress could constitute a link between sporadic and familial forms of ALS.

Neurodegeneration and Oxidative Stress in ALS

Loss of neurons in ALS could result from metal-mediated oxidative stress associated with excitotoxic stimulation and aggregation or dysfunction of proteins and genetic factors (Carri *et al.*, 2003).

Evidence for an Oxidative Stress in ALS Patients

Cells detoxify ROS via antioxidant defenses including enzymes such as superoxide dismutase (SOD), glutathione peroxidase (GSH-Px), glutathione reductase (GR) and catalase, but also nonenzymatic systems such as vitamins E and C, carotenoids, glutathione...(Figure 1). Besides lowered antioxidant defenses, ROS-induced damage on cellular targets can be classically assessed by three kinds of oxidative stress markers, i.e. markers of lipid peroxidation, protein oxidation and DNA oxidation (Thérond *et al.*, 2000). Nevertheless, besides direct harmful oxidizing properties, ROS (i.e., hydrogen peroxide, hydroxyl and superoxide radicals, lipid hydroperoxides) are now demonstrated as signaling mediators under subtoxic conditions. It is recognized that redox regulation involving ROS is able to modulate critical cellular functions, such as mitogen-activated protein (MAP) kinase cascade activation, ion transport, calcium mobilization or apoptosis activation. Cells have adaptative responses to oxidative stress, such as activation of genes incoding defense enzymes, transcription factors or structural proteins (Halliwell and Gutteridge, 1999; Cassarino and Bennett, 1999). Thus, ROS modulate various biological functions by stimulating distinct signal transduction mechanisms (Suzuki *et al.*, 1997), some of which being possibly involved in the pathogenesis of ALS, especially in apoptotic phenomenons.

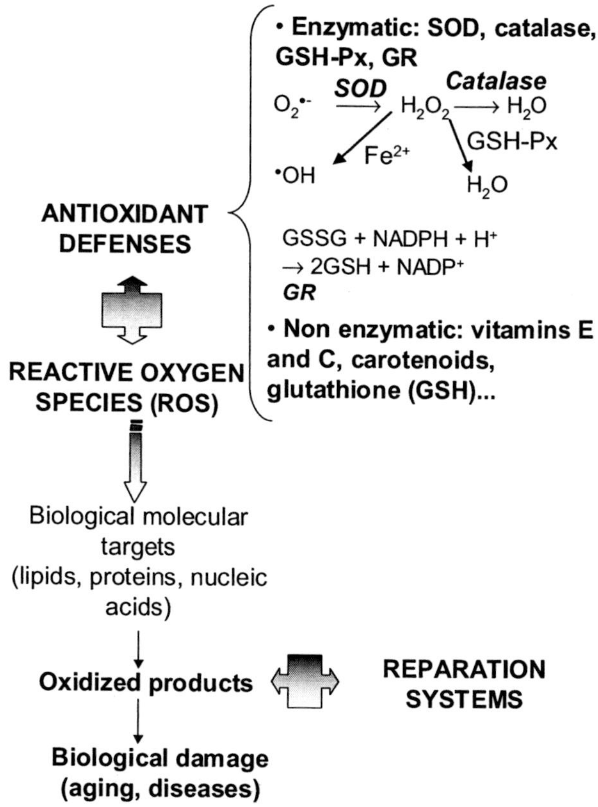

Figure 1. Detoxification of the ROS (especially those derived from $O_2^{\bullet-}$ produced by the mitochondrial electron transport chain) by enzymatic and nonenzymatic systems.

Table I. Markers of oxidative damage in ALS

Marker	Variation	Organism	MEDIUM	Reference
3-nitrotyrosine	↑	Transgenic mice with G37R SOD1 mutation	Spinal cord	Bruijn *et al.*, 1997
Malondialdehyde	↑	Transgenic mice with G93A SOD1 mutation	Spinal cord	Hall *et al.*, 1998
Protein carbonyl	↑	Transgenic mice with G93A SOD1 mutation	Spinal cord	Andrus *et al.*, 1998
•OH free radicals	↑ →	Transgenic mice with G93A SOD1 mutation Mice overexpressing wild-type human SOD1	Striatum	Bogdanov *et al.*, 1998
Free radicals	↑	Transgenic mice with G93A SOD1 mutation	Spinal cord	Liu *et al.*, 1998
H_2O_2 and •OH free radicals	↑	Transgenic mice with G93A SOD1 mutation	Dialysates collected from the CSF	Liu *et al.*, 1999
Protein carbonyl	↑	SALS patients	Frontal cortex	Bowling *et al.*, 1993
Protein carbonyl	↑	SALS patients	Spinal cord	Shaw *et al.*, 1995
Free radicals	↑	SALS patients	Erythrocytes	Ihara *et al.*, 1995
TBARS (and TBARS/α-tocopherol)	↑	SALS patients	Plasma	Oteiza *et al.*, 1997
3-nitrotyrosine	↑	FALS and SALS patients	Spinal cord	Beal *et al.*, 1997
Protein carbonyl	↑ →	SALS patients FALS patients	Motor cortex	Ferrante *et al.*, 1997a
8-OHdG	↑ →	SALS patients FALS patients	Motor cortex	Ferrante *et al.*, 1997a
Malondialdehyde	↑	FALS and SALS patients	Motor cortex	Ferrante *et al.*, 1997a
3-nitrotyrosine	↑	SALS patients	CSF	Tohgi *et al.*, 1999
TBARS	↑	SALS patients	Plasma	Bonnefont-Rousselot *et al.*, 2000
8-OHdG	↑	ALS patients	Plasma, urines and CSF	Bogdanov *et al.*, 2000
Hydroxynonenal-lysine and crotonaldehyde-lysine (markers of lipid peroxidation); N-ε-carboxymethyl-lysine (marker of glycoxidation)	↑	SALS patients	Spinal cord	Shibata *et al.*, 2001
Lipoperoxides	↑	ALS patients	Blood	Siciliano *et al.*, 2002

↑: elevated level; →: normal level; CSF: cerebrospinal fluid; FALS: familial ALS; SALS : sporadic ALS; 8-OHdG: 8-hydroxydeoxyguanosine.

The central nervous system is particularly sensitive to ROS attack, since it contains high contents of polyunsaturated fatty acids which are good substrates for oxidative damage. The cells of the adult brain use approximately 20% of the oxygen utilized by the body, although the brain only comprise 2% of the body weight (Dringen *et al.*, 2000). Moreover, antioxidant enzymes (i.e., catalase and glutathione peroxidase) are poorly represented (Martilla *et al.*, 1988; Halliwell, 1992), making central nervous system more susceptible to ROS-induced damage. Therefore, ROS, which are continuously produced during oxidative metabolism, are generated at high rates within the brain.

Table II. Antioxidant defences in ALS

Marker	Variation	Organism	Medium	Reference
Cu,Zn-SOD (SOD1)	↓ → →	FALS patients with SOD1 mutation FALS patients without SOD1 mutation SALS patients	Frontal cortex	Bowling *et al.*, 1993
Selenodependent GSH-Px	↑	FALS patients	Spinal cord	Ince *et al.*, 1994
Cu,Zn-SOD	→	SALS patients	Erythrocytes	Puymirat *et al.*, 1994
Cu,Zn-SOD	↑	SALS patients	Erythrocytes	Ihara *et al.*, 1995
Cu,Zn-SOD	↓ → →	FALS patients with SOD1 mutation FALS patients without SOD1 mutation SALS patients	Erythrocytes	Przedborski *et al.*, 1996a
Catalase	→	FALS and SALS patients	Erythrocytes	Przedborski *et al.*, 1996a
GSH-Px	→	FALS and SALS patients	Erythrocytes	Przedborski *et al.*, 1996a
Cu,Zn-SOD	→	SALS patients	Erythrocytes	Oteiza *et al.*, 1997
α-tocopherol	→	SALS patients	Erythrocytes	Oteiza *et al.*, 1997
β-carotene	→	SALS patients	Erythrocytes	Oteiza *et al.*, 1997
Ubiquinol (coenzyme Q10)	→	SALS patients	Erythrocytes	Oteiza *et al.*, 1997
Cu,Zn-SOD	↓	SALS patients	Erythrocytes	Apostolski et al., 1998
GSH-Px	↓	SALS patients	Erythrocytes	Apostolski et al., 1998
Cu,Zn-SOD	↑	SALS patients	Erythrocytes	Bonnefont-Rousselot *et al.*, 2000
GSH-Px	→	SALS patients	Erythrocytes	Bonnefont-Rousselot *et al.*, 2000
α-tocopherol	→	SALS patients	Plasma	Bonnefont-Rousselot *et al.*, 2000
β-carotene	→	SALS patients	Plasma	Bonnefont-Rousselot *et al.*, 2000
Vitamin A	→	SALS patients	Plasma	Bonnefont-Rousselot *et al.*, 2000
Total glutathione	↓	ALS patients	Substantia nigra	Schulz *et al.*, 2000
Total antioxidant status	↑	ALS patients	Serum	Ilzecka, 2003

FALS: familial ALS; SALS : sporadic ALS; ↑: elevated activity or level; →: normal activity or level; ↓: decreased activity or level.

Several studies reported high levels of oxidative stress markers in both forms of ALS in animal models (Bruijn *et al.*, 1997; Liu *et al.*, 1998; Hall *et al.*, 1998; Andrus *et al.*, 1998; Bogdanov *et al.*, 1998; Liu *et al.*, 1999) and in humans (Bowling *et al.*, 1993; Ihara *et al.*,

1995; Shaw *et al.*, 1995; Beal *et al.*, 1997; Ferrante *et al.*, 1997a; Oteiza *et al.*, 1997; Tohgi *et al.*, 1999; Bogdanov *et al.*, 2000; Bonnefont-Rousselot *et al.*, 2000; Shibata *et al.*, 2001; Siciliano *et al.*, 2002). Reactive nitrogen species (RNS), especially $^{\bullet}NO$-derived products such as peroxynitrite ($ONOO^-$) also react on molecular targets, resulting in a "nitrosative" stress (Table I).

As an example, detection of elevated concentrations of carbonylated proteins in cortex motor neurons and spinal cord of patients results from the interaction of ROS and peroxynitrite ($ONOO^-$) with proteins. Similarly, nitrotyrosine and inducible NO synthase (NOS2) have been immunohistochemically detected. In addition, DNA oxidation is revealed by increased levels of 8-hydroxydeoxyguanosine (8-OHdG) in plasma, urine and cerebrospinal fluid (CSF) (Bogdanov *et al.*, 2000). We assessed the blood oxidative stress status in 167 ALS patients (without SOD1 mutation) among whom two groups were defined: a first group of 43 patients without treatment (26 males and 17 females, aged 60 ± 14 years) and a second group of 124 patients (71 males and 53 females, aged 59 ± 12 years) treated with riluzole (100 mg riluzole per day, in 50 mg tablets) for 481 ± 308 days (Bonnefont-Rousselot *et al.*, 2000). Riluzole (2-amino-6-trifluoromethoxybenzothiazole) has been shown to significantly decrease the rate of death in ALS patients (Bensimon *et al.*, 1994; Lacomblez *et al.*, 1996). In our study, ALS patients were compared with age- and sex-matched healthy control subjects. We observed in blood of ALS patients an increase of plasma TBARS levels with no deficiency in plasma lipophilic antioxidants (vitamin E, vitamin A and β-carotene), confirming the existence of an oxidative stress in ALS patients with an enhancement of the free radical production.

Enzymatic and non enzymatic defense systems have also been studied in ALS patients (Table II), especially Cu,Zn-SOD activity, this latter point being reported above (paragraph "Oxidative stress and gain of toxic function related to mutations in the Cu,Zn-SOD (or SOD1) gene"). As an example, the activities of Cu,Zn- and Mn-SOD, catalase, selenodependent GSH-Px and glutathione reductase have been determined in spinal cord section of sporadic ALS patients and of control subjects (Ince *et al.*, 1994). This study showed only significant differences in GSH-Px activity with an increase in the selenium level of the spinal cord of the patients which might result from an oxidative stress-induced increase in the selenodependent GSH-Px. However, another study did not report any change in GSH-Px and catalase activities (Przedborski *et al.*, 1996a). In our study (Bonnefont-Rousselot *et al.*, 2000), erythrocyte Cu,Zn-SOD activity was significantly increased in ALS patients without treatment compared to healthy control patients and to ALS patients treated with riluzole. Since patients treated with riluzole exhibited an erythrocyte Cu,Zn-SOD activity intermediate between the elevated SOD activity of ALS patients without treatment and that of controls, a possible activity of riluzole on oxidative stress could be suggested. The total antioxidant status (TAS), that is an evaluation of the peroxyl scavenging capacity, has been determined in the serum of ALS patients in comparison with healthy control subjects. TAS level has been shown elevated in ALS patients; this may be the result of endogenous protection mechanisms against oxidative stress, but it was not a marker of ALS duration, clinical state or type of onset (Ilzecka, 2003).

Involvement of Mitochondria in the ROS-Induced Cell Damage and in Neurodegeneration

Significant mitochondrial abnormalities are reported in ALS and might underlie the oxidative stress observed in this disease (Bowling and Beal, 1995) even in sporadic cases which are the majority of ALS patients (Cassarino and Bennett, 1999). In ALS as in other neurodegenerative diseases (Alzheimer's disease, Parkinson's disease), there is evidence for both electron chain transport impairment and free radical-mediated cellular damage (Beal, 1995). Electron transport chain dysfunction acts as a free radical generator by blocking the normal passage of electrons down the chain until the ultimate reduction of molecular oxygen to water. This can be clearly shown by using inhibitors of this transport chain, such as N-methylpyridinium ion (MPP^+) (inhibitor of the complex I) or azide (inhibitor of complex IV), these inhibitors leading to an increased generation of free radicals (Smith and Bennett, 1997).

Neurodegeneration in ALS can be related to apoptotic cell death of motor neurons, which can be induced by ROS (Fleury *et al.*, 2002). Indeed, ROS-induced mitochondrial damage has been shown in both forms of ALS and could precede apoptotic process (Beal, 2000). Mitochondria damaged by oxidative stress could be implied in apoptosis. Lipid oxidation products such as malondialdehyde, 4-hydroxynonenal, 4-hydroxyhexenal, and free fatty acids produced by phospholipase A_2 may lead to the opening of the mitochondrial permeability transition pore (MPTP) (Broekemeier and Pfeiffer, 1995; Kristal *et al.*, 1996). Activation of MPTP allows a free diffusion of molecules lower than 1500 Da between the mitochondrial matrix and the cytosol. Among the factors released from mitochondria are cytochrome c, the apoptosis factor (AIP) and caspases. The formation of the MPTP can trigger a dissipation of the mitochondrial transmembrane potential and depletion of ATP, but also free radical formation (Jordan *et al.*, 2003). Cytochrome c (located in the mitochondrial electron transport chain required for ATP synthesis) can trigger the caspase chain when it is released from mitochondria and thus initiate apoptosis as programmed cell death.

Evidence for mitochondrial dysfunction in ALS has been reported by Vielhaber *et al.* (2000) on muscle biopsies of patients, with a heterogeneous distribution of the respiratory chain defect correlated with the presence of cytochrome c oxidase-negative muscle fibers histologically detected. These authors also reported diminished levels or multiple deletions of mitochondrial DNA. These abnormalities seemed to be related to a decreased activity of mitochondrial Mn-SOD that plays a key-role in ROS detoxification. Therefore, its deficiency, associated with the fact that the major site of ROS generation is the mitochondrial respiratory chain (Skulachev *et al.*, 1996), could result in an increase of the mitochondrial ROS concentrations and could explain the deletions observed in mitochondrial DNA (mtDNA) and the low levels of intact mtDNA. In addition, mtDNA has only poor repair capacity (Shoubridge *et al.*, 1990), which leads to exacerbate ROS-induced molecular damages.

Involvement of mitochondria in the pathogenesis of ALS is supported by several observations. Mitochondria-derived vacuoles in axons and dendrites have been described in the spinal cord of mouse models carrying mutations in Cu,Zn-SOD (Dal Canto and Gurney, 1994; Wong *et al.*, 1995; Mourelatos *et al.*, 1996; Kong and Xu, 1998). Such mutations were associated with autosomal dominant inherited familial ALS (Rosen *et al.*, 1993). Moreover, abnormal mitochondria have been described in anterior horn neurons of patients with sporadic form of ALS (Sasaki *et al.*, 1996). Bowling *et al.* (1993) also reported increased ROS-induced damage in post-mortem brain tissue from patients with sporadic ALS and altered mitochondrial energy metabolism (increased complex I activity) in brain tissue from patients with familial ALS. Finally, Klivenyi *et al.* (1999) demonstrated a neuroprotective effect of creatine administration to mice carrying a Cu,Zn-SOD mutation, which reinforces the fact that a defect in energy metabolism is involved in the pathogenesis of ALS. Nevertheless, Bendotti *et al.* (2001) reported microvacuoles in the cytoplasm and swelling of the mitochondria in motor neurons of mice carrying a mutant SOD, but without any change in the histochemical reactivity of cytochrome oxidase, suggesting that partial neuronal activity was maintained despite altered mitochondria.

Oxidative Stress and Gain of Toxic Function Related to Mutations in the Cu,Zn-SOD (or SOD1) Gene

Mutations in the Cu,Zn-SOD gene have been found in about 20% of the familial forms of ALS (Bowling *et al.*, 1993; Rosen et al., 1993; Borchelt *et al.*, 1994; Wong *et al.*, 1995; Bowling and Beal, 1995; Przedborski *et al.*, 1996b). The remaining 80% are probably in relation with unknown mutations in other genes. A tight linkage was found between the disease in several ALS families and the SOD1 gene (located on the chromosome region 21q22.1). Direct sequencing of this gene revealed the presence of 11-point mutations in 13 families (Rosen *et al.*, 1993). Further investigations revealed that over 50 missense mutations occurred in patients with familial ALS (Rainero *et al.*, 1994). This supported a defective handling of oxidative stress in ALS. Nevertheless, the selective degeneration of motor neurons is yet unexplained since SOD1 is present in almost all cell systems.

Cu,Zn-SOD is a cytosolic ubiquitous enzyme that catalyzes the conversion of superoxide radicals (intracellularly generated during oxidation of various compounds, such as hypoxanthine to xanthine via xanthine oxidase) to hydrogen peroxide (H_2O_2) and oxygen:

$$O_2^{\bullet-} + O_2^{\bullet-} \xrightarrow{2H^+} H_2O_2 + O_2$$

The reaction is a dismutation (or dispropornation, that is an oxidation coupled with a reduction) and H_2O_2 is further detoxified by catalase or glutathione peroxidase. A copper atom at the active site of SOD1 mediates catalysis.

More than 60 mutations of Cu,Zn-SOD have been described in familial ALS in different cell lines. Mutations in SOD1 that impair the antioxidant functions of the enzyme could lead to toxic accumulation of superoxide (Deng *et al.*, 1993; Bowling *et al.*, 1993). Elevated superoxide levels may lead to the production of very oxidant hydroxyl radicals by the metal-catalyzed Haber-Weiss reaction (Halliwell, 1989). As an example, Ghadge *et al.* (1997) reported that expression of mutant SOD1 in PC12 cells was associated with higher rates of superoxide production under various conditions. Hall *et al.* (1998) also detected an increase in spinal cord lipid peroxidation in transgenic mice with SOD mutations, whereas increased protein carbonyl levels were found in the spinal cord of patients with sporadic motor neuron disease (Shaw *et al.*, 1995), thus indicating oxidative damage in these patients.

However, the hypothesis of this loss-of-function of SOD1 was not supported by the observation that the overexpression of mutant SOD1 G93A (i.e. in which alanine at position 93 of SOD1 has been substituted for glycine) in mice resulted in motor neuron disease despite an elevated SOD1 activity (Gurney *et al.*, 1994). Conversely, mice knocked out for SOD1 exhibited a total inactivation of the enzyme but without any motor neuron disaese (Reaume *et al.*, 1996).

These observations lead to suggest that SOD1 mutations should cause the disease by a toxic gain of function, rather than by the loss of the scavenging activity of SOD1. According to this theory, the mutant SOD1 could enhance its reactivity towards abnormal substrates (Rowland and Shneider, 2001). Thus, while normal reaction of SOD1 is to catalyze dismutation of $O_2^{\bullet-}$ according to the reaction:

$$\text{SOD1-Cu}^{2+} + O_2^{\bullet-} \rightarrow \text{SOD1-Cu}^{+} + O_2$$
$$\text{SOD1-Cu}^{+} + O_2^{\bullet-} \rightarrow \text{SOD1-Cu}^{2+} + H_2O_2,$$

Mutations in the SOD1 gene could reverse this reaction, leading to an abnormal production of $^{\bullet}OH$ free radicals through use of H_2O_2 as a substrate (Wiedau-Pazos *et al.*, 1996; Yim *et al.*, 1996):

$$\text{SOD1-Cu}^{2+} + H_2O_2 \rightarrow \text{SOD1-Cu}^{+} + O_2^{\bullet-} + 2H^{+}$$
$$\text{SOD1-Cu}^{+} + H_2O_2 \rightarrow \text{SOD1-Cu}^{2+} + {}^{\bullet}OH + OH^{-}$$

Similarly, mutant SOD1 could use peroxynitrite as abnormal substrate, thereby favoring nitration of proteins (Beckman *et al.*, 1993), especially neurofilaments:

$$\text{SOD1-Cu}^{2+} + \text{ONOO}^{-} \rightarrow \text{SOD1-CuO-...NO}_2^{+}$$
$$\text{SOD1-CuO-...NO}_2^{+} + \text{Tyr} \rightarrow \text{SOD1-Cu}^{2+} + OH^{-} + NO_2\text{-Tyr}$$

Thus, SOD1-catalyzed nitration of neurofilament-L might play a role in the ALS pathogenesis (Crow *et al.*, 1997a). As a consequence of this abnormal activity of mutant SOD1, 3-nitrotyrosine used as marker of protein nitration has been found at enhanced levels in the spinal cord of ALS patients (Beal *et al.*, 1997) and in transgenic mice with SOD1 mutation (Ferrante *et al.*, 1997b).

Some SOD1 mutations have been shown to structurally weaken the enzyme, which indirectly decreases its affinity for zinc (Estevez *et al.*, 1999; Beckman *et al.*, 2001) that plays a role in the stability of the normal enzyme. Such decreased affinity for zinc also favours tyrosine nitration (Crow *et al.*, 1997b). This Zn-deficient SOD is able to induce apoptosis through a mechanism involving peroxinitrite. Since Zn-deficient wild-type SOD exhibits a toxicity that is similar to that of Zn-deficient ALS mutant SOD, this suggests that the loss of Zn in wild-type SOD could be involved in the majority of ALS cases (without any SOD mutation detected).

In addition, the copper binding affinities were decreased in the mutant SOD1, which could result in a release of potentially prooxidant copper ions (Eum and Kang, 1999); this could be due to an unstability of the enzyme, but also to glycation which causes fragmentation of SOD1 (Takamiya *et al.*, 2003).

It has been observed that a misfolding of mutant SOD1 could result in a toxic gain-of-function of the enzyme by triggering abnormal protein aggregates (Durham *et al.*, 1997; Bruijn *et al.*, 1998; Cleveland and Liu, 2000; Valentine and Hart, 2003). Zinc-deficient wild-type SOD1 and SOD1 mutants are very prone to form aggregates upon oxidation as compared with normal wild-type SOD1 (Olsen *et al.*, 2001; Rakhit *et al.*, 2002).

Besides, in patients with ALS as well as in mice with SOD1 mutation (Hirano *et al.*, 1984; Rouleau *et al.*, 1996), neurofilaments accumulate in the cells and proximal axons of motor neurons, impeding the axonal transport of molecules. These aggregates are probably the results from the toxic effects of mutant SOD1 since axonal neurofilaments appear as potential targets of mutant SOD1. Another intermediate filament called peripherin has been found associated with neurofilaments in the neuronal inclusions of patients with sporadic ALS (Corbo and Hays, 1992) and in mice with mutant SOD1 (Tu *et al.*, 1996). Its overexpression in mice induces degeneration of motor neurons (Beaulieu *et al.*, 1999). The development of axonal intermediate filament inclusions might block transport and transgenic mice expressing the G93A mutation on SOD1 exhibited similar alterations in the neuronal cytoskeleton as ALS patients (Tu *et al.*, 1996; Beaulieu and Julien, 2003).

In patients with familial ALS, mutant SOD1 could lead to excitotoxic neuronal injury by inactivation of a glutamate transporter called EAAT2 (Trotti *et al.*, 1999). This glutamate excitotoxicity involves an excessive entry of extracellular calcium and was suggested in all patients with ALS (Rothstein, 1995; Shaw and Ince, 1997), which represents another link between familial and sporadic forms of ALS.

It is of interest to note the effects of increased oxidative stress on energy metabolism and thus to show the linkage between mitochondrial dysfunction and SOD1 mutant enzyme. Browne *et al.* (1998) reported that ALS patients with SOD1 mutations exhibited significant increases in the mitochondrial complex I and II-III activities. The same observation was reported in transgenic mice overexpressing human mutant SOD1 (Browne *et al.*, 1998). These abnormalities involving mitochondrial energy metabolism could reflect an adaptation to an enhanced energy demand.

Therapeutic Perspectives in Relation with Oxidative Stress and Other Related Pathophysiological Hypotheses

As a global conclusion on the pathophysiology of ALS, neurodegeneration may arise by converging pathways (Figure 2), such as:

- ROS-induced damage of cellular targets (triggered, in the case of mutant SOD1, by a misfolding resulting in a deficient copper binding);

- disorganisation of intermediate filaments;
- triggering of inflammation;
- glutamate-mediated excitotoxicity and other abnormalities of intracellular calcium regulation in a process that may involve mitochondrial damage and apoptosis.

These pathophysiological hypotheses lead to supplementations conducted on cell lines transfected with mutant SOD1 genes, on transgenic mice and in humans (Cookson and Shaw, 1999). These therapeutic trials were based on:

- antioxidants: vitamin E, N-acetylcysteine (Andreassen *et al.*, 2000), selenium, coenzyme Q10. In transgenic mice carrying the G93A mutation in SOD1 (model of ALS), chronic administration of vitamin E delayed the onset of the disease when treatment was initiated while the animals were presymptomatic (Gurney *et al.*, 1996). It is interesting to note that coenzyme Q10 protects *in vitro* against glutamate toxicity and acts as an acceptor of electrons coming from complexes I and III of the mitochondrial transport chain. In its reduced form, it acts as antioxidant in mitochondria and cell membrane (Matthews *et al.*, 1998);
- glutamate antagonists such as riluzole or gabapentine. To date, the only efficient treatments are those carried with riluzole that increases survival time (Bensimon *et al.*, 1994; Lacomblez *et al.*, 1996). As regards gabapentin, after a promising phase II trial (Miller *et al.*, 1996), a phase III trial did no show evidence for a beneficial effect on disease progression or symptoms (Miller *et al.*, 2001).
- apoptosis inhibitors such as Bcl-2 or penicillamine. Bcl-2 protein could inhibit the opening of the mitochondrial transition pore and the activity of caspases that are proapototic cytoplasmic proteins, and could normalize the activity of Cu,Zn-SOD (Kostic *et al.*, 1997);
- creatine, since a deficit of ATP production in mice carrying mutant SOD1 has been hypothesized. Creatine and creatine phosphate could play a role by giving energy and by limitating the opening of the mitochondrial transition pore (Klivenyi *et al.*, 1999). However in a recent study, creatine has been shown to have no clear effect in ALS patients (Groeneveld *et al.*, 2003). In the transgenic G93A mouse model of ALS, administration of cyclooxygenase 2 (COX-2) inhibitors (antiinflammatory drugs) associated with creatine produced additive effects and extended survival by about 30% (Klivenyi *et al.*, 2004); COX-2 inhibitors resulted in a protection of anterior horn motor neurons and association with creatine enhance this effect; this is related to the observation that mutant SOD1 transgenic mice exhibited an upregulation of genes related to inflammation (such as TNFα) together with changes in apoptosis-related genes (such as caspase 1) (Yoshihara *et al.*, 2002).

In animal, vitamin E, selenium and bcl-2 protein increased the phase preceding the appearance of the disease, but they did not modify the survival. In contrast, glutamate antagonists, coenzyme Q10 and creatine did not modify the lag phase, but increased survival (Gurney *et al.*, 1996; Brown, 1996; Kostic *et al.*, 1997; Mathews *et al.*, 1998). Supplementation of animals with creatine also improved their motricity, reduce the concentration of 3-nitrotyrosine, increased glutamate neuronal reuptake and protected against motor neuron disappearance (Klivenyi *et al.*, 1999).

These data suggested that oxidative stress and glutamate toxicity are probably intricate. Similarly, our observation that patients treated with riluzole exhibited an erythrocyte Cu,Zn-SOD activity intermediate between the elevated SOD activity of ALS patients without treatment and that of controls (Bonnefont-Rousselot *et al.*, 2000) suggests a possible activity of the drug on the oxidative stress.

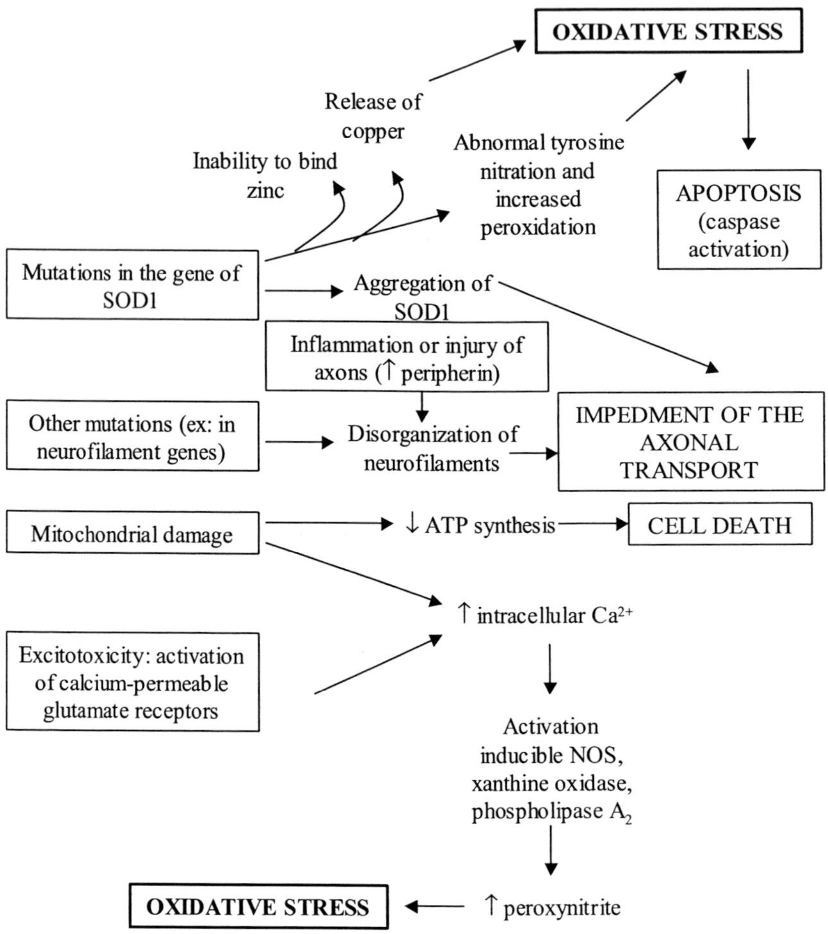

Figure 2. Mechanisms contributing to the neurodegeneration in ALS (from Rowland and Shneider, 2001).

Some current treatments (antioxidant compounds, anti apoptotic compounds, anti inflammatory drugs) are under trials. A recently tested association of riluzole and vitamin E in 288 ALS patients resulted in a less severe evolution after one year of treatment, compared to non treated patients, when using the ALS Health State scale (Desnuelle *et al.*, 2001). In this study, TBARS levels of patients receiving α-tocopherol for 12 months were restored to those observed in normal young adults. Nevertheless, this placebo-controlled randomized clinical trial provided no evidence for a beneficial effect of traetment with α-tocopherol on the rate of functional deteriration as measured with the Norris scale, nor on survival.

Although not the only factors involved in cell death in neurodegeneration, free radicals nonetheless seem to contribute to neuronal damage and eventual death. Antioxidant could thus be an interesting way of research in preventing and/or treating these diseases. As a whole, results suggest that combinations of therapies targeting different disease mechanisms may be a useful strategy in the treatment of ALS. Reliable biological markers are needed in ALS, especially indicators for oxidative damage that could detect the disease in its pre-clinical or early clinical stage, would help early diagnosis and follow-up of clinical trials and epidemiological studies (Dib, 2003).

References

Andreassen OA, Dedeoglu A, Klivenyi P, Beal MF, Bush AI. N-acetyl-L-cysteine improves survival and preserves motor performance in an animal model of familial amyotrophic lateral sclerosis. *Neuroreport* 2000; 11: 2491-2493.

Andrus PK, Fleck TJ, Gurney ME, Hall ED. Protein oxidative damage in a transgenic mouse model of familial amyotrophic lateral sclerosis. *J Neurochem* 1998; 71: 2041-2048.

Beal MF. Aging, energy, and oxidative stress in neurodegenerative diseases. Ann Neurol 1995; 38: 357-366.

Beal MF. Mitochondria and the pathogenesis of ALS. *Brain* 2000; 123: 1291-1292.

Beal MF, Ferrante RJ, Browne SE, Matthews RT, Kowall NW, Brown RH Jr. Increased 3-nitrotyrosine in both sporadic and familial amyotrophic lateral sclerosis. *Ann Neurol* 1997; 42: 644-654.

Beaulieu JM, Julien JP. Peripherin-mediated death of motor neurons rescued by overexpression of neurofilament NF-H proteins. *J Neurochem* 2003; 85: 248-256.

Beaulieu JM, Robertson J, Julien JP. Interactions between peripherin and neurofilaments in cultured cells: disruption of peripherin assembly by the NF-M and NF-H subunits. *Biochem Cell Biol* 1999;77(1):41-45.

Beckman JS, Carson M, Smith CD, Koppenol WH. ALS, SOD and peroxynitrite. *Nature* 1993; 364: 584 (letter).

Beckman JS, Estevez AG, Crow JP, Barbeito L. Superoxide dismutase and the death of motoneurons in ALS. *Trends Neurosci* 2001; 24 (Suppl.): S15-S20.

Bendotti C, Calvaresi N, Chiveri L, Prelle A, Moggio M, Braga M, Silani V, De Biasi S. Early vacuolization and mitochondrial damage in motor neurons of FALS mice are not associated with apoptosis or with changes in cytochrome oxidase histochemical reactivity. *J Neurol Sci* 2001; 191: 25-33.

Bensimon G, Lacomblez L, Meininger V, the ALS/Riluzole Study Group. A controlled trial of riluzole in amyotrophic lateral sclerosis. *N Engl J Med* 1994; 330: 585-591.

Bogdanov MB, Ramos LE, Xu Z, Beal MF. Elevated « hydroxyl radical » generation in vivo in an animal model of amyotrophic lateral sclerosis. *J Neurochem* 1998; 71: 1321-1324.

Bogdanov M, Brown RH Jr, Matson W, Smart R, Hayden D, O'Donnell H, Beal MF, Cudkowicz M. Increased oxidative damage to DNA in ALS patients. *Free Radic Biol Med* 2000; 29: 652-658.

Bonnefont-Rousselot D, Lacomblez L, Jaudon MC, Lepage S, Salachas F, Bensimon G, Bizard C, Doppler V, Delattre J, Meininger V. Blood oxidative stress in amyotrophic lateral sclerosis. *J Neurol Sci* 2000; 178: 57-62.

Borchelt DR, Lee MK, Slunt HS, Guarnieri M, Xu ZS, Wong PC, Brown RH Jr, Price DL, Sisodia SS, Cleveland DW. Superoxide dismutase 1 with mutations linked to familial amyotrophic lateral sclerosis possesses significant activity. *Proc Natl Acad Sci USA* 1994; 91: 8292-8296.

Bowling AC, Beal MF. Bioenergetic and oxidative stress in neurodegenerative diseases. *Life Sci* 1995; 56: 1151-1171.

Bowling AC, Schulz JB, Brown RH Jr, Beal MF. Superoxide dismutase activity, oxidative damage, and mitochondrial energy metabolism in familial and sporadic amyotrophic lateral sclerosis. *J Neurochem* 1993; 61: 2322-2325.

Broekemeier KM, Pfeiffer DR. Inhibition of the mitochondrial permeability transition by cyclosporin A during long time frame experiments: relationship between pore opening and the activity of mitochondrial phospholipases. *Biochemistry* 1995; 34: 16440-16449.

Brown RH. Superoxide dismutase and familial amyotrophic lateral sclerosis: new insights into mechanisms and treatments. *Ann Neurol* 1996; 39: 145-146.

Browne SE, Bowling AC, Baik MJ, Gurney M, Brown RH Jr, Beal MF. Metabolic dysfunction in familial, but not sporadic, amyotrophic lateral sclerosis. *J Neurochem* 1998; 71: 281-287.

Bruijn LI, Beal MF, Becher MW, Schulz JB, Wong PC, Price DL, Cleveland DW. Elevated free nitrotyrosine levels, but not protein-bound nitrotyrosine or hydroxyl radicals, throughout amyotrophic lateral sclerosis (ALS)-like disease implicate tyrosine nitration as an aberrant in vivo property of one familial ALS-linked superoxide dismutase 1 mutant. *Proc Natl Acad Sci USA* 1997; 94: 7606-7611.

Bruijn LI, Houseweart MK, Kato S, Anderson KL, Anderson SD, Ohama E, Reaume AG, Scott RW, Cleveland DW. Aggregation and motor neuron toxicity of an ALS-linked SOD1 mutant independent from wild-type SOD1. *Science* 1998; 281: 1851-1854.

Carri MT, Ferri A, Cozzolono M, Calabrese L, Rotilio G. Neurodegeneration in amyotrophic lateral sclerosis: the role of oxidative stress and altered homeostasis of metals. *Brain Res Bull* 2003; 61: 365-374.

Cassarino DS, Bennett JP Jr. An evaluation of the role of mitochondria in neurodegenerative diseases: mitochondrial mutations and oxidative pathology, protective nuclear responses, and cell death in neurodegeneration. *Brain Res Rev* 1999; 29: 1-25.

Cleveland DW, Liu J. Oxidation versus aggregation - how do SOD1 mutants cause ALS? *Nat Med* 2000; 6: 1320-1321.

Cookson MR, Shaw PJ. Oxidative stress and motor neuron disease. *Brain Pathol* 1999; 39: 158-165.

Corbo M, Hays AP. Peripherin and neurofilament protein coexist in spinal spheroids of motor neuron disease. *J Neuropathol Exp Neurol* 1992; 51: 531-537.

Crow JP, Ye YZ, Strong M, Kirk M, Barnes S, Beckman JS. Superoxide dismutase catalyzes nitration of tyrosines by peroxynitrite in the rod and head domains of neurofilament-L. *J Neurochem* 1997a; 69: 1945-1953.

Crow JP, Sampson JB, Zhuang Y, Thompson JA, Beckman JS. Decreased zinc affinity of amyotrophic lateral sclerosis-associated superoxide dismutase mutants leads to enhanced catalysis of tyrosine nitration by peroxynitrite. *J Neurochem* 1997b; 69: 1936-1944.

Dal Canto MC, Gurney ME. Development of central nervous system pathology in a murine transgenic model of human amyotrophic lateral sclerosis. *Am J Pathol* 1994; 145: 1271-1279.

Deng HX, Hentati A, Tainer JA, Iqbal Z, Cayabyab A, Hung WY, Getzoff ED, Hu P, Herzfeldt B, Roos RP *et al.* Amyotrophic lateral sclerosis and structural defects in Cu,Zn superoxide dismutase. *Science* 1993; 261: 1047-1051.

Desnuelle C, Dib M, Garrel C, Favier A. A double-blind, placebo controlled randomised clinical trial of α-tocopherol (vitamin E), in the treatment of amyotrophic lateral sclerosis. *Amyotrophic Lateral Scler Other Motor Neuron Disord* 2001; 2: 9-18.

Dib M. Amyotrophic lateral sclerosis: progress and prospects for treatment. *Drugs* 2003;63(3):289-310.

Dringen R, Gutterer JM, Hirrlinger J. Glutathione metabolism in brain metabolic interaction between astrocytes and neurons in the defense against reactive oxydgen species. *Eur J Biochem* 2000; 267: 4912-4916.

Durham HD, Roy J, Dong L, Figlewicz DA. Aggregation of mutant Cu/Zn superoxide dismutase proteins in a culture model of ALS. *J Neuropathol Exp Neurol* 1997; 56: 523-530.

Estevez AG, Crow JP, Sampson JB, Reiter C, Zhuang Y, Richardson GJ, Tarpey MM, Barbeito L, Beckman JS. Induction of nitric oxide-dependent apoptosis in motor neurons by zinc-deficient superoxide dismutase. *Science* 1999; 286: 2498-2500.

Eum WS, Kang JH. Release of copper ions from the familial amyotrophic lateral sclerosis-associated Cu,Zn-superoxide dismutase mutants. *Mol Cells* 1999; 9: 110-114.

Ferrante RJ, Browne SE, Shinobu LA, Bowling AC, Baik MJ, Mac Gravey U, Kowall NW, Brown RH Jr, Beal MF. Evidence of increased oxidative damage in both sporadic and familial amyotrophic lateral sclerosis. *J Neurochem* 1997a; 69: 2064-2074.

Ferrante RJ, Shinobu LA, Schulz JB, Matthews RT, Thomas CE, Kowall NW, Gurney ME, Beal MF. Increased 3-nitrotyrosine and oxidative damage in mice with a human copper/zinc superoxide dismutase mutation. *Ann Neurol* 1997b; 42: 326-334.

Fleury C, Mignotte B, Vayssière JL. Mitochondrial reactive oxygen species in cell death signaling. *Biochimie* 2002; 84: 131-141.

Ghadge GD, Lee JP, Bindokas VP, Jordan J, Ma L, Miller RJ, Roos RP. Mutant superoxide dismutase-1-linked familial amyotrophic lateral sclerosis: molecular mechanisms of neuronal death and protection. *J Neurosci* 1997; 17: 8756-8766.

Groeneveld GJ, Veldink JH, van der Tweel I, Kalmijn S, Beijer C, de Visser M, Wokke JH, Franssen H, van den Berg LH. A randomized sequential trial of creatine in amyotrophic lateral sclerosis. *Ann Neurol.* 2003; 53: 437-445.

Gurney ME, Pu H, Chiu AY, Dal Canto MC, Polchow CY, Alexander DD, Caliendo J, Hentati A, Kwon YW, Deng HX, Chen W, Zhai P, Sufit R, Siddique T. Motor neuron degeneration in mice that express a human Cu,Zn superoxide dismutase mutation. *Science* 1994; 264: 1772-1775.

Gurney ME, Cutting FB, Zhai P, Doble A, Taylor CP, Andrus PK, Hall ED. Benefit of vitamin E, riluzole, and gabapentin in a transgenic model of familial amyotrophic lateral sclerosis. Ann Neurol 1996; 39: 147-157.

Hall ED, Andrus PK, Oostveen JA, Fleck TJ, Gurney ME. Relationship of oxygen radical-induced lipid peroxidative damage to disease onset and progression in transgenic model of familial ALS. *J Neurosci Res* 1998; 53: 66-77.

Halliwell B. Oxidants and the central nervous sytem, some fundamental questions. Is oxidant damage relevant to Parkinson's disease, Alzheimer's disease, traumatic injury or stroke? *Acta Neurol Scand* 1989; 126: 23-33.

Halliwell B. Reactive oxygen species and the central nervous system. *J Neurochem* 1992; 59: 1609-1623.

Halliwell B, Gutteridge JMC, editors. *Free radicals in biology and medicine.* New York : Oxford University Press, 1999, 3rd Ed.

Hand CK, Rouleau GA. Familial amyotrophic lateral sclerosis. *Muscle Nerve* 2002; 25: 135-159.

Hirano A, Donnenfeld H, Sasaki S, Nakano I. Fine structural observations of neurofilamentous changes in amyotrophic lateral sclerosis. *J Neuropathol Exp Neurol* 1984;43: 461-470.

Hurko O, Walsh FS. Novel drug development for amyotrophic lateral sclerosis. *J Neurol Sci* 2000; 180:21-28.

Ihara Y, Mori A, Hayabara T, Kawai M, Namba R, Nobukuni K, Sato K, Kibata M. Superoxide dismutase and free radicals in sporadic amyotrophic lateral sclerosis: relationship to clinical data. *J Neurol Sci* 1995; 134: 51-56.

Ikeda K, Kinoshita M, Iwasaki Y, Tagaya N, Shiojima T. Lecithinized superoxide dismutase retards wobbler mouse motoneuron disease. *Neuromuscul Disord* 1995; 5: 383-390.

Ilzecka J. Total antioxidant status is increased in the serum of amyotrophic lateral sclerosis patients. *Scand J Clin Lab Invest* 2003; 63: 297-302.

Ince PG, Shaw PJ, Candy JM, Mantle D, Tandon L, Ehmann WD, Markesbery WR. Iron, selenium and glutathione peroxidase activity are elevated in sporadic motor neuron disease. *Neurosci Lett* 1994; 182: 87-90.

Jordan J, Cena V, Prehn JH. Mitochondrial control of a neuron death and its role in neurodegenerative disorders. *J Physiol Biochem* 2003; 59: 129-141.

Klivenyi P, Ferrante RJ, Matthews RT, Bogdanov MB, Klein AM, Andreassen OA, Mueller G, Wermer M, Kaddurah-Daouk R, Beal MF. Neuroprotective effects of creatine in a transgenic animal model of amyotrophic lateral sclerosis. *Nature Med* 1999; 5: 347-350.

Klivenyi P, Kiaei M, Gardian G, Calingasan NY, Beal MF. Additive neuroprotective effects of creatine and cyclooxygenase 2 inhibitors in a transgenic mouse model of amyotrophic lateral sclerosis. *J Neurochem* 2004; 88: 576-582.

Kong J, Xu Z. Massive mitochondrial degeneration in motor neurons triggers the onset of amyotrophic lateral sclerosis in mice expressing a mutant SOD1. *J Neurosci* 1998; 18: 3241-3250.

Kostic V, Jackson-Lewis V, De Bilbao F, Dubois-Dauphin M, Przedborski S. Bcl2-prolonging life in a transgenic mouse model of familial amyotrophic lateral sclerosis. *Science* 1997; 277: 559-562.

Kristal BS, Park BK, Yu BP. 4-Hydroxyhexenal is a potent inducer of the mitochondrial permeability transition. *J Biol Chem* 1996; 271: 6033-6038.

Lacomblez L, Bensimon G, Leigh PN, Guillet P, Meininger V. Dose-ranging study of riluzole in amyotrophic lateral sclerosis. Amyotrophic Lateral Sclerosis/Riluzole Study Group II. *Lancet* 1996; 347: 1425-1431.

Liu R, Althaus JS, Ellerbrock BR, Becker DA, Gurney ME. Enhanced oxygen radical production in transgenic mouse model of familial amyotrophic lateral sclerosis. *Ann Neurol* 1998; 44: 763-770.

Liu D, Wen J, Liu J, Li L. The roles of free radicals in amyotrophic lateral sclerosis: reactive oxygen species and elevated oxidation of protein, DNA, and membrane phospholipids. *FASEB J* 1999; 13: 2318-2328.

Marttila RJ, Lorentz H, Rinne UK. Oxygen toxicity protecting enzymes in Parkinson's disease. Increase of superoxide dismutase-like activity in the substantia nigra and basal nucleus. *J Neurol Sci* 1988; 86: 321-331.

Matthews RT, Yang L, Browne S, Baik M, Beal MF. Coenzyme Q10 administration increases brain mitochondrial concentrations and exerts neuroprotective effects. *Proc Natl Acad Sci USA* 1998; 95: 8892-8897.

Miller RG, Moore D, Young LA, Armon C, Barohn RJ, Bromberg MB, Bryan WW, Gelinas DF, Mendoza MC, Neville HE, Parry GJ, Petajan JH, Ravits JM, Ringel SP, Ross MA. Placebo-controlled trial of gabapentin in patients with amyotrophic lateral sclerosis. WALS Study Group. Western Amyotrophic Lateral Sclerosis Study Group. *Neurology* 1996; 47:1383-1388.

Miller RG, Moore DH 2nd, Gelinas DF, Dronsky V, Mendoza M, Barohn RJ, Bryan W, Ravits J, Yuen E, Neville H, Ringel S, Bromberg M, Petajan J, Amato AA, Jackson C, Johnson W, Mandler R, Bosch P, Smith B, Graves M, Ross M, Sorenson EJ, Kelkar P, Parry G, Olney R; Western ALS Study Group. Phase III randomized trial of gabapentin in patients with amyotrophic lateral sclerosis. *Neurology* 2001; 56: 843-848.

Mourelatos Z, Gonatas NK, Stieber A, Gurney ME, Dal Canto MC. The Golgi apparatus of spinal cord motor neurons in transgenic mice expressing mutant Cu,Zn superoxide dismutase gene becomes fragmented in early, preclinical stages of the disease. *Proc Natl Acad Sci USA* 1996; 93: 5472-5477.

Olsen MK, Roberds SL, Ellerbrock BR, Fleck TJ, McKinley DK, Gurney ME. Disease mechanisms revealed by transcription profiling in SOD1-G93A transgenic mouse spinal cord. *Ann Neurol* 2001; 50: 730-740.

Oteiza PI, Uchitel OD, Carrasquedo F, Dubrovski AL, Roma JC, Fraga CG. Evaluation of antioxidants, protein, and lipid oxidation products in blood from sporadic amyotrophic lateral sclerosis patients. *Neurochem Res* 1997; 22: 535-539.

Przedborski S, Donaldson DM, Murphy PL, Hirsch O, Lange D, Naini AB, McKenna-Yasek D, Brown RH Jr. Blood superoxide dismutase, catalase and glutathione peroxidase activities in familial and sporadic amyotrophic lateral sclerosis. *Neurodegeneration* 1996a; 5: 57-64.

Przedborski S, Donaldson D, Jakowec M, Kish SJ, Guttman M, Rosoklija G, Hays AP. Brain superoxide dismutase, catalase, and glutathione peroxidase activities in amyotrophic lateral sclerosis. *Ann Neurol* 1996b; 39: 158-165.

Puymirat J, Cossette L, Gosselin F, Bouchard JP. Red blood cell Cu/Zn superoxide dismutase activity in sporadic amyotrophic lateral sclerosis. *J Neurol Sci* 1994; 127: 121-123.

Rainero I, Pinessi L, Tsuda T, Vignocchi MG, Vaula G, Calvi L, Cerrato P, Rossi B, Bergamini L, McLachlan DR, *et al.* SOD1 missense mutation in an Italian family with ALS. *Neurology* 1994; 44: 347-349.

Rakhit R, Cunningham P, Furtos-Matei A, Dahan S, Qi XF, Crow JP, Cashman NR, Kondejewski LH, Chakrabartty A. Oxidation-induced misfolding and aggregation of superoxide dismutase and its implications for amyotrophic lateral sclerosis. *J Biol Chem* 2002; 277: 47551-47556.

Reaume AG, Elliott JL, Hoffman EK, Kowall NW, Ferrante RJ, Siwek DF, Wilcox HM, Flood DG, Beal MF, Brown RH Jr, Scott RW, Snider WD. Motor neurons in Cu/Zn superoxide dismutase-deficient mice develop normally but exhibit enhanced cell death after axonal injury. *Nat Genet* 1996; 13: 43-47.

Rosen DR, Siddique T, Patterson D, Figlewicz DA, Sapp P, Hentati A Donaldson D, Goto J, O'Regan JP, Deng HX, *et al.* Mutations in Cu/Zn superoxide dismutase gene are associated with familial amyotrophic lateral sclerosis. *Nature* 1993; 362: 59-62.

Rothstein JD. Excitotoxic mechanisms in the pathogenesis of amyotrophic lateral sclerosis. *Adv Neurol* 1995; 68: 7-20.

Rouleau GA, Clark AW, Rooke K, Pramatarova A, Krizus A, Suchowersky O, Julien JP, Figlewicz D. SOD1 mutation is associated with accumulation of neurofilaments in amyotrophic lateral sclerosis. *Ann Neurol* 1996; 39: 128-131.

Rowland LP, Shneider NA. Amyotrophic lateral sclerosis. *N Engl J Med* 2001; 344: 1688-1700.

Sasaki S, Iwata M. Ultrastructural study of synapses in the anterior horn neurons of patients with amyotrophic lateral sclerosis. *Neurosci Lett* 1996; 204: 53-56.

Schulz JB, Lindenau J, Seyfried J, Dichgans J. Glutathione, oxidative stress and neurodegeneration. *Eur J Biochem* 2000; 267: 4904-4911.

Shaw PJ, Ince PG. Glutamate, excitotoxicity and amyotrophic lateral sclerosis. *J Neurol* 1997; 244: S3-S14.

Shaw PJ, Ince PG, Falkous G, Mantle D. Oxidative damage to protein in sporadic motor neuron disease spinal cord. *Ann Neurol* 1995; 38: 691-695.

Shibata N, Nagai R, Uchida K, Horiuchi S, Yamada S, Hirano A, Kawaguchi M, Yamamoto T, Sasaki S, Kobayashi M. Morphological evidence for lipid peroxidation and protein glycoxidation in spinal cords from sporadic amyotrophic lateral sclerosis patients. *Brain Res* 2001; 917: 97-104.

Shoubridge EA, Karpati G, Hastings KE. Deletion mutants are functionnly dominant over wild-type mitochondrial genomes in skeletal muscle fiber segments in mitochondrial disease. *Cell* 1990; 62: 43-49.

Siciliano G, D'Avino C, Del Corona A, Barsacchi R, Kusmic C, Rocchi A, Pastorini E, Murri L. Impaired oxidative metabolism and lipid peroxidation in exercising muscle from ALS patients. *Amyotroph Lateral Scler Other Motor Neuron Disord* 2002; 3: 57-62.

Skulachev VP. Role of uncoupled and non-coupled oxidations in maintenance of safety low levels of oxygen and its one-electron reductants. *Q Rev Biophys* 1996; 29: 169-202.

Smith TS, Bennett JP Jr. Mitochondrial toxins in models of neurodegenerative diseases. I: In vivo brain hydroxyl radical production during systemic MPTP treatment or following microdialysis infusion of methylpyridinium or azide ions. *Brain Res* 1997;765:183-188.

Suzuki YJ, Forman HJ, Sevenian A. Oxidants as stimulators of signal transduction. *Free Radic Biol Med* 1997; 22: 269-285.

Takamiya R, Takahashi M, Myint T, Park YS, Miyazawa N, Endo T, Fujiwara N, Sakiyama H, Misonou Y, Miyamoto Y, Fujii J, Taniguchi N. Glycation proceeds faster in mutated Cu,Zn-superoxide dismutases related to familial amyotrophic lateral sclerosis. *FASEB J* 2003; 17: 938-940.

Thérond P, Bonnefont-Rousselot D, Davit-Spraul A, Conti M, Legrand A. Biomarkers of oxidative stress: an analytical approach. *Curr Opin Clin Nutr Metab Care* 2000; 3: 373-384.

Tohgi H, Abe T, Yamazaki K, Murata T, Ishizaki E, Isobe C. Remarkable increase in cerebrospinal fluid 3-nitrotyrosine in patients with sporadic amyotrophic lateral sclerosis. *Ann Neurol* 1999; 46: 129-131.

Trotti D, Rolfs A, Danbolt NC, Brown RH Jr, Hediger MA. SOD1 mutants linked to amyotrophic lateral sclerosis selectively inactivate a glial glutamate transporter. *Nat Neurosci* 1999; 2: 848.

Tu PH, Raju P, Robinson KA, Gurney ME, Trojanowski JQ, Lee VM. Transgenic mice carrying a human mutant superoxide dismutase transgene develop neuronal cytoskeletal pathology resembling human amyotrophic lateral sclerosis lesions. *Proc Natl Acad Sci USA* 1996; 93: 3155-3160.

Valentine JS, Hart PJ. Misfolded CuZnSOD and amyotrophic lateral sclerosis. *Proc Natl Acad Sci USA* 2003; 100: 3617-3622.

Vielhaber S, Kunz D, Winkler K, Wiedemann FR, Kirches E, Feistner H, Heinze HJ, Elger CE, Schubert W, Kunz WS. Mitochondrial DNA abnormalities in skeletal muscle of patients with sporadic amyotrophic lateral sclerosis. *Brain* 2000; 123: 1339-1348.

Wiedau-Pazos M, Goto JJ, Rabizadeh S, Gralla EB, Roe JA, Lee MK, Valentine JS, Bredesen DE. Altered reactivity of superoxide dismutase in familial amyotrophic lateral sclerosis. *Science* 1996; 271: 515-518.

Wong PC, Pardo CA, Borchelt DR, Lee MK, Copeland NG, Jenkins NA, Sisodia SS, Cleveland DW, Price DL. An adverse property of a familial ALS-linked SOD1 mutation causes motor neuron disease characterized by vacuolar degeneration of mitochondria. *Neuron* 1995; 14: 1105-1116.

Yim MB, Kang JH, Yim HS, Kwak HS, Chock PB, Stadtman ER. A gain-of-function of an amyotrophic lateral sclerosis-associated Cu,Zn-superoxide dismutase mutant: an enhancement of free radical formation due to a decrease in Km for hydrogen peroxide. *Proc Natl Acad Sci USA* 1996; 93: 5709-5714.

Yoshihara T, Ishigaki S, Yamamoto M, Liang Y, Niwa J, Takeuchi H, Doyu M, Sobue G. Differential expression of inflammation- and apoptosis-related genes in spinal cords of a mutant SOD1 transgenic mouse model of familial amyotrophic lateral sclerosis. *J Neurochem* 2002; 80: 158-167.

In: Amyotrophic Lateral Sclerosis: New Research
Editor: Christine A. Murray, pp. 155-178 ISBN 1-59454-179-5

Chapter VI

Excitability and Potentials of Human Fibres in Amyotrophic Lateral Sclerosis: Model Investigations

D. I. Stephanova*
Institute of Biophysics, Bulgarian Academy of Sciences,
Acad.G. Bontchev St., Bl 21, Sofia 1113, Bulgaria.

Abstract

The excitability and potentials (intracellular and electrotonic) of human motor and sensory axons in amyotrophic lateral sclerosis (ALS) types (termed as ALS1, ALS2 and ALS3, respectively) can be reliably studied using double cable models of the fibres. The intracellular potentials can be then used as input to a line source model that allows the calculation of the corresponding spatial and temporal distributions of the extracellular potentials at various radial distances in the surrounding volume conductor. The potentials and indices of the axonal excitability delivered from single or pairs of threshold stimuli, such as strength-duration and charge-duration curves, strength-duration time constants, rheobasic currents and recovery cycles depend on the methods of fibre stimulation. Two cases of fibre stimulation are considered in the present investigations. The first case of point application of current intra-axonally at the center of the first node closely approximates the effects of point application of current extra-axonally at the node and realizes a point fibre polarization. The second case of simultaneous intracellular current application at the midpoints of all available internodal segments closely approximates the effects of external surface stimulation with a large electrode and realizes a periodic kind of uniform fibre polarization. Each of these investigations also depends on the electrophysiological cable characteristics of the axons. Together they can provide new information about thc pathophysiology underlying abnormalitics in the excitability and potentials of the human fibres in ALS. Simulated results indicate that the used models are

* Correspondence concerning this article should be addressed to Dr. Stephanova D.I. Institute of Biophysics, Bulgarian Academy of Sciences, Acad.G. Bontchev St., Bl 21, Sofia 1113, Bulgaria.

rather promising tools in studying the prominent feature (fasciculation) of ALS which up till now has not been sufficiently well understood.

Keywords: Amyotrophic lateral sclerosis, computational neuroscience, strength-duration properties, recovery cycles, potentials.

Introduction

Amyotrophic lateral sclerosis (ALS) is a progressive and fatal neurodegenerative disorder involving the neurons of the motor system in the brain and spinal cord. The primary clinical symptom of ALS is progressive muscle weakness. The weakness spreads to involve the muscles of the trunk and abdomen, and the bulbar muscles of the face, mouth and throat. The involved muscles also show both upper and lower motor neuron findings. The upper motor neuron findings include spasticity and hyperreflexia. The lower motor neuron findings consist of fasciculations and atrophy. The fasciculations due to spontaneous motor unit discharges may be regarded as a consistent feature of ALS (Forster and Alpers 1944; Trojaborg and Buchthal 1965; Lambert 1969; Wettstein 1979; Condradi et al. 1982; Layzer 1982; Sobue et al. 1983; Roth 1982, 1984; Finsterer et al. 1997; Roswinska et al. 1997). ALS is also characterized by the simultaneous dying of motor neurons. The increased axonal excitability is a prelude to cell death in ALS (Trojaborg and Buchthal 1965; Guiloff and Modarres-Sadeghi 1992; Murray 1994). Another feature of ALS is the motor nerve conduction slowing. Amplitude-dependent slowing of the velocity is obtained in ALS (Sobue et al. 1983; Nakanishi et al. 1989; Wirguin et al. 1992; Arasaki and Tamaki 1998; Feinberg et al. 1999). The hypothesis for the major mechanism of conduction slowing is the loss of large, fast-conducting fibres. Using a threshold-tracing system (non-invasive technique of threshold electrotonus), the strength-duration properties of motor and sensory human axons are recorded from patients with ALS, and compared with those of healthy subjects (Mogyoros et al. 1998). The studies on the ion channel dysfunction in ALS (Bostock et al. 1995) show that the human axons in ALS patients respond abnormally to subthreshold depolarizing currents. These abnormal responses are consistent with a loss of functional sodium and potassium (fast and slow) channels and the authors propose that this ion channel dysfunction could also be responsible for the motor neuron degeneration in this disease. To analyze the nature of the abnormalities in the excitability and potentials in and around active human fibres in ALS, we have applied the method of mathematical modeling. This chapter reviews some of the simulations of the electrogenesis underlying the membrane properties of myelinated human fibres that can also be studied in vivo in healthy subjects and patients with ALS.

Method of Mathematical Modeling

Studies continue to reveal more information regarding the complex anatomical and diverse electrophysiological properties of the myelinated human nerve fibre. At the node of Ranvier, the dynamics of nodal sodium and potassium (fast and slow) channels in the human fibre have been studied (Schwarz et al. 1995; Vogel and Schwarz 1995; Bostock and Rothwell 1997; Reid et al. 1999). Direct evidence for the presence of different types of ion channels in the internodes of mammalian (including human) myelinated axons has come from voltage clamp studies of acutely demyelinated internodal axolemma (Roper and Schwarz 1989; Scholz et al. 1993; Safronov et al. 1993; Vogel and Schwarz 1995). Mathematical models (one cable, double cable and multi-layered) are developed to examine the possible influence of anatomical and electrical properties (normal or abnormal) on the functional behavior of the myelinated fibres (Fitzhugh 1962; Frankenhaeuser and Huxley 1964; Goldman and Albus 1968; Smith and Koles 1970; Waxman et al. 1979; Wood et al. 1982a, b; Stephanova 1988a, b, c, 1989a, b, 1990 - one cable models; Blight 1985; Awiszus 1990; Halter and Clark 1991; Stephanova and Kossev 1996; Stephanova and Chobanova 1997; Stephanova and Daskalova 2003a, b - double cable models; Stephanova 2001- multi-layered model).

Double-Cable Models

The electrogenesis of myelinated human motor and sensory axons can be studied successfully using the double cable models of these fibres (Stephanova and Bostock 1995, 1996; Stephanova and Mileva 2000). The interested reader is referred to Fig.1 of Stephanova and Bostock (1995) for an electrical equivalent circuit representation of a human motor fibre. The electrical equivalent circuit is based on the nodal and internodal channels in a previous, two-component model of human motor axons (Bostock et al. 1991), added to a complex extended double cable structure of nodal, paranodal and internodal segments. The double cable model assumes a high-resistance myelin sheath and a leakage pathway to the internodal axolemma via the paranodal seal resistance and periaxonal space. The parameter values of the model are adjusted to match the recordings of threshold electrotonus in human motor fibres (Bostock et al. 1991). Kirchoff's current law is used to derive a system of partial differential equations for the electrical equivalent circuit. The same double cable model is used for human sensory fibres (Stephanova and Mileva 2000), however the parameter values of this model are adjusted to math the recordings of threshold electrotonus in human sensory fibres (Bostock et al. 1994, 1998). Threshold electrotonus responses from patients with ALS are found to be variable to subthreshold depolarizing currents (Bostock et al. 1995). Some responses are found to have a fairly normal shape, but others show decreases or rapid increases in threshold to 40% depolarizing currents. Abnormal potentials (intracellular and electrotonic) defined as ALS1, ALS2 and ALS3 types, respectively, are simulated for the human motor and sensory fibres (Daskalova and Stephanova 2001) based on their double cable models. The simulated potential abnormalities resemble in some respects the experimental data of Bostock et al. (1995) and the effects of blocked potassium channels on the intracellular potentials, accommodation, adaptation and anode break excitation in normal human motor and sensory fibres (Stephanova and Mileva 2000). The simulated ALS types are consistent with a dysfunction of the axonal membrane parameters (Table 1). The other membrane and geometric parameter values for the fibres are the same as described earlier (Stephanova and Bostock 1995, 1996; Stephanova and Mileva 2000) and in brief, the model fibres comprise 20 nodes and 19 internodes. Each space between the nodes is divided into two paranodal and five internodal segments. All calculations are carried out for fibres with an axon diameter of 12.5 μm and a myelin thickness of 2.4 μm, giving an external diameter of 17.3 μm. The lengths of node, paranode and nodal center to nodal center are 1.5 μm, 200 μm and 1400 μm, respectively.

Table 1. Membrane parameter values characteristic for the human motor and sensory fibres in the normal and ALS1, ALS2, and ALS3 cases: R_{ax} (axoplasmic resistance); R_{pn}(paranodal resistance); maximum channel permeabilities where P_{Na} (sodium), P_{Kf} (fast potassium), P_{Ks} (slow potassium), P_{IR} (inward rectifier), P_{LK} (leak) and * denotes an internodal quantity. The selected membrane parameter values, which provide major indication for the given ALS type, are underlined. From Daskalova and Stephanova (2001), with permission.

	motor				sensory			
	normal	ALS1	ALS2	ALS3	normal	ALS1	ALS2	ALS3
R_{ax}[MΩ]	8	10	10	10	8	10	10	10
R_{pn}[MΩ]	125	145	145	145	145	145	145	145
$P_{Na}.10^{-9}[sm^3s^{-1}]$	9	7	7	7	10	8	8	8
$P_{Kf}.10^{-9}[sm^3s^{-1}]$	0.07	0	0.07	0.07	0.13	0	0	0
$P_{Ks}.10^{-9}[sm^3s^{-1}]$	0.26	0.13	0	0	0.2	0.3	0.2	0.2
$P_{Kf}*.10^{-9}[sm^3s^{-1}]$	27	24.3	0	0	10	9	0	0
$P_{Ks}*.10^{-9}[sm^3s^{-1}]$	2	1.8	0.6	0	2	1.8	0.5	0
$P_{IR}*.10^{-11}[sm^3s^{-1}]$	0.8	0.8	0.8	0.8	2	2	2	2
$P_{Lk}*.10^{-11}[sm^3s^{-1}]$	0.64	0.54	0.5	0.5	0.56	0.56	0.54	0.54

The nodal and internodal axolemmal capacitances are 1 pF and 350 pF, respectively and the temperature is 37° C. The double cable models can describe the intracellular and electrotonic potentials of the normal and abnormal human motor and sensory fibres in response to both short (0.025-1 ms) and long-lasting (100-300 ms) current pulses. The accommodation, adaptation and anode break excitation in the fibres can also be predicted in a satisfactory manner by the models. The systems of differential equations are solved by numerical integration (Euler method) with a fixed time increment, usually 0.0001 ms. Non-uniform spatial step sizes are used in accordance with the complex structure of the fibres.

Line-Source Model

The extracellular recordings provide information about the bioelectric activity of a specific region of tissue. In that sense, the description of the extracellular potential field of a single myelinated fibre in an extensive conducting media is of great interest in the field of the electrophysiology. Since recordings of neuroactivity are always performed at some distance from the nerve fibre, the volume conductor always plays an important part in the interpretation of the extracellular potential fields in terms of their sources. Using the double cable models of the human motor and sensory fibres in the normal and ALS cases, the spatial and temporal distributions of the intracellular potentials are calculated. The intracellular potential models comprise 25 nodes and 24 internodes and each space between the nodes is divided into 2 paranodal and 17 internodal segments. Such spatial step size was found to be accurate enough for the calculation of the extracellular potentials. The model-generated spatial and temporal intracellular potentials are then used as input to a line source model that allows the calculation of the corresponding spatial and temporal distributions of the extracellular potentials at various radial distances in the surrounding volume conductor. The fibres are assumed to be circular cylinders. The chosen coordinate system is cylindrical with radial and axial coordinates of the field point in the surrounding infinite volume conductor. The interested reader is referred to the paper of Stephanova et al. (1989) for a system of equations representing the line source model (approximate solution of Laplace's equation). The line source model is the most frequently used for the unmyelinated (Clark and Plonsey, 1968, 1970; Rosenfalck, 1969; Plonsey 1974; Stegeman et al., 1979; Altman and Plonsey, 1990; Trayanova et al. 1990) and myelinated fibres (Ganapathy and Clark, 1987; Stephanova et al., 1989; Gydikov et al. 1990; Struijk, 1997; Meler et al., 1998).

Methods of Stimulation

To make accurate inferences about the anatomical structures or physiological mechanisms involved in electrical stimulation, one must know which elements are stimulated. Two cases of fibre stimulation are considered. The first case of point application of current intra-axonally at the center of the first node realizes a point fibre polarization. The second case of simultaneous intracellular current application at the midpoints of all available internodal segments realizes a periodic kind of uniform fibre polarization. This polarization is first simulated in the human motor electrotonus model (Stephanova and Bostock 1996), since the in vivo situation for recording threshold electrotonus in man, where current is applied to the peripheral nerve via its high-resistance sheath and a 1-cm diameter surface electrode (Bostock et al. 1991), is thought to correspond more closely to periodic kind of uniform polarization than point polarization of the fibre. [Note that in the case of periodic kind of uniform polarization, the total internodal membrane (approximately 99.9% of axonal membrane) is stimulated]. The studies on the spatial distributions of the extracellular potentials of human myelinated fibre indicate (i) that the first case of intracellular stimulation closely approximates the effects of external stimulation with a needle electrode, and (ii) that the second case of intracellular stimulation closely approximates the effects of external surface stimulation with a large electrode (Fig. 1). In both cases of intracellular stimulation, the discontinuous nature of the fibre is well manifested in the extracellular potentials close to the fiber membrane. With the increase of the radial distance, the potentials become smoother, and at given radial distances, the local extrema are no longer present in the potentials. However, the extracellular potential profiles are substantially different, because of the difference between the corresponding intracellular potentials obtained for both intracellular stimulations. In the first case, the smoothed longitudinal profiles of the extracellular potentials (at r = 5.0 mm, Fig. 1A, A1) are very similar to the spatial extracellular profiles typical of the case of point application of current extra-axonally at the node. In the second case, the smoothed longitudinal profiles of the extracellular potentials (at r = 5.0 mm, Fig. 1B, C), along the fibre length, are very similar to the spatial extracellular profiles typical of the case of external surface stimulation with a large electrode as obtained by Rattay (1988, 1989). The results also confirm the claim that the large surface electrode uniformly polarizes the axon.

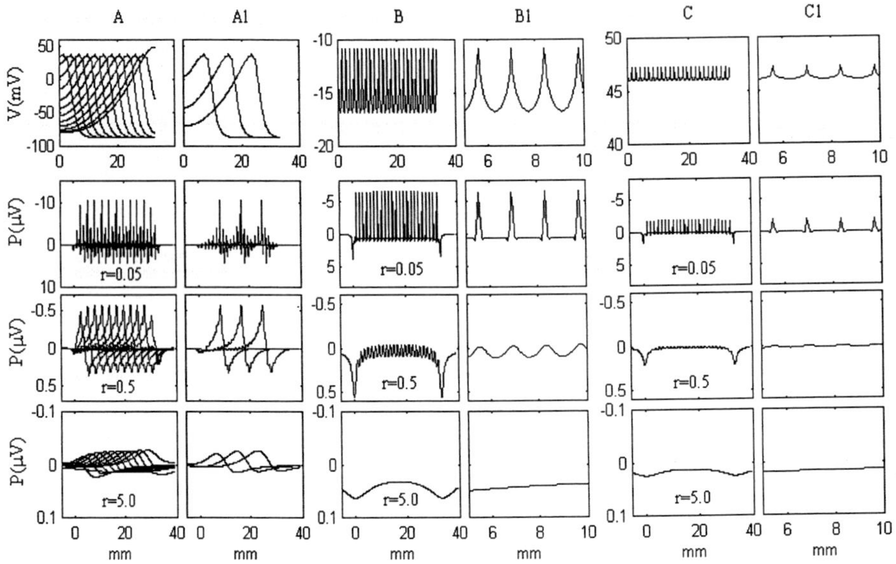

Figure 1. Spatial distributions of the intracellular potentials (V) and their corresponding extracellular potentials (P) in the cases of point (A, A1) and periodic kind of uniform (B, B1, C, C1) polarization of human motor fibre. The intracellular potentials are in response to 0.1ms threshold current pulses. In A case the spatial intracellular potentials are at the times of potential maxima at each second node from the 2nd to the 24th, whereas in A1 case they are at the times of potential maxima at the 6th, 12th and 18th nodes only. In B and C cases the spatial intracellular potentials are at the times of 2 ms and 2.23 ms, respectively, along the fibre length. In B1 and C1 cases the figures from B and C cases are repeated on expanded scales (5-10 mm). The extracellular potentials are given for three radial distances (r = 0.05, 0.5 and 5.0 mm). From Stephanova and Daskalova (2003b), with permission.

Axonal Excitability Depends on the Methods of Stimulation

The electrical excitability of an axon is defined by the threshold current that excites it. The study of the mechanisms underlying the generation of the intracellular potential shows that the axonal excitability depends on the methods of stimulation. Figure 2Aa illustrates the temporal intracellular potentials at each node, from the 1st to the 10th in the case of point fibre polarization in response to a threshold (4 nA x 0.1ms) stimulus. In the case of periodic kind of uniform fibre polarization (Fig. 2Ba), the temporal intracellular potentials are not only for nodes from the 1st to the 10th, but they are also for each segment between them in response to a threshold (0.99 nA x 0.1ms) stimulus. Because of the periodic kind of uniform fibre polarization, each node and internode behaves identically, and an overlap of the potentials at the nodes and internodal segments is obtained. The double cable models permit decomposition of the intracellular potential into its transaxonal and transmyelin components. We can also distinguish between the membrane currents across the nodal or internodal axolemma and the external membrane current, which are usually not the same, since current can flow longitudinally in the periaxonal space.

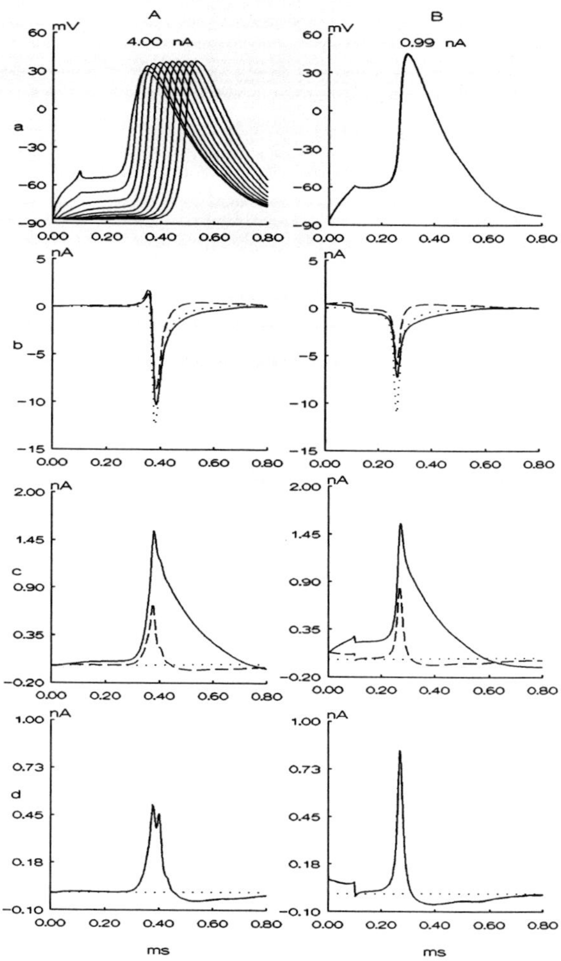

Figure 2. Temporal distributions of the intracellular potentials (a) and the kinetics of currents at node 5 (b), paranode next to node 5 (c) and mid-internode between nodes 5 and 6 (d), in the cases of point (A) and periodic kind of uniform (B) polarization of human motor fibre. The potentials are in response to 0.1 ms pulses with threshold current values given at the top. In Aa case the temporal intracellular potentials are at each node, from the 1st to the 10th, whereas in Ba case they are at each node, from the 1st to the 10th and at each internodal segment between them. Currents: total ionic currents (· ·), membrane currents across the nodal / internodal axolemma (—) and external membrane currents (- -).

For both cases of fibre stimulation, the externally recorded nodal current is less than the current across the nodal axolemma, because of short-circuiting through the paranodal seal resistance (Fig. 2AB,b). Similarly, considerably more outward current flows across the paranodal axolemma than is apparent from the current flowing across the myelin (Fig.2AB, c). At the mid-internode, the recorded currents across the internodal axolemma and myelin sheath are equal (Fig. 2AB, d). (In the paranodal and internodal segments, the external membrane current is equal to the transmyelin current). The total nodal ionic currents are similar (Fig. 2AB, b), but the total internodal ionic currents do not change significantly either at the paranode or mid-internode (see straight lines in Fig. 2AB, cd). In the case of periodic kind of uniform polarization, the total internodal membrane being stimulated and depolarized decreases the minimal threshold value for excitation of the fibre. In this case, the current across the nodal axolemma (Fig. 2Bb) after the end of the smaller depolarizing currents will be generally smaller than the same current recorded in the case of point fibre polarization. The results indicate that the model normal axon is much less sensitive to the point application of intracellular current (4.00 nA x 0.1 ms) at the node than to the simultaneous application of intracellular current (0.99 nA x 0.1 ms) at the total internodal axolemma (with return path via the external medium). The threshold current, which defined the axonal excitability, is sensitive to membrane potential at the site of stimulation, and provides information to the axonal conduction studies.

Abnormalities in the Potentials of ALS Fibres

As mentioned above, the double cable models can describe the intracellular and electrotonic potentials of the human fibres in ALS. A comparison between these potentials for the normal and ALS1, ALS2 and ALS3 cases is presented for the motor (Fig. 3) and sensory (Fig. 4) fibres. Compared with the normal cases, the peaks of the intracellular potentials are of lower amplitude for the ALS types. The afterpotential amplitudes are larger than normal (Figs. 3A, 4A, abc). The abnormal intracellular potentials are consistent with the nodal ion channel dysfunction and with the dysfunction of the passive axonal (R_{ax}, R_{pn}) parameters (see Table 1). The changed parameters are adjusted to reproduce the conduction slowing in the human fibres as it is obtained in ALS (Sobue et al. 1983; Nakanishi et al. 1989; Wirguin et al. 1992; Arasaki and Tamaki 1998; Feinberg et al. 1999). There is almost no difference in the electrotonic potentials between the ALS1 types and normal cases for the motor and sensory fibres (Figs. 3Ba and 4Ba), because the internodal channel permeabilities in the ALS1 cases are adjusted to match the normal potentials to the subthreshold depolarizing and hyperpolarizing pulses. ALS2 types are simulated using the previous types, but the reduced permeabilities of the nodal and internodal potassium (fast, slow) channels in these types are adjusted to reproduce spontaneous discharges (fasciculations) during the early depolarization of the axonal membrane (Figs. 3Bb, 4Bb). Such ALS1 and ALS2 types typical of the threshold electrotonic responses from patients with ALS are recorded by Bostock et al. (1995). The electrotonic potentials are most abnormal in the ALS3 types of the axons (Figs. 3Bc and 4Bc). In these ALS3 cases, the axons are excited easily and reproduce fasciculations at the offset of the subthreshold hyperpolarizing currents as well as at the onset of the subthreshold depolarizing currents. The spontaneous discharges to the subthreshold hyperpolarizing currents are consistent with the simultaneous removal of the internodal potassium channels under the myelin sheath. Because there are many different ways in which channels could be altered to achieve these effects in the simulated ALS types, we are unable to be specific about the nature of the channel abnormality in ALS. However, the used models confirm that the obtained abnormalities (fasciculations) in the electrotonic potentials to the subthreshold depolarizing and hyperpolarizing current pulses are consistent with the loss of functional potassium channels involving both the fast and slow potassium channel types.

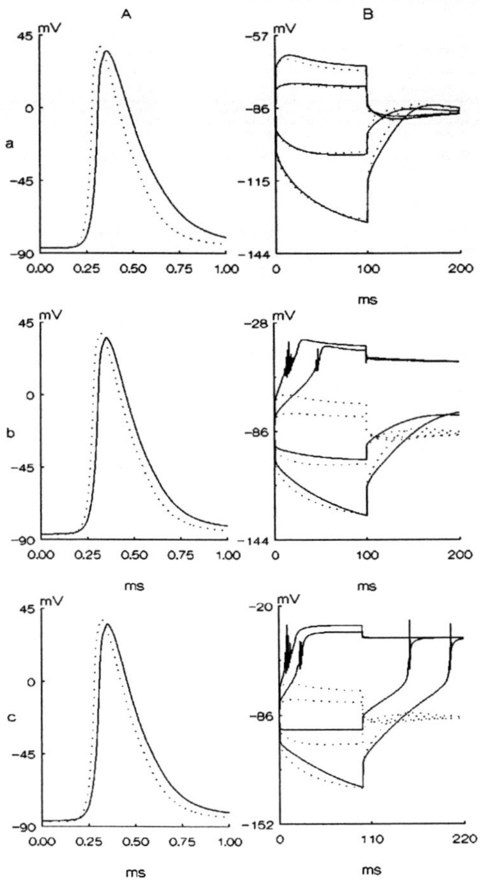

Figure 3. Comparison between the intracellular (A) and electrotonic (B) potentials of human motor fibre in the normal (*dotted lines*), ALS1 (a), ALS2 (b) and ALS3 (c) (*continued lines*) cases, respectively. The intracellular potentials in response to 0.1ms threshold pulses are presented at the tenth node only. The electrotonic potentials in response to 100-ms current pulses (±40, ±80% of threshold) are presented at the first node only.

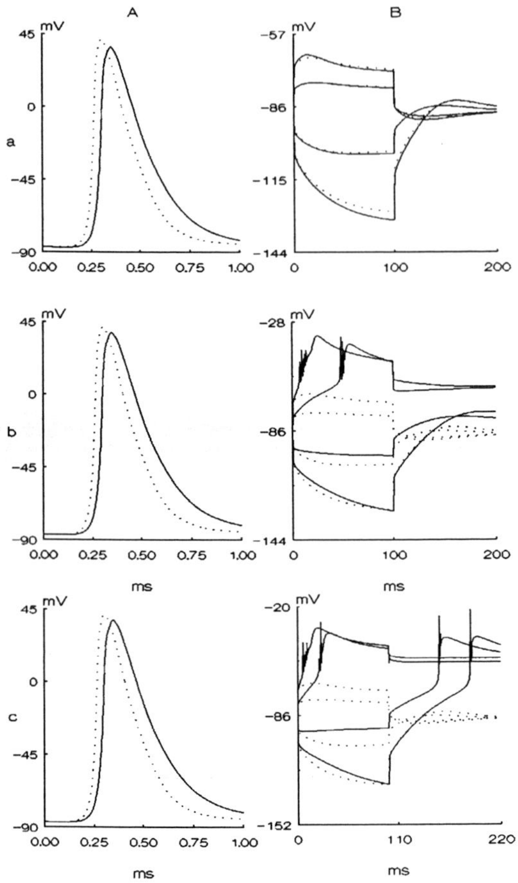

Figure 4. Comparison between the intracellular (A) and electrotonic (B) potentials of human sensory fibre in the normal (*dotted lines*), ALS1 (a), ALS2 (b) and ALS3 (c) (*continued lines*) cases, respectively. The intracellular potentials in response to 0.1ms threshold pulses are presented at the tenth node only. The electrotonic potentials in response to 100-ms current pulses (±40, ±80% of threshold) are presented at the first node only.

The spatial distributions of the extracellular potentials of the normal and ALS1 type fibres are almost identical (Fig.5), because the reduced peak-to-peak amplitudes in the normal and ALS1 cases are negligible. For the normal and abnormal cases, close to the fibre membrane the discontinuity of the intracellular potential propagation is reflected in the spatial extracellular potentials, while further in the volume conductor the potentials are smoothed.

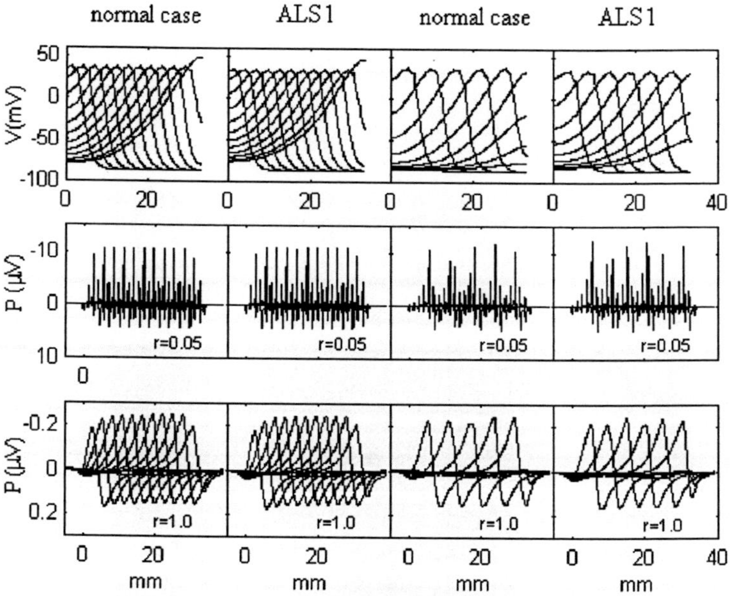

Figure 5. Spatial distributions of the intracellular potentials (V) and their corresponding extracellular potentials (P) of human motor fibre in the normal and ALS1 cases. The intracellular potentials in the first and second columns are at the times of the potential maxima at each second node from the 2nd to the 24th, whereas in the third and fourth columns they are in the time interval from 0.2 ms to 1.0 ms at increments of 0.1 ms, respectively. The extracellular potentials are given for two radial distances (r = 0.05 and 1.0 mm). From Stephanova and Daskalova (2002).

The temporal extracellular potentials of the normal and ALS type fibres show that they are again almost identical (Fig. 6). However, these potentials are different from the spatial extracellular ones, because of the difference between their corresponding temporal and spatial intracellular potentials. In the case of adaptation, the temporal intracellular and their corresponding extracellular potentials, of the normal and abnormal ALS fibres, are also illustrated (Fig. 7). The case of fibre adaptation is simulated by applying a long-lasting threshold depolarizing pulse realizing the periodic kind of uniform fibre polarization. When the normal case is compared with the three ALS cases, the obtained differences are the repetitive activities. In contrast to the normal case, in the ALS cases, after the onset of the spike initiation there is a short train of spontaneous discharges (fasciculations). Increasing the degree of ALS causes an increase of the number of the spontaneous potentials. Their amplitudes are smaller than that of the first potential. The intervals between the fasciculations decrease until the repetitive activity dies out and this is better shown on the expanded scale (see third row in the figure). The shown temporal extracellular potentials of the normal and ALS fibres are very similar to the clinical electromyograms (EMG) from healthy subjects and ALS patients as reported in the literature (Finsterer et al., 1997; Rowinska-Marcinska et al., 1997). The fasciculations due to the spontaneous discharges within the compound action potential EMG are a characteristic feature of ALS and these spontaneous discharges in the EMG are probably based on the potential fasciculations of the single myelinated fibres.

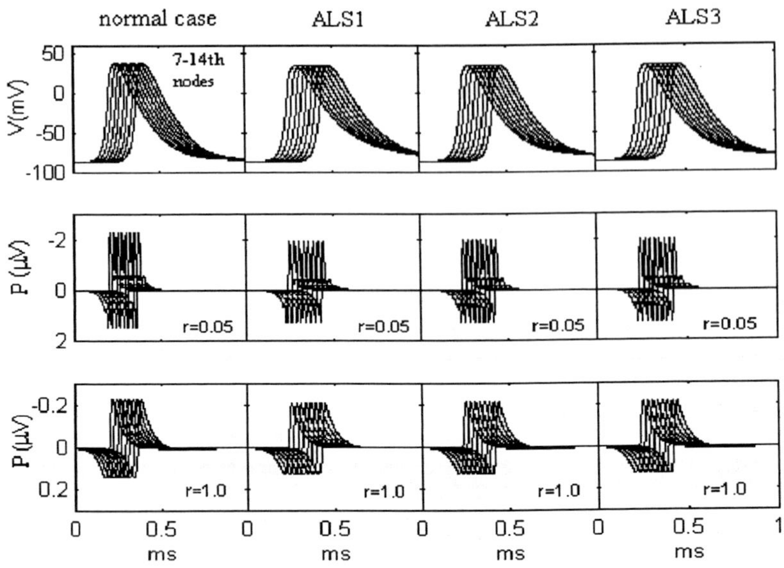

Figure 6. Temporal distributions of the intracellular potentials (V) and their corresponding extracellular potentials (P) of human motor fibre in the normal and three ALS cases. The intracellular potentials are at each node from the 7th to the 14th, respectively. The extracellular potentials are given for two radial distances (r = 0.05 and 1.0 mm). From Stephanova and Daskalova (2002).

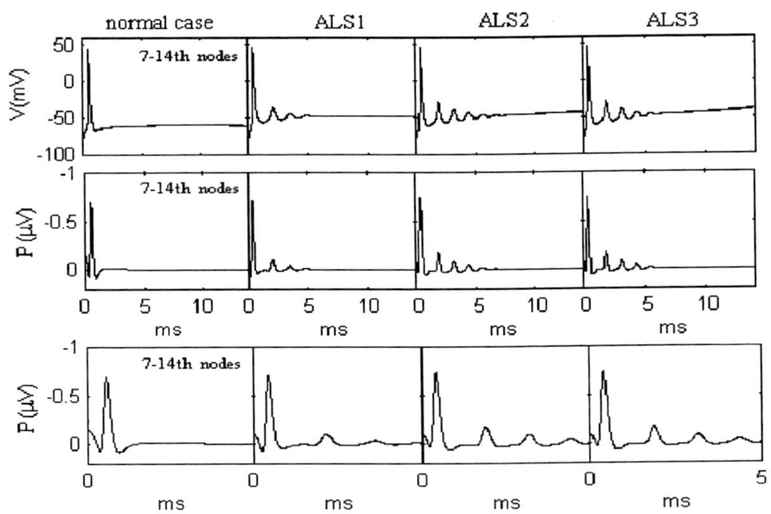

Figure 7. Temporal distributions of the intracellular potentials (V) and their corresponding extracellular potentials (P) of the normal and three ALS types in the case of adaptation of the motor human fibre. The intracellular potentials are at each node from the 7th to the 14th. The extracellular potentials are given for a radial distance r =1.0 mm. The extracellular potentials are repeated in the third line on an expanded (0-5 ms) scale. From Stephanova and Daskalova (2002).

Abnormalities in the Excitability of ALS Fibres

The threshold current, which defined the axonal excitability usually, provides little information. More information is provided by excitability properties obtained from threshold stimuli of different duration (i.e. strength-duration and charge-duration curves, strength-duration time constants and rheobasic currents) or obtained by comparing pairs of threshold stimuli (e.g. recovery cycles). From axonal excitability properties and the changes in these properties it is possible to infer information about the membrane potential and biophysical properties of the normal and abnormal myelinated human axons.

Strength-Duration time Constant and RHEOBASIC CURRENTS

The study of the relationship between the strength and the duration of a threshold stimulus to nerves is subject of early observations (Cole et al. 1955; Cooley et al. 1965; Noble and Stein 1966). The strength-duration time constant depends on the techniques used

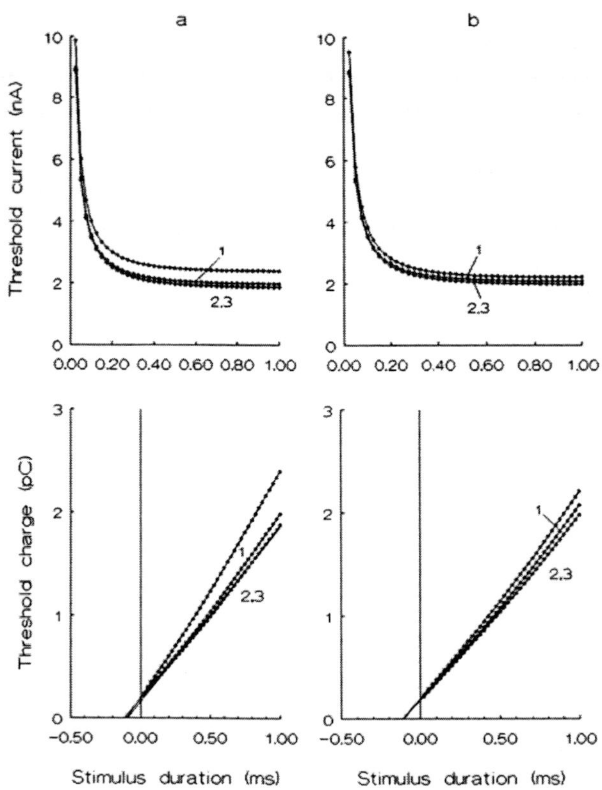

Figure 8. Strength-duration and charge-duration curves for the motor (a) and sensory (b) fibres in the normal (*unnumbered line*) and ALS1 (1), ALS2 (2) and ALS (3) cases, respectively. The threshold currents are determined in the case of point polarization of the fibres.

to make measurements and calculations. Weiss (1901) has proposed a simple linear formula for fitting the charge-duration data obtained from frog nerves and the classical hyperbolic strength-duration equations of Lapicque (1907) and Hill (1936) are based on the models of the excitable processes. The strength-duration time constants and rheobasic currents are investigated for healthy subjects (Bostock 1983; Mogyoros et al. 1996; McIntyre and Grill 1998; Wesselink et al. 1999) and patients with ALS (Mogyoros et al. 1998).

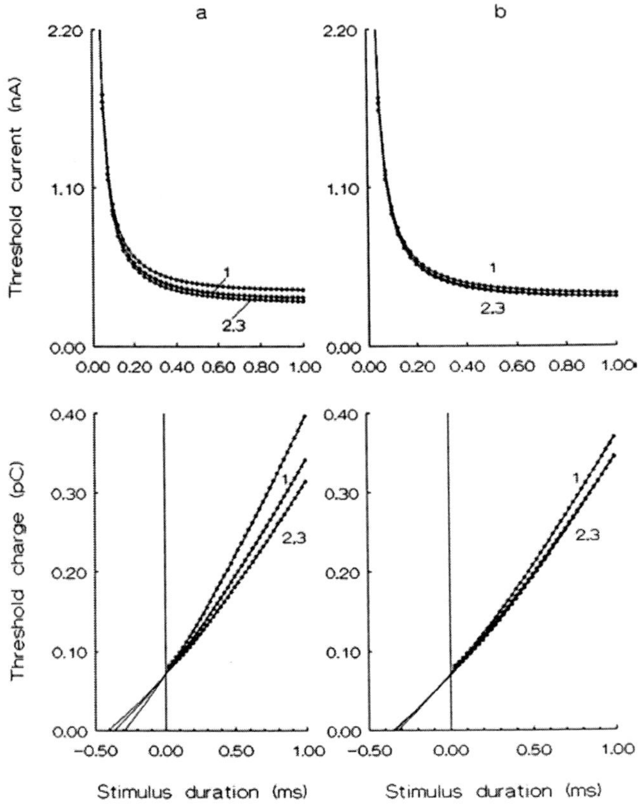

Figure 9. Strength-duration and charge-duration curves for the motor (a) and sensory (b) fibres in the normal (*unnumbered line*) and ALS1 (1), ALS2 (2) and ALS (3) cases, respectively. The threshold currents are determined in the case of periodic kind of uniform polarization of the fibres.

Results concerning the strength-duration time constants and rheobasic curves are also presented here for the human fibres in ALS. To show that these excitability properties depend on the methods of fibre stimulation, both methods of intracellular stimulation are used for the threshold determination. The stimulus duration is increased in 0.025-ms steps from 0.025-ms to 1-ms and the threshold strength-duration and charge-duration curves are illustrated for the cases of point polarization (Fig. 8) and periodic kind of uniform polarization (Fig.9) of the motor and sensory fibres in the normal and the three ALS cases. A polynomial function of degree 2 (transfer standard parabola), which relates threshold charge (Q) to stimulus duration (t), provides an accurate fit of the fibre data: $Q = a_2[t^2+(a_1/a_2).t + a_0/a_2]$, where a_0, a_1, a_2 are the polynomial coefficients. The strength-duration time constant is defined as the absolute value of the smallest square root of the function (i.e. only one of the both direct intercepts of the regression curve on the duration axis has a biophysical sense and only this direct intercept is shown on the given figures). The rheobase is defined as the final decreased threshold value, after which the potential generation is not obtained with the increase of the stimulus duration. The strength-duration time constants and rheobasic currents are termed as nodal when the case of point polarization is realized, whereas the strength-duration time constants and rheobasic currents are termed as internodal when the case of periodic kind of uniform polarization is realized for the fibres. (The quantities 'nodal/ internodal strength-duration time constants' are first introduced by Bostock et al. 1983). To provide a better illustration of the results, histograms are also used (Fig. 10).

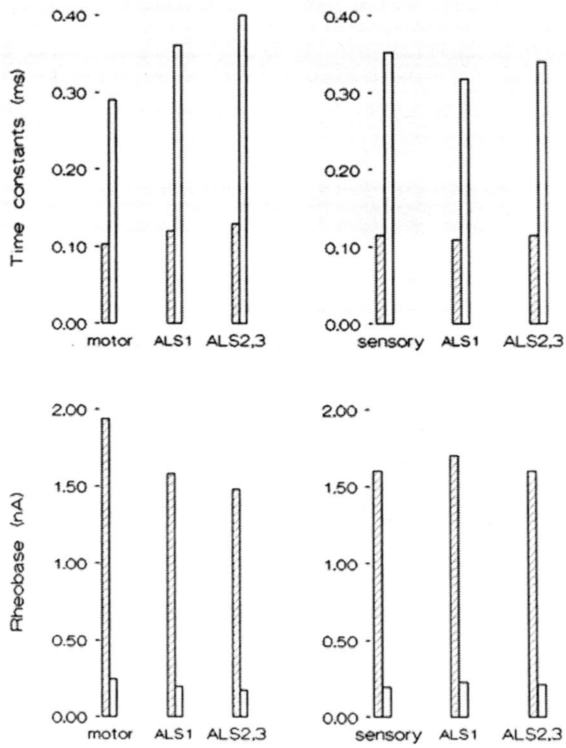

Figure 10. Comparison between the nodal (*shadowed histograms*) and internodal (*no shadowed histograms*) strength-duration time constants and rheobasic currents for the motor and sensory fibres in the normal and three ALS cases. From Daskalova and Stephanova (2001), with permission.

The values are also summarized in Table 2. For the motor axons, the internodal /nodal strength-duration time constants of the ALS types are substantially longer than these of normal case. For the sensory axons, the internodal/nodal time constants are slightly lower for the ALS1 case and almost no changed for the ALS2 and ALS3 cases than for the normal case. The strength-duration time constants of the ALS2 and ALS3 types are equal. There is an inverse relationship between the strength-duration time constants and rheobases of the axons, and this is the same for their three ALS cases (see also Table 2). The results also indicate that the nodal and internodal strength-duration time constants and nodal and internodal rheobasic currents are considerably different for the normal and ALS cases. The nodal strength-duration time constant of 0.115 ms of the sensory fibre is fairly close to the chronaxie 0.119 ms calculated by Wesselink et al. (1999) for afferent fibres where the case of point fibre stimulation is realized. However, the internodal strength-duration time constant of 0.352 ms of the same fibre is close to the mean values of 0.349; 0.318; 0.369 ms obtained by Panizza et al. (1994, 1998) for compound sensory action potentials. Moreover, there is a close resemblance between the internodal strength-duration time constants of the motor and sensory axons in the ALS cases and those experimentally obtained by Mogyoros et al. (1998) where the case of external surface stimulation with a large electrode is realized. The study shows that the nodal strength-duration time constants for both fibre types are not so different, but the internodal strength-duration time constants are greater in the sensory than in the motor fibres and this is the same for the abnormal ALS cases. The study also demonstrates that the charge-duration data from single axons are best described by a parabola than a linear Weiss's formula used for the calculation of the strength-duration time constants from human compound action potentials (Mogyoros et al. 1996, 1998). A likely explanation for this discrepancy is the different method used for the threshold current determination. In the latter papers, the threshold currents are determined, as currents required to produce a compound action potential of 30-40% of maximum.

Table 2. Values of the nodal (τ_n) / internodal (τ_{in}) strength-duration time constant and nodal (I_{rhn}) / internodal (I_{rhin}) rheobase current for the motor and sensory fibres in the normal and ALS cases

	motor			sensory		
	normal	ALS1	ALS2 ALS3	normal	ALS1	ALS2 ALS3
τ_n[ms]	0.103	0.120	0.130	0.115	0.109	0.115
τ_{in}[ms]	0.291	0.361	0.406	0.352	0.318	0.340
I_{rhn}[nA]	2.4012	1.9852	1.8782	1.9802	2.0760	1.9810
I_{rhin}[nA]	0.3875	0.3206	0.3006	0.3384	0.3568	0.3272

Recovery Cycles

When two equal pulses are used in pairs, the response of second (testing) pulse in the refractory period may be greater or less than the response of the first (conditioning) pulse, depending on the conditioning-testing intervals. The studies on the recovery cycles of axonal excitability show that the properties of motor and sensory human axons are not identical and their responses to nerve disorders may therefore differ (Potts et al. 1994; Kiernan et al. 1996,

1997, 2000; Shefner et al. 1996; Burke et al. 1998; Mogyoros et al. 1998, 2000; Feinberg 1999; Kuwabara et al. 2000).

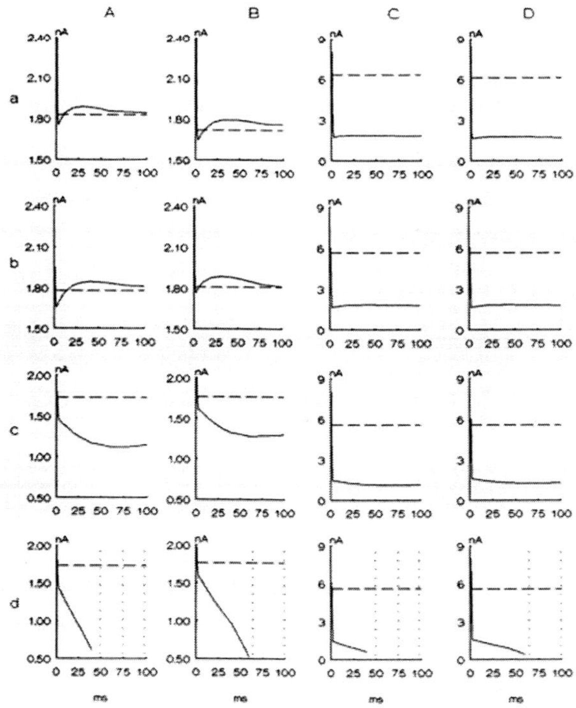

Figure 11. Threshold currents for the testing pulses as a function of the conditioning-testing intervals for the human motor (A, C) and sensory (B, D) nerve fibres, during 100 ms recovery cycles, in the normal (a), ALS1 (b), ALS2 (c) and ALS3 (d) cases, respectively. The conditioning and testing pulses are with a 0.05 ms duration. The recovery cycles are for the case of uniformly polarized axons (A, B) and for the case of point polarized axons (C, D). The *dashed lines* indicate the threshold intensities of the conditioning pulses. The *dotted vertical lines* indicate the abnormalities of the recovery cycles in the ALS3 axonal types. From Stephanova et al. (2001), with permission.

The excitability changes of the human motor and sensory axons in the normal and ALS cases during 100 ms recovery cycles are illustrated (Fig.11). In the cases of periodic kind of uniform polarization (Fig. 11A,B) and point polarization (Fig.11C, D) of the fibres, the recovery cycles show that the excitability changes of the axons are similar, when the conditioning-testing intervals are below 1-2 ms. Both axonal types in the normal and ALS cases are initially unexcitable, then excitable with a raised threshold and after about 2 ms they are superexcitable. In the unexcitable case, the axons are absolutely refractory for 0.05-1.0 ms, during which they cannot generate second intracellular potential no matter how strong the testing depolarizing pulses are. The axons are then relatively refractory for 1-2 ms, during which a stronger testing stimulus than conditioning depolarizing stimulus is required to generate second intracellular potential. In the superexcitable case, the testing stimulus necessary to generate second intracellular potential is less than the conditioning stimulus. The recovery cycles are considerably different above 2 ms conditioning-testing intervals. For the uniformly polarized axons in the normal and ALS1 cases, the superexcitable period usually followed by a late subnormal period (Fig. 11AB, ab). For the ALS2 types, in the case of uniformly polarized axons (Fig. 11AB,c), the superexcitability of the axons increases markedly and the axons remain superexcitable to the end of the 100 ms period. The similar superexcitable periods are found for the normal, ALS1 and ALS2 types in the case of point polarized axons (Fig. 11CD, a-c). Abnormalities in the recovery cycles are obtained for the ALS3 axonal types, when the interpulse intervals are above 50-60 ms (see vertical lines in Fig.11A-D, d). In these ALS3 cases a block of generation of the second (testing) intracellular potential is achieved.

The temporal distributions of the intracellular potentials of the sensory fibres as a function of the conditioning-testing intervals for the normal and ALS cases are also presented (Figs. 12). The second potentials are at each node from the 1st to the 10th, and only when the conditioning-testing intervals correspond to 2 ms, they are compared with the first potentials (Fig.12A-D, a). With increasing the degree of ALS, the length-dependent second potentials propagate with complex, desynchronized amplitudes and velocities, and as an extreme consequence, a conduction block is obtained for the ALS3 type, when the conditioning-testing intervals are above 50-60 ms (Fig. 12D, c-d). In these cases, the regenerative depolarization caused by the first (conditioning) afterpotentials triggers spontaneous discharges and the generation of the second (testing) intracellular potentials is blocked.

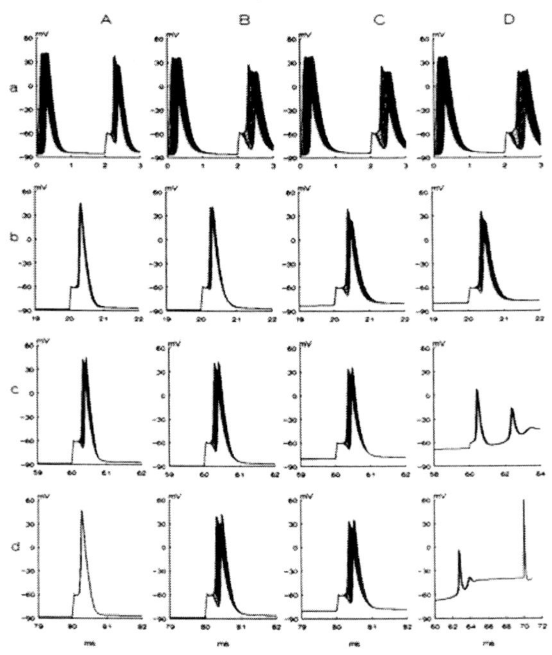

Figure 12. Temporal distributions of the intracellular potentials of sensory axons in the normal (A), ALS1 (B), ALS2 (C) and ALS3 (D) cases, when the testing stimulus is applied as a function of the conditioning-testing intervals corresponding to 2 ms (a), 20 ms (b), 60 ms (c) and 80 ms (d), respectively. The second (testing) potentials are at each node from the 1st to the 10th and only in the case of 2 ms conditioning-testing intervals the potentials are compared with those of the first (conditioning) potentials. The latter are also at each node from the 1st to the 10th. From Stephanova et al. (2001), with permission.

Discussion

Nerve conduction studies remain the basic method for the clinician investigating nerve function. However, the measurements of compound action potential amplitude, latency and conduction velocity are not always indicators of the disease mechanisms, such as the mechanisms of conduction block and spontaneous impulse activity. Such information can be obtained from the simultaneous measurements of the potentials (electrotonic, intracellular, extracellular) and excitability properties of the axons. In patients with ALS, there is evidence for decreased potassium conductances (Bostock et al. 1995), longer strength-duration time constants of the abnormal motor axons and shorter strength-duration time constants of the abnormal sensory axons (Mogyoros et al. 1998). In recent years, the method of mathematical modeling has been used as a promising tool for studying the mechanisms of neuropathic disorders. With this method we show that the abnormalities of the intracellular potentials are mainly based on the nodal ion channel dysfunction, whereas the fasciculations in the electrotonic and extracellular potentials in the case of adaptation are based on the dysfunction of the potassium (fast and slow) ion channels. Decreasing the potassium channel permeabilities causes an increase of the axonal superexcitability. The results also show that there is much in common in the conduction processes during the recovery cycle, when the interpulse intervals are up to 2 ms, independently of the axonal types. However, the extent of axonal superexcitability varies with the degree of ALS and can reproduce a conduction block in the axons. The results are consistent with the interpretation that the considerably different behavior of human motor and sensory axons in ALS cases depend not only on the cable properties of the axons, but also on the methods of fibre stimulation. The obtained here changes in the potential and excitability properties of the axons in ALS cases are specific indicators of the pathophysiology of this disease. The results could be used to analyze the pathophysiology and for diagnosis of ALS.

References

Altman KW, Plonsey R (1990) Point source nerve bundle stimulation: effects of fiber diameter and depth on simulated excitation. *IEEE Trans Biomed Eng 37*:688-698

Arasaki K, Tamaki M (1998) A loss of functional spinal alpha motor neuronal in amyotrophic lateral sclerosis. *Neurology 51*:603-605

Awiszus F (1990) Effects of paranodal potassium permeability on repetitive activity of mammalian myelinated nerve fiber models. *Biol Cybern 64*:69-76

Blight A (1985) Computer simulation of action potentials and afterpotentials in mammalian myelinated axons: the case for a lower resistance myelin sheath. *Neuroscience 15*:13-31

Bostock H (1983) The strength-duration relationship for excitation of myelinated nerve: computed dependence on membrane parameters. *J Physiol (Lond) 341*:59-74

Bostock H, Baker M, Reid G (1991) Changes in excitability of human motor axons underlying post-ischaemic fasciculations: evidence for two stable states. *J Physiol (Lond) 441*:537-557

Bostock H, Rothwell JC (1997) Latent addition in motor and sensory fibres of human peripheral nerve. *J Physiol (Lond) 498*:277-294

Bostock H, Sears TA, Sherratt RM (1983) The spatial distribution of excitability and membrane current in normal and demyelinated mammalian nerve fibres. *J Physiol (Lond) 341*: 41-58

Bostock H, Burke D, Hales JP (1994) Differences in behavior of sensory and motor axons following release of ischaemia. *Brain 117*:225-234

Bostock H, Cikurel K, Burke D (1998) Threshold tracking techniques in the study of human peripheral nerve. *Muscle Nerve 21*:137-158

Bostock H, Sharief MK, Reid G, Murray NMF (1995) Axonal ion channel dysfunction in amyotrophic lateral sclerosis. *Brain 118*: 217-225

Burke D, Mogyoros I, Vagg R, Kiernan MC (1998) Quantitative description of the voltage dependence of axonal excitability in human cutaneous afferents. *Brain 121*:1975-1983

Clark JW, Plonsey R (1968) The extracellular potential field of the single active nerve fiber in a volume conductor. *Biophys J* 8:842-864

Clark JW, Plonsey R (1970) A mathematical study of nerve fiber interaction. *Biophys J 10*:973-957

Cole KS, Antosiewicz HA, Rabinowitz P (1955) Automatic computation on nerve excitation. *J Soc Ind Appl Math 3*:153-172

Conradi S, Grimby L, Lundemo G (1982) Pathophysiology of fasciculations in ALS as studied by electromyography of single motor units. *Muscle Nerve 5*:202-208

Cooley J, Dodge F, Cohen H (1965) Digital computer solutions for excitable membrane models. *J Cell Comp Physiol 66*, Suppl 2:99-108

Daskalova M, Stephanova D (2001) Strength-duration properties of human myelinated motor and sensory axons in normal case and in amyotrophic lateral sclerosis. *Acta Physiol Pharmacol Bulg 26*:11-14

Feinberg DM, Preston DC, Shefner JM, Logigian EL (1999) Amplitude-dependent slowing of conduction in amyotrophic lateral sclerosis and polyneuropathy. *Muscle Nerve 22*:937-940

Finsterer J, Fuglsang-Frederiksen A, Mamoli B (1997) Needle EMG of the tongue: motor unit action potential versus peak ratio analysis in limb and bulbar onset amyotrophic lateral sclerosis. *J Neurol Neurosurg Psychiatry 63*:175-180

Fitzhugh R (1962) Computation of impulse initiation and saltatory conduction in a myelinated nerve fiber. *Biophys J* 2:11-21

Forster FM, Alpers BJ (1994) Site of origin of fasciculations in voluntary muscle. *Arch Neurol Psychiatry 51*:264-267

Frankenhaeuser B, Huxley AF (1964) The action potential in the myelinated nerve fiber of Xenopus Laevis as computed on the basis of voltage clamp data. *J Physiol (Lond) 171*:302-315

Ganapathy N, Clark JW (1987) Extracellular currents and potentials of the active myelinated nerve fiber. *Biophys J 52*: 749-761

Gidikov A, Kossev A, Trayanova N, Stephanova D (1990) Electrotonic potentials of myelinated nerve fibers. *Electromyogr Clin Neurophysiol 30*:47-51

Goldman L, Albus JS (1968) Computation of impulse conduction in myelinated fibers: theoretical basis of velocity-diameter relation. *Biophys J 8*:596-607

Guiloff RJ, Modarres-Sadeghi H (1992) Voluntary activation and fiber density of fasciculations in motor neuron disease. *Ann Neurol 31*:416-424

Halter J, Clark J (1991) A distributed-parameter model of the myelinated nerve fiber. *J Theor Biol 148*:345-382

Hill AV (1936) Excitation and accommodation in nerve. *Prec R Soc B 119*:305-355

Kiernan MC, Mogyoros I, Burke D (1996) Differences in the recovery of excitability in sensory and motor axons of human median nerve. *Brain 119*:1099-1105

Kiernan MC, Burke D, Andersen KV, Bostock H (2000) Multiple measures of axonal excitability: a new approach in clinical testing. *Muscle Nerve 23*:399-409

Kiernan MC, Mogyoros I, Hales JP, Gracies JM, Burke D (1997) Excitability changes in human cutaneous afferents induced by prolonged repetitive axonal activity. *J Physiol (Lond) 500*:255-264

Kuwabara S, Cappelen-Smith C, Lin CS, Mogyoros I, Bostock H, Burke D (2000) Excitability properties of median and peroneal motor axons. *Muscle Nerve 23*:1365-1373

Lambert EH (1969) *Electromyography in amyotrophic lateral sclerosis.* In: Norris FH, Kirland LT (ed) Motor neuron diseases: research on amyotrophic lateral sclerosis and related disorders. Grune and Stratton, New York, pp 135-153

Lapicque L (1907) Recherches quantitatives sur I'excitation électrique des nerfs traitée comme une polaresation. *J Physiol (Paris) 9*:622-635

Layzer RB (1982) *Diagnostic implications of clinical fasciculation and cramps*. In: Rowland LP (ed) Human motor neuron diseases. Raven Press, New York, pp 23-29

Meler JH, Rutten WL, Boom HB (1998) Extracellular potentials from active myelinated fiber inside insulated and noninsulated peripheral nerve. *IEEE Trans Biomed Eng 45*:1146-1153

McIntyre CC, Grill WM (1998) Sensitivity analysis of a model of mammalian neural membrane. *Biol Cybern 79*:29-37

Mogyoros I, Kiernan MC, Burke D (1996) Strength-duration properties of human peripheral nerve. *Brain 119*:439-447

Mogyoros I, Kiernan MC, Burke D, Bostock H (1998) Strength-duration properties of sensory and motor axons in amyotrophic lateral sclerosis. *Brain 121*,851-859

Mogyoros I, Lin C, Dowla S, Grosskreutz J, Burke D (2000) Reproducibility of indices of axonal excitability in human subjects. *Clin Neurophysiol 111*:23-28

Murray NMF (1994) *Neurophysiology*. In: Williams AC (ed) Motor neuron disease. Chapman and Hall, London, pp 171-190

Nakanishi T, Tamaki M, Arasaki K (1989) Maximal and minimal motor nerve conduction velocity in amyotrophic lateral sclerosis. *Biology 39*:580-583

Noble D, Stein B (1966) The threshold conditions for initiation of action potentials by excitable cells. *J Physiol 187*:129-162

Panizza M, Nilsson J, Roth BJ, Rothwell J, Hallett M (1994) Time constants of motor and sensory peripheral nerve fibers measured with the method of latent addition. Electroenceph. *Clin Neurophysiol 93*:147-154

Panizza M, Nilsson J, Roth BJ, Grill SE, Demiiirci M, Hallett M (1998) Differences between the strength-duration time constants of sensory and motor peripheral nerve fibers: further studies and considerations *Muscle & Nerve 21*:48-54

Plonsey R (1974) The active fiber in a volume conductor. *IEEE Trans Biomed Eng 21*:371-381

Potts F, Young RR, Shefner JM (1994) Long lasting excitability changes in human peripheral nerve. *Muscle Nerve 17*:74-79

Rattay F (1988) Modeling the excitation of fibers under surface electrodes. *IEEE Transactions on Biomedical Engineering 35 (3)*:199-202

Rattay F (1989) Analysis of models for extracellular fiber stimulation. *IEEE Transactions on Biomedical Engineering 36 (7)*:676-682

Reid G, Scholz A, Bostock H, Vogel W (1999) Human axons contain at least 5 types of voltage-dependent potassium channels. *J Physiol (Lond) 518*:681-696

Rosenfalck P (1969) Intra- and extracellular potential fields of active nerve and muscle fibers. *Acta Physiol Scand Suppl 321*:1-168

Roper J, Schwarz JR (1989) Heterogeneous distribution of fast and slow potassium channels in myelinated rat nerve fibres. *J Physiol (Lond) 416*:93-110

Roth G (1982) The origin of fasciculations. *Ann Neurol 12*:542-547

Roth G (1984) Fasciculations and their F-response. Localization of their axonal origin. *J Neurol Sci 63*:299-306

Rowinska-Marcinska K, Ryniewicz B, Hansmanowa-Petrusewicz I, Karvanska A (1997) Diagnostic values of satellite potentials in clinical EMG. *Electromyogr Clin Neurophysiol 37*:483-489

Safronov BV, Kampe K, Vogel W (1993) Single voltage-dependent potassium channels in rat peripheral nerve membrane. *J Physiol (Lond) 460*: 675-691

Scholz A, Reid G, Vogel W, Bostock H (1993) Ion channels in human axons. *J Neurophysiol 70*:1274-1279

Schwarz JR, Reid G, Bostock H (1995) Action potentials and membrane currents in the human node of Ranvier. *Pflügers Arch 430*:283-292

Shefner JM, Preston DC, Logigian EL (1996) Activity-dependent conduction in single motor units. *Neurology 46*:1387-1390

Smith RS, Koles ZJ (1970) Myelinated nerve fibers: Computed effect of myelin thickness conduction velocity. *Am J Physiol 219*:1256-1258

Sobue G, Hashizume Y, Sahashi K, Takahashi A, Mukai E, Matsuoka Y, Mukoyama M (1983) Amyotrophic lateral sclerosis. Lack of central chromatolytic response of motor neurocytons corresponding to active axonal degeneration. *Arch Neurol 40*:306-309

Stegeman DF, de Weerd JPC, Eijkman EGJ (1979) A volume conductor study of compound action potentials of nerves in situ: the forward problem. *Biol Cybern 33*:97-111

Stephanova DI (1988a) Systematic paranodal demyelination of nerve fibres: computer simulations. *Electromyogr Clin Neurophysiol 28*:107-110

Stephanova DI (1988b) Reorganization of the axonal membrane in a demyelinated nerve fibre: computer simulation. *Electromyogr Clin Neurophysiol 28*:101-105

Stephanova DI (1988c) The effect of temperature on a simulated systematically paranodally demyelinated nerve fibre. *Biol Cybern 60*:73-77

Stephanova DI (1989a) Model investigations of the temperature dependence of demyelinated and reorganized axonal membrane. *Biol Cybern 60*:439-443

Stephanova DI (1989b) Conduction along myelinated and demyelinated nerve fibres during the recovery cycle: model investigations. *Biol Cybern 62*:83-87

Stephanova DI (1990) Conduction along myelinated and demyelinated nerve fibres with a reorganized axonal membrane during the recovery cycle: model investigations. *Biol Cybern 64*:129-134

Stephanova DI (2001) Myelin as longitudinal conductor: a multi-layered model of the myelinated human motor nerve fibre. *Biol Cybern 84*:301-308

Stephanova DI, Bostock H (1995) A distributed-parameter model of the myelinated human motor nerve fibre: temporal and spatial distributions of action potentials and ionic currents. *Biol Cybern 73*:275-280

Stephanova DI, Bostock H (1996) A distributed-parameter model of the myelinated human motor nerve fibre: temporal and spatial distributions of electrotonic potentials and ionic currents. *Biol Cybern 74*:543-547

Stephanova DI, Chobanova M (1997) Action potentials and ionic currents through paranodally demyelinated human motor nerve fibres: computer simulations. *Biol Cybern 76*:311-314

Stephanova DI, Daskalova M (2002) Extracellular potentials of human motor myelinated nerve fibers in normal case and in amyotrophic lateral sclerosis. *Electromyogr Clin Neurophysiol 42*:443-448

Stephanova DI, Daskalova M (2003a) Abnormalities in the axonal excitability and potentials of demyelinated human motor fibres. *Comptes rendus de l'Academie bulgare des Sciences 56 (9)*:113-118

Stephanova DI, Daskalova M (2003b) Nodal and internodal strength-duration time constants and rheobase currents for human myelinated motor and sensory nerve axons. *Comptes rendus de l'Academie bulgare des Sciences 56 (10)*:113-118

Stephanova DI, Kossev A (1997) Action potentials and ionic currents through internodally demyelinated human motor nerve fibres: computer simulations. *Comptes rendus de l'Academie bulgare des Sciences 50 (3)*:107-110

Stephanova DI, Mileva K (2000) Different effects of blocked potassium channels on action potentials, accommodations, adaptation and anode break excitation in human motor and sensory myelinated nerve fibres: computer simulations. *Biol Cybern 83*:161-167

Stephanova DI, Daskalova M, Kristev I (2001) Excitability changes during the recovery cycle of human myelinated motor and sensory axons in normal case and in amyotrophic lateral sclerosis. *Acta Physiol Pharmacol Bulg 26*:41-44

Stephanova DI, Trayanova N, Gidikov A, Kossev A. (1989) Extracellular potentials of a single myelinated nerve fiber in an unbounded volume conductor. *Biol. Cybern 61*:205-210

Struijk JJ (1997) The extracellular potential of a myelinated nerve fiber in an unbounded medium and in nerve cuff models. *Biophys J 72*:2457-2469

Trayanova N, Henriques CZ, Plonsey R (1990) Limitations of approximate solutions for computing the extracellular potentials of single fibers and bundle equivalents. *IEEE Trans Biomed Eng 37*:22-35

Trojaborg W, Buchthal F (1965) Malignant and bening fasciculations. *Acta Neurol Scand Suppl 13*: 251-254

Vogel W, Schwarz JR (1995) *Voltage-clamp studies in axons: macroscopic and single-channel currents.* In: Waxman SG, Kocsis JD, Stys PK (eds) The axon. Oxford University Press, New York, pp 257-280

Waxman SG, Kocsis JD, Brill MH, Swadlow HA (1979) Dependence of refractory period measurements on conduction distance: a computer simulation analysis. *Electroencephalogr Clin Neurophysiol 47*:717-724

Weiss G. (1901) Sur la possibilité de rendre comparables entre eux les appareils servant à l'excitation électrique. *Arch Ital Biol 35*:413-446

Wesselink WA, Holsheimer J, Boom HBK (1999) A model of the electrical behavior of myelinated sensory nerve fibres based on human data. *Med Biol Eng Comput 37*:228-235

Wettstein A (1979) The origin of fasciculations in motoneuron disease. *Ann Neurol 5*:295-300

Wirguin I, Brenner T, Argov Z, Steiner I (1992) Multifocal motor nerve conduction abnormalities in amyotrophic lateral sclerosis. *J Neurol Sci 112*:199-203

Wood SL, Waxman SG (1982a) Conduction in demyelinated nerve fibers: Computer simulations of the effects of variation in voltage sensitive conductances, in: *Proc IV Ann IEEE Frontiers of Engineering in Health Care 11*.7.1: 424

Wood SL, Waxman SG, Kocsis J (1982b) Conduction of trains of impulses in uniform myelinated fibers: Computer dependence on stimulus frequency. *Neuroscience 7*:423-430.

In: Amyotrophic Lateral Sclerosis: New Research
Editor: Christine A. Murray, pp. 179-196

ISBN 1-59454-179-5

Chapter VII

On the Origin of the Degenerated Fibers in the White Matter of the Spinal Cord in Amyotrophic Lateral Sclerosis

Kiyomitsu Oyanagi[1,*], *Mineo Yamazaki*[1,2], *Emiko Kawakami*[1], *Takashi Morita*[3], *Takao Makifuchi*[4] *and Hitoshi Takahashi*[5]

[1]Department of Neuropathology, Tokyo Metropolitan Institute for Neuroscience, Tokyo, Japan,
[2]Department of Neurology, Nippon Medical University, Tokyo, Japan,
[3]Department of Pathology, Shinrakuen Hospital, Niigata, Japan,
[4]Department of Neuropathology, National Saigata Hospital, Niigata, Japan,
[5]Department of Pathology, Brain Research Institute, Niigata University, Niigata, Japan.

ABSTRACT

The characters of the degeneration of the white matter of the spinal cord of amyotrophic lateral sclerosis (ALS) were examined, and the origins of the degenerated fibers were discussed.

1. The degree of large myelinated fiber loss in the lateral corticospinal tract (l-CST) did not correlate with either the duration of their illness or their history of respirator use. Direct correlation of disease mechanism was absent between the anterior horn cells and the l-CST in classic ALS.

2. The patients who required respirator support showed more severe degeneration of the anterolateral funiculus (ALF) in the ALS than those who required none, and the degree of myelinated fiber loss in the l-CST did not correspond with either the illness duration

* Correspondence to: Kiyomitsu Oyanagi, MD, PhD, Department of Neuropathology, Tokyo Metropolitan Institute for Neuroscience, 2-6 Musashidai, Fuchu, Tokyo 183-8526, Japan ; Tel.: +81-42-325-3881 Ext. 4711; Fax: +81-42-321-8678; e-mail: k123ysm@tmin.ac.jp.

or the history of respirator use. Thus the large myelinated fibers in the l-CST and ALF degenerate independently in classic ALS.
3. The large myelinated fibers in the ALF of the mid-cervical spinal cord of humans originate from the tegmentum of the brain stem and the lower cervical spinal cord, not from the cerebrum, or the thoracic or lumbar spinal cord. The origin of the large myelinated fibers in the ALF of the spinal cord in humans, is considered to be the long-descending neurons in the brain stem tegmentum and the propriospinal neurons in the spinal cord.

Keywords: Amyotrophic lateral sclerosis, Anterolateral funiculus, Corticospinal tract, Middle root zone, Morphometry, Spinal neurons.

Introduction

Amyotrophic lateral sclerosis (ALS) is a motor neuron disease occurring in adults mainly involving the upper and lower motor neurons with relative sparing of the abducens and oculomotor nerve nuclei, and of the autonomic and sensory neurons in the brain stem and spinal cord. About 90% of ALS patients have been reported to be sporadic, and the sporadic ALS are roughly classified into classic ALS, "multi-system type ALS" [Hayashi & Kato 1989, Mizutani et al. 1992], and ALS with temporal lobe involvement [Yuasa 1970, Mitsuyama & Takamatsu 1971, Nakano et al. 1992]. Among the familial ALS patients with inheritance, superoxide dismutase (SOD)-1 gene mutation was revealed in about 20% of the patients [Shaw 2001].

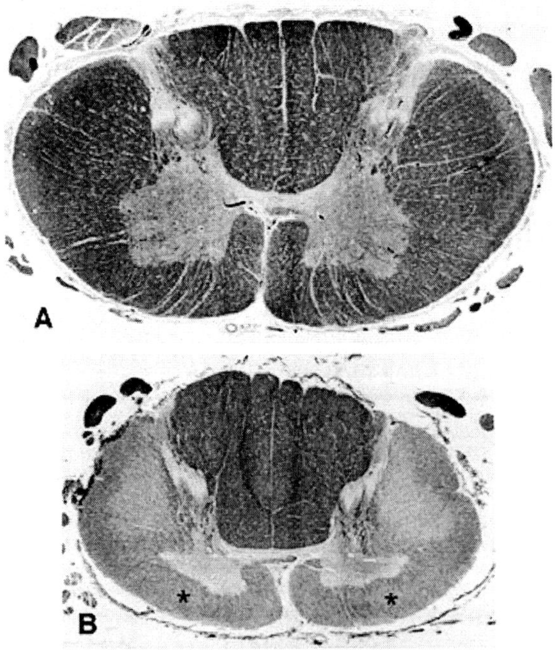

Figure 1. Cervical cord of a control subject (A) and a patient with classic ALS (B). Asterisks indicate ALF. Klüver-Barrera preparation.

In the spinal cord of ALS, degeneration of the corticospinal tract (CST), lateral and anterior, is commonly obvious. In addition to this, since being proposed by Charcot [1880], it has been reported repeatedly that degeneration of the anterolateral funiculus (ALF) occurs in the spinal cord of patients with classic ALS (Fig. 1) [Holmes 1909, Ikuta et al. 1979, 1982, Lawyer & Netsky 1953, Smith 1960]. The posterior funiculus was scarcely/occasionally involved in the classic ALS, but severely deteriorated in the "multi-system type ALS" [Hayashi & Kato 1989, Mizutani et al. 1992]. Some cases of familial ALS with or without superoxide dismutase (SOD)-1 mutation show degeneration of the posterior funiculus and spinocerebellar and spinothalamic tracts in addition to the CST degeneration.

In the present paper, the characteristic patterns of the degeneration of the white matter of the spinal cord of ALS patients were analyzed, and the origins of the degenerated fibers was discussed, based on the observation by the authors and the literature review.

Materials and Methods

1. Examined Subjects

The control subjects and patients with sporadic and familial ALS examined by the authors were Japanese, and none of them had had cardiac arrest, hypoglycemic episodes, or severe liver dysfunction. Neuropathological findings of many of the cases were previously reported by the authors [Ikuta et al. 1979, 1982, Makifuchi & Ikuta 1977, Oyanagi et al. 1983, 1989, 1995, 1999, Takahashi et al. 1992, 1993a, 1993b, 1994].

2. Light Microscopic Examination

Serial 6-μm-thick sections of the brains and spinal cords were made from 10% formalin- or 4 % paraformaldehyde in phosphate buffer-fixed-paraffin embedded blocks, and stained with hematoxylin-eosin, Klüver-Barrera, Bodian, Gallyas, phosphotungustic acid hematoxylin, periodic acid Schiff and other preparations, and examined light microscopically. Other sections (also 6 μm thick) were subjected to immunohistochemical staining using the avidin-biotin-peroxidase complex (ABC) method, using a Vectastain ABC kit (Vector, Burlingame, CA, USA). The primary antibodies used were: rabbit anti-cow ubiquitin polyclonal antibody (dilution 1:150; Dakopatts A/S, Glostrup, Denmark), a rabbit anti-cystatin C (dilution 1:1000; DAKO, Denmark), a rabbit anti-Cu/Zn superoxide dismutase (SOD; dilution 1:10000, a gift from Dr. K. Asayama, Yamanashi Medical School, Yamanashi, Japan), a mouse anti-phosphorylated neurofilament protein (SMI-31; dilution 1:10000, Sternberger Monoclonals, Baltimore, Md, USA), a rabbit anti-glial fibrillary acidic protein (GFAP) polyclonal antibody (dilution 1:500; Dakopatts A/S, Glostrup, Denmark), rabbit anti-human tau polyclonal antibody [dilution 1:1000; a gift from Prof. Y. Ihara, Tokyo University, Tokyo, Japan], anti-tau monoclonal antibody AT8 (dilution 1:1000) (Innogenetics, Belgium), and anti-α-synuclein monoclonal antibody LB509 [gift from Prof. T. Iwatsubo, Tokyo University, Tokyo, Japan]. Antigenicity was increased for ubiquitin immunostaining by pretreating the sections with 0.025% trypsin for 15 min at room temperature, and for α-synuclein immunohistochemistry by pretreating the sections with hydrated autoclaving (121°C, 15 min). Nonspecific binding of the biotin/avidin system reagents was blocked by pretreating the sections with a blocking solution from the kit (Vector), and then incubating them with the required primary antibody overnight at 4°C. The sections were then incubated with the secondary reagent containing biotinylated anti-rabbit, or anti-mouse IgG (diluted 1:200) for 2 h, and finally with the ABC solution for 1 h. The sections were subjected to the peroxidase reaction using freshly prepared 0.02% 3,3'-diaminobenzidine-tetrahydrochloride and 0.005% hydrogen peroxide in 0.05 M Tris-HCl buffer, pH 7.6, for 10 min at room temperature. As antibody controls, the primary antisera were either omitted or were replaced with normal rabbit or mouse serum. Several specimens of neural and non-neural tissue from the patients served as positive or negative tissue controls.

3. Topographic and Quantitative Study of the Neurons in the Spinal Cord

Tissues were embedded in paraffin, serially sectioned at 8 μm, and stained with thionine. The thickness of the sections was verified by manipulating the fine adjustment drum of the light microscope. Five serial sections each of the 5th cervical and of the 7th thoracic segment and 4 serial sections of the second sacral segment were examined. The entire spinal gray matter of each serial section was surveyed under 1000-fold magnification. Neurons were identified by the presence of Nissl substance and prominent nucleoli. The longest diameter of the nucleus (A) and the largest dimension perpendicular to the diameter (B) were measured with an ocular micrometer (4), and the nuclear area (S) was calculated according to the formula $S=\pi AB/4$. There was a significant positive correlation coefficient (r=0.97) between the area obtained by calculation and that obtained by counting 1 mm squares of section paper over the enlarged photograph of the nuclei.

The frequency distribution of nuclear areas by 10 μm^2 increments was obtained for each case, and it was represented in graphs as the nuclear area x n (number of nuclei) to show that the large nuclei, though fewer in number, cover a wider area.

Spinal neurons were classified into 14 groups according to their nuclear areas. The first group was composed of neurons whose nuclear areas were smaller than 40 μm^2. Neurons with nuclear area ranging from 41 to 150 μm^2 were divided into 11 groups (2nd to 12th) in 10 μm^2 increments. The 13th group consisted of neurons with nuclear areas of 151 to 200 μm^2, and the 14th, neurons with nuclear areas greater than 201 μm^2. Each of the neurons was expressed by dots of various sizes and was plotted on the trace of the spinal gray matter magnified 100 times.

4. Quantitative Examination of the Myelinated Fibers in the Lateral Corticospinal Tract (l-CST) and Anterolateral Funiculus (ALF) of the Spinal Cord

The fourth or fifth cervical segments of the spinal cord were fixed in 20% formalin in 0.1 M phosphate buffer (PB; pH 7.3) or 3% glutaraldehyde-1% paraformaldehyde in 0.1 M PB (pH 7.3). The right half of each segment was then fixed in 1% osmium tetroxide in 0.1 M PB (pH 7.3) followed by dehydration through a graded ethanol series and embedded in Epon 812. Sections (1 μm thick) were cut, stained with toluidine blue, and then examined with the aid of a light microscope.

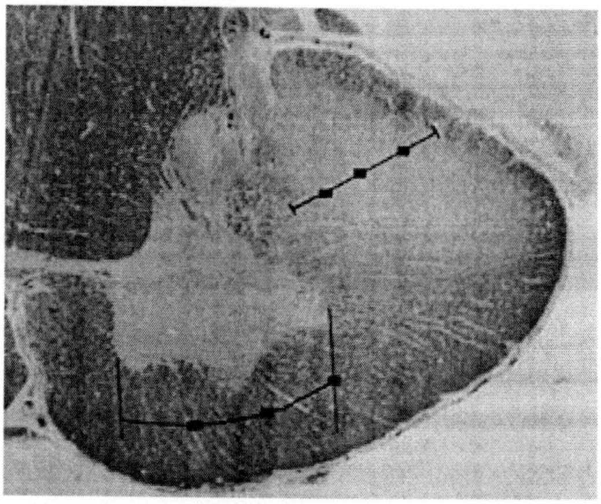

Figure 2. Photographs were taken at three points in both the anterolateral funiculusu (ALF) and lateral corticospinal tract (l-CST). For further details, see text. Cited from ref. Oyanagi et al. 1995.

Photographs (x200) were taken at three points in both the ALF and l-CST. The ALF was divided anteriorly into three equal parts from the medial to lateral margins of the anterior horn and photographs of the mid-medial, mid-lateral and lateral portions were taken (Fig. 2). Large bundles of myelinated fibers with diameters of 10-12 μm (thought to be the intramedullary portion of the anterior spinal root) crossing the ALF were avoided when taking the photographs. The l-CST was divided into four equal parts and photographs were taken at positions midway between the three dividing lines (mid-medial, medial and mid-lateral portions). Enlarged prints (x2285) were made and the mean diameter of the myelinated fibers was obtained, using a digitizer, by averaging the longest and shortest diameters (the latter was perpendicular to the former).

In the present study, in order to determine the origin of the large myelinated fibers in the ALF of the human spinal cord, the number of which is severely reduced in patients with ALS, myelinated fibers in the ALF of the mid-cervical spinal cord were examined quantitatively in five groups of subjects, including control subjects (Group I). The disease groups that were examined included patients with cerebral lesions showing complete degeneration of the unilateral/bilateral pyramis of the medulla oblongata (Group II), those with lesions of the pontine tegmentum (Group III), those with lesions of the lower cervical spinal cord (Group IV), and those with thoracic/lumbar lesions (Group V) (Fig. 3).

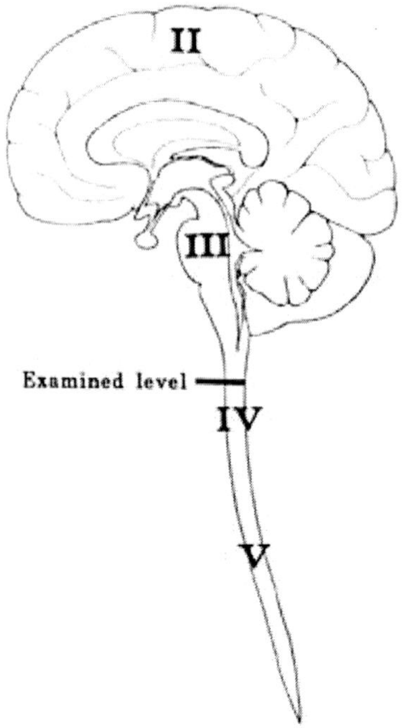

Figure 3. Myelinated fibers in the ALF of the mid-cervical spinal cord were examined quantitatively in five groups of subjects, including control subjects (Group I). The disease groups that were examined included patients with cerebral lesions showing complete degeneration of the unilateral/bilateral pyramis of the medulla oblongata (Group II), those with lesions of the pontine tegmentum (Group III), those with lesions of the lower cervical spinal cord (Group IV), and those with thoracic/lumbar lesions (Group V).

The data for the three areas in the ALF and l-CST of each patient and control subject were summed, and the frequency distribution of the myelinated fiber diameters, in 1-μm increments, was determined and represented on bar charts as the number of myelinated fibers (n) x πr^2 (r: half the mean diameter of the myelinated fibers), to show that the large myelinated fibers, although fewer in number, cover a wide area. The total area of the ALF and of the l-CST in each patient examined was 0.057 mm^2. For the control subjects, the average of each increment was expressed on the bar chars, and for the ALS cases, the data obtained for each patient and the average values for the patients with and without respirator-support were evaluated. Statistical evaluation was performed using the Mann-Whitney U test to compare the number of myelinated fibers with diameters of less than 3 μm (small), 3-6 μm (medium), and over 6 μm (large).

The myelinated fibers in the ALF and l-CST were quantitatively examined bilaterally in control subjects and in patients with cerebral lesions. Based on the obtained data that there was no difference in number between the myelinated fibers in the right and left side, those in the right side of the ALF and l-CST were examined in other groups.

Anatomic Definition of Nerve Fiber Tracts in the Spinal Cord

The white matter of the spinal cord contains bundles of various nerve fiber tracts. It has been reported that the anterolateral funiculus (ALF), which is the ventral part of the lateral funiculus [Nathan et al. 1996], contains, as long-descending tracts, the ventral pyramidal tract (human [Barnes 1901]), corticospinal tracts (human [Nathan et al. 1990]), reticulospinal tracts (cat, opossum and human [Ikuta et al, 1982, Iwamoto et al. 1990, Martin et al. 1979, Nathan et al. 1996, Nyberg-Hansen 1965, Parent 1996]), the vestibulospinal tract (cat and human [Parent 1996, Rose et al. 1996, Shinoda et al. 33]), and raphe spinal tracts (opossum [Martin et al. 1982]). In addition, the ALF contains, as long-ascending tracts, the spinothalamic tract (human [Kuru 1976, Parent 1996, Smith 1951, Smith 1957]), the spinoreticular tract (human [Parent 1996]), the spinocerebellar tract (human [Kuru 1976, Parent 1996]), and Helweg's triangular tract (human [Smith & Deacon 1981]). Propriospinal fibers (cat and human [Altermark et al. 1987, Giok 1958, Parent 1996]) have also been observed.

On the origin of these fibers, experimental studies of animals and human autopsy cases with various destructive lesions in the brain and spinal cord revealed the topographic localization of the neurons, however, the origin neurons of the above mentioned nerve tracts have not yet been completely ascertained in humans so far (Fig. 1).

Lateral Corticospinal Tract (l-CST) Degeneration and Spinal Neuron Loss

Patients with ALS of long course of the illness or on artificial respiration usually show severe loss of neurons in the spinal gray matter including anterior horn and intermediate zone (Fig. 4 & 5). On the contrary, the spinal cord of a housewife, who died at the age of 59 with 1 year-7 months-clinical course refusing the use of a respirator, and whose muscular strength was fairly well preserved up to death, shows only moderate loss of AHCs and quite well preserved neurons in the intermediate zone (Fig. 6). The findings indicate that the primary degeneration may occur in the AHCs and the neurons in the intermediate zone degenerate sequentially in the spinal gray matter in ALS (Fig. 7).

These findings indicate the occurrence of a sequential degeneration of the neurons in the intermediate zone (Rexed's [Rexed 1954] laminae V-VIII) of the spinal cord to loss of anterior horn cells (Rexed's lamina IX) in patients with ALS [Oyanagi et al. 1983, 1989]. Terao et al. [1994] also reported neuronal loss in the intermediate zone of the ALS spinal cord. Long-ascending neurons [Parent 1996], internuncial neurons [Parent 1996], and propriospinal neurons [Altermark et al. 1987, Molenaar & Kuypers 1978] have been shown to originate in the intermediate zone of the spinal cord.

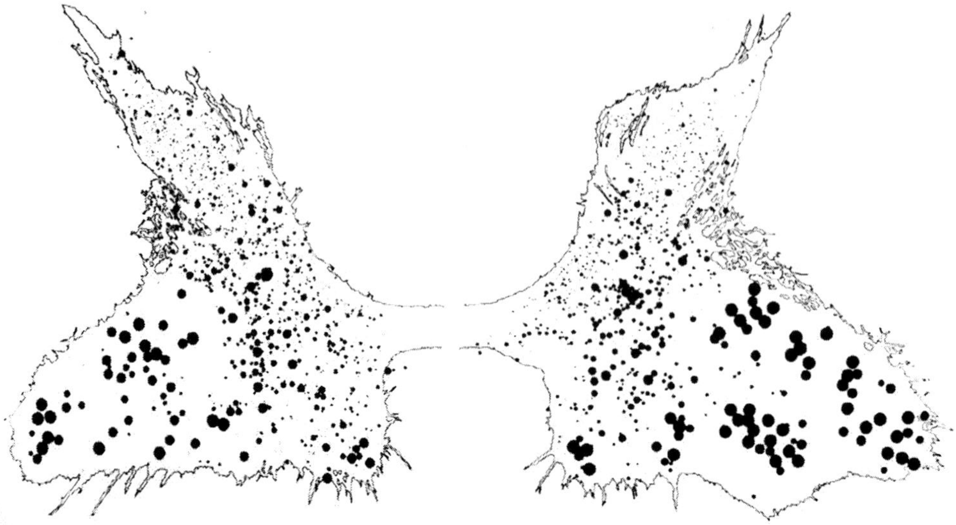

Figure 4. Size distribution of neurons in the cervical gray matter of a control subject. Large neurons, with a nuclear area greater than 151 μm^2, are located in lamina IX; middle sized neurons, 71 to 120 μm^2, in laminae IV-VIII; and numerous small neurons are distributed in laminae II, III and VII. This pattern of distribution seems to correspond to the laminar cell architecture of the cat reported by Rexed (1954). Cited from ref. Oyanagi et al. 1983.

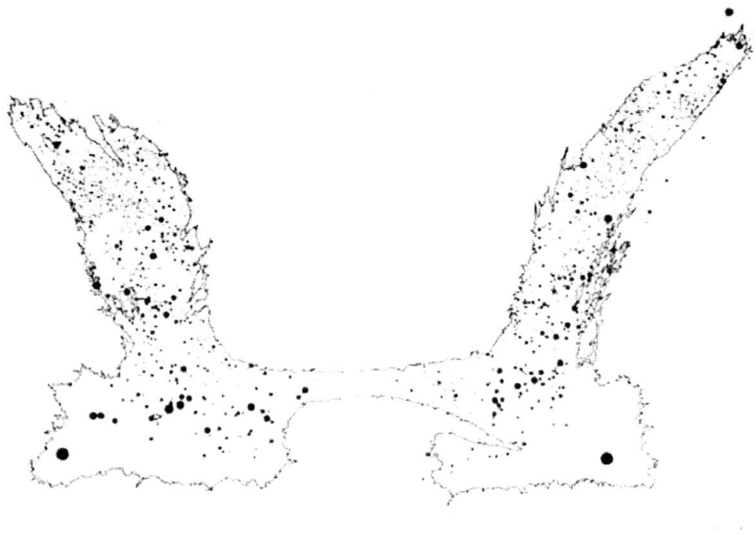

Figure 5. Size distribution of neurons in the cervical gray matter of an advanced ALS patient. The large neurons in lamina IX disappear almost completely. The middle-sized neurons located in laminae VI, VII, and VIII decrease markedly. However, the distribution of the small neurons appears the same as in the control subjects in all parts of the spinal gray matter. Cited from ref. Oyanagi et al. 1983.

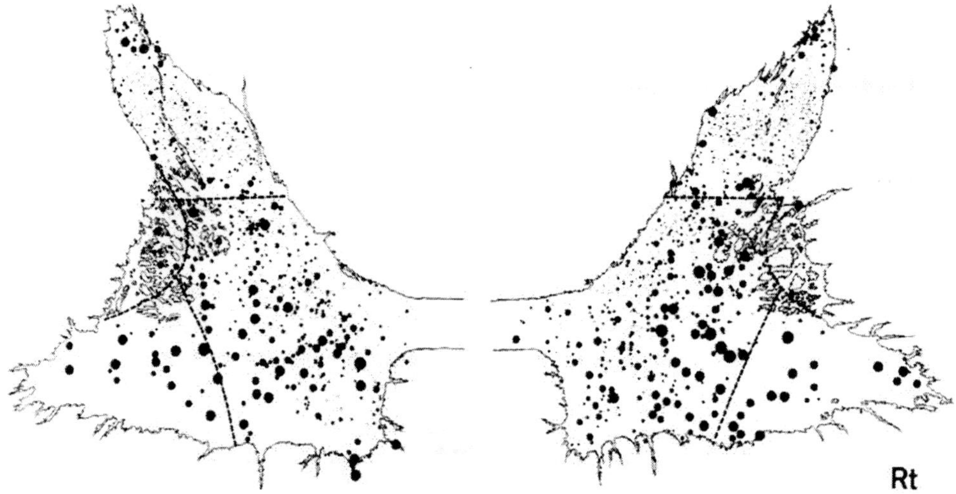

Figure 6. Size distribution of the neurons in the cervical gray matter of a ALS patient, whose muscular strength was fairly well preserved up to death. The large neurons, with a nuclear area greater than 151 μm^2, are severely decreased in Rexed's lamina IX. However, the degree of decrease of the neurons is not equal to that of advanced ALS patients. The neurons in the intermediate zone and posterior horn are quite well preserved. Cited from ref. Oyanagi et al. 1989.

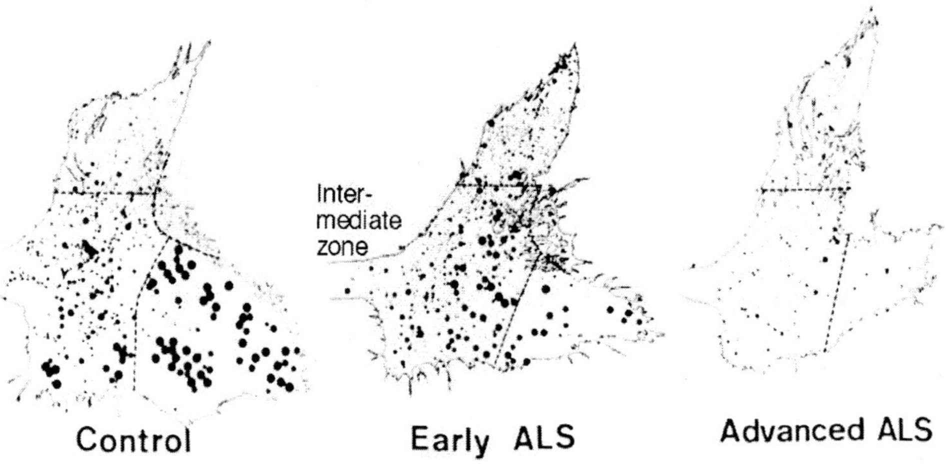

Figure 7. Progression pattern of neuronal loss in the spinal gray matter of ALS. The findings indicate that the primary degeneration may occur in the anterior horn cells and the neurons in the intermediate zone degenerate sequentially in the spinal gray matter in ALS.

It has been reported that the degeneration of the CST caused by hemispherectomy [Ikuta et al. 1982] and stroke [Terao et al. 1997] does not induce trans-synaptic degeneration in the AHCs in humans. Long duration of the illness and respirator use tend to cause severe degeneration of both the l-CST and marked loss of neurons in the spinal gray matter. However, some patients with marked loss of spinal neurons show only mild degeneration of the l-CST (Fig.8). Based on these findings, the degree of myelinated fiber loss in the l-CST did not completely correlate with either the duration of their illness or their history of respirator use [Oyanagi et al. 1995] These findings mean absence of direct correlation of disease mechanism between the AHCs and the l-CST in ALS.

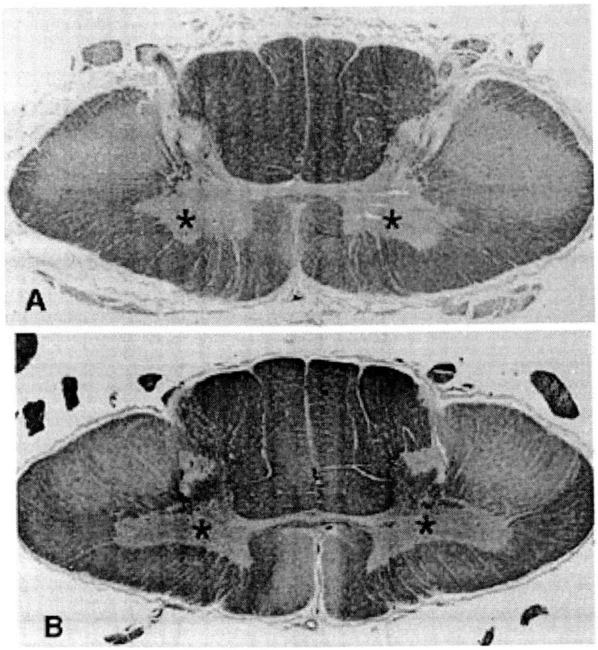

Figure 8. An ALS patient with relative preserved AHCs (asterisks) but severe degeneration of the l-CST (A). An ALS patient with marked loss of AHCs (asterisks) but relatively slight degeneration of the l-CST (B). Cervical cord. Klüver-Barrera preparation.

Laterality of Corticospinal Tract (CST) Degenerration in ALS: Proportion of Crossed and Uncrossed Fibers

Symptoms of most of the ALS patients occurs in unilateral extremity at the initiation. According to the course of the disease, muscle weakness usually progressed to the other extremity in the patients, and the neuropathological examination reveals symmetric or almost symmetric degeneration of the CST and loss of AHCs. However, occasionally, there have been reported asymmetric degeneration of the l-CST [Reuter 1931, Swash et al. 1988] and loss of AHCs [Mochizuki et al. 1995].

The proportion of the crossed (lateral) and uncrossed (anterior) CST should be considered, when asymmetric degeneration of the CST is present in the spinal cord, since dysproportion, probably developmental, of the crossed and uncrossed CST is observed occasionally in Japanese subjects in routine neuropathological examination. It has been observed that the apparent asymmetry of the CST degeneration was caused not by the severity of the degeneration, but by the dyspropotion of the nerve fibers of the crossed and uncrossed CST (Fig. 9).

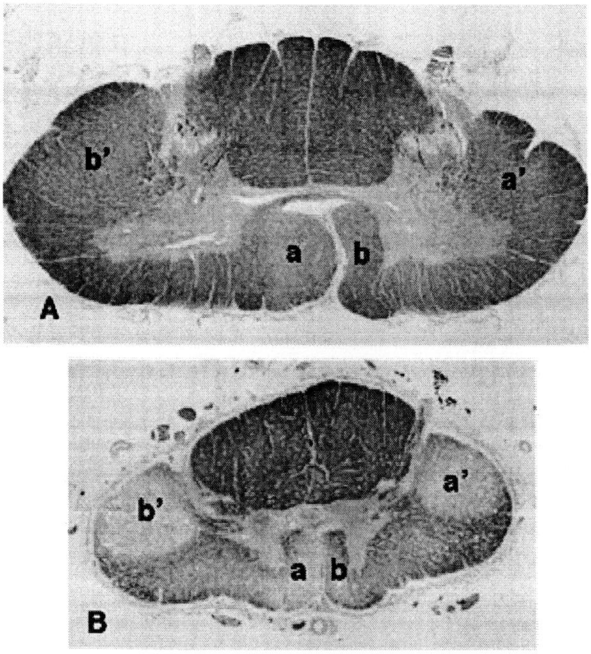

Figure 9. ALS patients showing asymmetry of the spinal white matter. Volume of the left anterior CST (a) is large, and that of right anterior CST (b) is small, but left lateral CST (b') is large, and right lateral CST (a') is small. This finding indicates a + a' = b + b'. A: cervical, B; thoracic of a different patient. Klüver-Barrera preparation.

Loss of Myelinated Fibers in the Anterolateral Funiculus (ALF) in Classic ALS

In the white matter of most the patients with sporadic ALS, the ALF degenerates along with the lateral and anterior CST [Charcot 1880, Holmes 1909, Ikuta et al. 1979, 1982, Lawyer & Netsky 1953, Oyanagi et al. 1995, Smith 1960]. In the present morphometric study on the myelinated fibers in the ALF and l-CST of the cervical segment revealed that: (1) marked and significant loss of large myelinated fibers in the ALF of ALS patients, (2) the patients who required respirator support showed more severe degeneration of the ALF in the ALS than those who required none, and (3) the degree of myelinated fiber loss in the l-CST did not correspond with either the illness duration or the history of respirator use, (4) large myelinated fibers in the l-CST and ALF degenerate independently in classic ALS [Oyanagi et al. 1995] (Fig. 10).

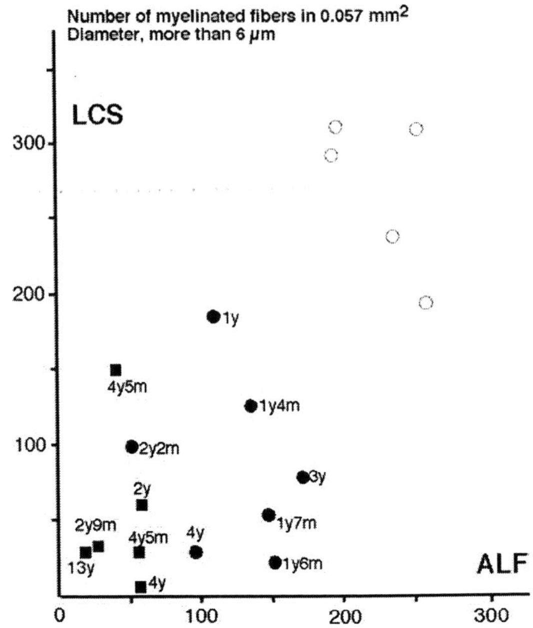

Figure 10. Evaluation of the ratio for the decrease in numbers of large myelinated fibers between the ALF and l-CST. Open circle; control subject, solid circle; ALS patient without respirator support, solid square; ALS patient with respirator support. Numbers indicate the duration of illness. Patients who required respirator support showed more severe degeneration of the ALF in the ALS than those who required none, and the degree of myelinated fiber loss in the l-CST did not correspond with either the illness duration or the history of respirator use. Cited from ref. Oyanagi et al. 1995.

Origin of the Degenerated Fibers of the ALF in Classic ALS

The neurons originating the reticulospinal tract, the neurons in the spinal cord [Ikuta et al. 1982], and the propriospinal neurons [Oyanagi et al. 1983, 1989] have been proposed as the origins of the degenerated fibers observed in the ALF of patients with ALS.

In the present study, in order to determine the origin of the large myelinated fibers in the ALF of the human spinal cord, the number of which is severely reduced in patients with ALS, myelinated fibers in the ALF of the mid-cervical spinal cord were examined quantitatively in five groups of subjects, including control subjects (Group I). The disease groups that were examined included patients with cerebral lesions showing complete degeneration of the unilateral/bilateral pyramis of the medulla oblongata (Group II), those with lesions of the pontine tegmentum (Group III), those with lesions of the lower cervical spinal cord (Group IV), and those with thoracic/lumbar lesions (Group V) (Fig. 3).

The results of the present study have revealed that: (1) large myelinated fibers in the ALF of the mid-cervical spinal cord originate from the tegmentum of the brain stem and from the lower cervical spinal cord, (2) large and medium-sized myelinated fibers in the ALF of the mid-cervical spinal cord are not corticospinal tracts, (3) nor are these fibers long-ascending tracts from the thoracic and lumbar spinal cord (Table 1).

A histological and quantitative study has revealed neither degenerative fibers, loss of myelinated fibers, nor atrophy of the ALF in patients with hemispherectomy [Ueki 1966]. The finding concurs with the results of the present study.

The number of large and medium-sized myelinated fibers in the ALF of the mid-cervical spinal cord in patients with complete transverse myelopathy at the thoracic level was not reduced. This indicates that the long-ascending tracts, such as the spinothalamic [Kuru 1976, Parent 1996, Smith 1951, Smith 1957], spinoreticular [Parent 1996], spinocerebellar [Kuru 1976, Parent 1996], and Helweg's triangular [Smith & Deacon 1981] tracts are either not composed of large or medium-sized myelinated fibers, or else do not pass through the areas investigated in the present study.

Table 1. The number of myelinated fibers in the ALF. The mean ± SD of the values are indicated. The examined area is 0.057 mm^2 in each subject or patient. Statistical evaluation was performed using the Mann-Whitney U test to compare the numbers of myelinated fibers with diameters of less than 3 μm, 3-6 μm and over 6 μm. In the patients with lesions of the pontine tegmentum (group III) and with lesions of the lower cervical cord (group IV), the number of myelinated fibers with a diameter of over 6 μm had decreased significantly. Cited from ref. Oyanagi et al. 1999

		Diameter		
		< 3.0 μm	3-6 μm	> 6.0 μm
I. Control	(n=5)	2645.2 +/- 247.6	605.2 +/- 62.8	158.4 +/- 11.6
II. Cerebral lesions	(n=4)	2335.5 +/- 400.9	627.0 +/- 83.6	183.0 +/- 91.6
III. Pontine tegmentum lesions	(n=5)	2745.4 +/- 607.6	620.2 +/- 54.5	56.4 +/- 19.3 *
IV. Lower cervical lesions	(n=5)	3472.4 +/- 802.8	519.2 +/- 117.9	88.6 +/- 23.6 *
V. Thoracic/lumbar lesions	(n=4)	2403.0 +/- 83.2	607.0 +/- 91.6	148.0 +/- 25.6

* P< 0.01

The result of the present study shows that a proportion of the large myelinated fibers in the ALF of the mid-cervical spinal cord originate from the lower cervical cord, and that the large myelinated fibers in the ALF are not long-ascending fibers from the thoracic and lumbar spinal cord. This finding suggests that the large myelinated fibers reduced in number in patients with lower cervical involvement are not long-ascending fibers, but propriospinal fibers connecting neighboring segments. The present study has also revealed that the large myelinated fibers in the ALF of the mid-cervical segment originate from the tegmentum of the brain stem and the lower cervical spinal cord, and their origins are considered to be reticulo-, vestibulo- and/or raphe-spinal neurons, and propriospinal neurons.

In advanced ALS patients who require the long-term use of a respirator, an extensive reduction in the number of neurons other than motor neurons has been observed in addition to complete loss of the anterior horn cells [Hayashi & Kato 1989, Mizutani et al. 1992]. It has also been noted that the tegmentum of the brain stem and the intermediate zone of the spinal cord exhibit extremely severe atrophy and neuronal loss, and that the ALF degenerates markedly in these ALS patients [Hayashi & Kato 1989, Mizutani et al. 1992]. Bunina bodies and ubiqutin-immunopositive inclusions have been observed in the neurons of the reticular formation of the medulla oblongata in patients with ALS [Bergmann 1993, Nakano et al. 1993]. This indicates that an ALS specific disease process exists in the neurons in the reticular formation.

It has been shown that propriospinal neurons at the cervical segment are located in laminae V-VII (cat and monkey [Molenaar and Kuypers 1978]) of Rexed [Rexed 1954], and that these neurons play roles in movement control and sensorimotor integration of the extremities [Martin 1996, Pierrot-Deseilligny 1996]. The reticulospinal and propriospinal tracts terminate in laminae V-VIII in the cervical cord (cat [Barilari & Kuypers 1969]). Thus, the reticulospinal neurons in the brain stem and propriospinal neurons in the spinal cord are considered to be closely linked to the degeneration of the ALF in classic ALS.

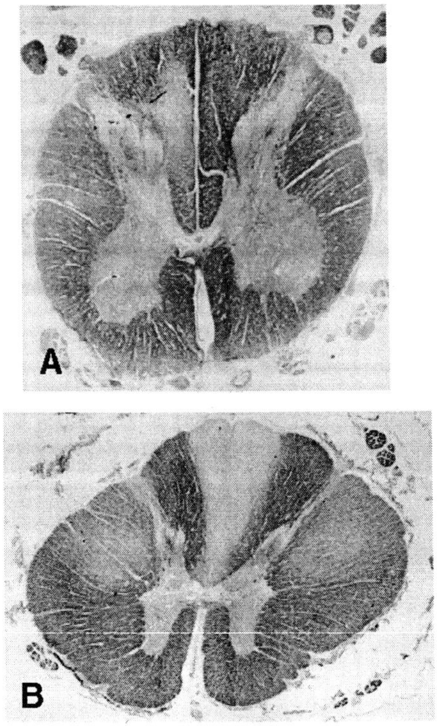

Figure 11. A familial ALS patient with SOD-1 gene mutation showing a degeneration of the left middle root zone (A) of the 12th thoracic segment. Mid-thoracic cord of a patient with SMON (B). Klüver-Barrera preparation.

Mechanism of the Middle Root Zone Degeneration in Familial ALS

Some patients of familial ALS with or without SOD-1 gene mutation show degeneration of the posterior funiculus, that is “middle root zone degeneration” (Fig. 11A) [Makifuchi and Ikuta 1977, Takahashi et al. 1994]. The pattern is quite different from that of the Wallerian degeneration of the transverse myelopathy, or the subacute myelo-optico-neuropathy (SMON), an intoxication of clioquinol (hydoxyquinoline), which primarily involves the spinal ganglia and the axons [Tateishi J et al. 1972, 1973] (Fig, 11B). On the pathomechanism of this finding, Ikuta et al. (1982) reported a retrograde trans-synaptic degeneration of the afferent fibers to the degenerated Clarke's column, based on the findings of marked loss of neurons in the Clarke's column at the severely degenerated side of the posterior funiculus (Fig. 11A).

Acknowledgments

The authors are indebted to Emeritus Professor Fusahiro Ikuta, Niigata University, Niigata, Japan, and the Brain Research Center, Niigata Neurosurgical Hospital, Niigata, Japan, to proceed the research. This work was supported in part by grants from the Japanese Ministry of Education, Science, Sports and Culture (#14580735 to KO and # 14657376 to EK), and the Japanese Ministry of Health, Labor and Welfare (Research on Psychiatric and Neurological Diseases (H16-kokoro-017) to KO).

References

Altermark B, Lundberg A, Pinter M, Sasaki S (1987) Long C_3-C_5 propriospinal neurons in the cat. *Brain Res 404*: 382-388

Barilari MG, Kuypers HGJM (1969) Propriospinal fibers interconnecting the spinal enlargements in the cat. *Brain Res 14*: 321-330

Barnes S (1901) Degenerations in hemiplegia: with special reference to a ventrolateral pyramidal tract, the accessory fillet and Pick's bundle. *Brain 24*: 463-501

Bergmann M (1993) Motor neuron disease/amyotrophic lateral sclerosis-lesson from ubiquitin. *Path Res Pract 189*: 902-912

Charcot JM (1880) *Lecons sur les maladies du systeme nerveuz faites á la Salpetriere*. vol 2, 3rd edn. Delahaye, Paris, pp 213-226

Giok SP (1958) The fasciculus intermediolateralis of Loewenthal in man. Brain 81: 577-587

Hayashi H, Kato S (1989) Total manifestation of amyotrophic lateral sclerosis. ALS in the totally locked-in state. *J Neurol Sci 93*: 19-35

Holmes G (1909) The pathology of amyotrophic lateral sclerosis. *Rev Neurol Psychiatry 7*: 693-725

Ikuta F, Makifuchi T, Ichikawa T(1979) *Comparative studies of tract degeneration in ALS and other disorders*. In Tsubaki T, Toyokura Y (eds) Amyotrophic lateral sclerosis. University of Tokyo Press, Tokyo, pp 177-200

Ikuta F, Makifuchi T, Ohama E, Takeda S, Oyanagi K, Nakashima S, Motegi T (1982) Tract degeneration of the human spinal cord: Some observations on ALS and hemispherectomized humans. *Shinkei Kenkyu no Shinpo 26*: 710-736

Iwamoto Y, Sasaki S, Suzuki I (1990) Input-output organization of reticulospinal neurones, with special reference to connections with dorsal neck motoneurones in the cat. *Exp Brain Res 80*: 260-276

Kuru, M (1976) Sensory paths in the spinal cord and brain stem of man. Kimura Shoten, Tokyo

Lawyer, T Jr, Netsky MG (1953) Amyotrophic lateral sclerosis. A clinicoanatomic study of fifty-three cases. *Arch Neurol Psychiatry 69*: 171-192

Makifuchi T, & Ikuta F (1977) Degeneration of the accessory cuneate nucleus in familial ALS with the "middle root zone" involvement. *No to Shinkei 29*: 1332-1334

Martin GF, Humbertson AO Jr, Laxson LC, Panneton WM, Tschismadia I (1979) Spinal projections from the mesencephalic and pontine reticular formation in the North American opossum: A study using axonal transport techniques. *J Comp Neurol 187*: 373-400

Martin GF, Cabana T, Ditirro FJ, Ho RH, Humbertson AO Jr (1982) Raphespinal projections in the North American opossum: evidence for connectional heterogeneity. *J Comp Neurol 208*: 67-84

Martin JH (1996) Differential spinal projections from the forelimb areas of the rostral and caudal subregions of primary motor cortex in the cat. Exp Brain Res 108: 191-205

Mitsuyama Y, Takamatsu I (1971) An autopsy case of presenile dementia with motor neuron disease. *No to Shinkei 23*: 409-416

Mizutani T, Sakamaki S, Tsuchiya N, Kamei S, Kohzu H, Horiuchi R, Ida M, Shiozawa R, Takasu T (1992) Amyotrophic lateral sclerosis with ophthalmoplegia and multisystem degeneration in patients on long-term use of respirators. *Acta Neuropathol 84*: 372-377

Mochizuki Y, Mizutani T, Takasu T (1995) Amyotrophic lateral sclerosis with marked neurological asymmetry: clinicopathological study. *Acta Neuropathol 90*: 44-50

Molenaar I, Kuypers HGJM (1978) Cells of origin of propriospinal fibers and of fibers ascending to supraspinal levels. A HRP study in cat and rhesus monkey. *Brain Res 152*: 429-450

Nakano I, Iwatsubo T, Hashizume Y, Mizutani T, Mannen T (1992) Amyotrophic lateral sclerosis with dementia –lesions in the apical cortex and some deeper structures of the temporal lobes. *Neuropathol 12*: 69-77

Nakano I, Iwatsubo T, Hashizume Y, Mizutani T (1993) Bunina bodies in neurons of the medullary reticular formation in amyotrophic lateral sclerosis. *Acta Neuropathol 85*: 471-474

Nathan PW, Smith MC, Deacon P (1990) The corticospinal tracts in man. Course and location of fibres at different segmental levels. *Brain 113*: 303-324

Nathan PW, Smith M, Deacon P (1996) Vestibulospinal, reticulospinal and descending propriospinal nerve fibres in man. *Brain 119*: 1809-1833

Nyberg-Hansen R (1965) Sites and mode of termination of reticulo-spinal fibers in the cat. An experimental study with silver impregnation methods. *J Comp Neurol 124*: 71-100

Oyanagi K, Ikuta F, Horikawa Y (1989) Evidence for sequential degeneration of the neurons in the intermediate zone of the spinal cord in amyotrophic lateral sclerosis: a topographic and quantitative investigation. *Acta Neuropathol 77*: 343-349

Oyanagi K, Kawakami E, Morita T, Takahashi H (1999) Pursuit of the origin of the large myelinated fibers of the anterolateral funiculus in the spinal cord in humans in relation to the pathomechanism in amyotrophic lateral sclerosis. *Acta Neuropathol 98*: 635-640

Oyanagi K, Makifuchi T, Ikuta F (1983) A topographic and quantitative study of neurons in human spinal gray matter, with special reference to their changes in amyotrophic lateral sclerosis. *Biomed. Res 4*: 211-224

Oyanagi K, Makifuchi T, Ikuta F (1995) The anterolateral funiculus in the spinal cord in amyotrophic lateral sclerosis. *Acta Neuropathol 90*: 221-227

Parent A (1996) Carpenter's Human Neuroanatomy, 9th ed. Williams & Wilkins, Baltimore, pp 325-417

Pierrot-Deseilligny E (1996) Transmission of the cortical command for human voluntary movement through cervical propriospinal premotoneurons. *Prog Neurobiol 48*: 489-517

Reuter A (1931) Zur pathogenese der amyotrophischen Lateralsklerose. Deutz Nervenheilk 122: 237-254

Rexed B (1954) The cytoarchitectonic organization of the spinal cord in the cat. *J Comp Neurol 96*: 415-496

Rose PK, Tourond JA, Donevan AH (1996) Morphology of single vestibulospinal collaterals in the upper cervical spinal cord of the cat: III Collaterals originating from axons in the ventral funiculus ipsilateral to their cells of origin. *J Comp Neurol 364*: 16-31

Shaw PJ (2001) Genetic inroads in familial ALS. *Nature Gen 29*: 103-102

Shinoda Y, Ohgaki T, Futami T (1986) The morphology of single lateral vestibulospinal tract axons in the lower cervical spinal cord of the cat. *J Comp Neurol 249*: 226-241

Smith MC (1951) The use of Marchi staining in the later stages of human tract degeneration. *J Neurol Neurosurg Psychiatry 14*: 222-225

Smith M (1957) Observations on the topography of the lateral column of the human cervical spinal cord. *Brain 80*: 263-272

Smith MC (1960) Nerve fibre degeneration in the brain in amyotrophic lateral sclerosis. *J Neurol Neurosurg Psychiatry 23*: 269-282

Smith MC, Deacon P (1981) Helweg's triangular tract in man. *Brain 104*: 249-277

Swash M, Scholtz CL, Vowles G, Ingram DA (1988) Selective and asymmetric vulnerability of corticospinal and spinocerebellar tracts in motor neuron disease. *J Neurol Neurosurg Pshchiatr 51*: 785-789

Takahashi H, Makifuchi T, Nakano R, Sato S, Inuzuka T, Sakimura K, Mishina M, Honma Y, Tsuji S, Ikuta F (1994) Familial amyotrophic lateral sclerosis with a mutation in the Cu/Zn superoxide dismutase gene. *Acta Neuropathol 88*: 185-188

Takahashi H, Oyanagi K, Ikuta F (1993a) The intermediolateral nucleus in sporadic amyotrophic lateral sclerosis. *Acta Neuropathol 86*: 190-192

Takahashi H, Oyanagi K, Ikuta F, Tanaka M, Yuasa T, Miyatake T (1993b) Widespread multiple system degeneration in a patient with familial amyotrophic lateral sclerosis. *J Neurol Sci 120*: 15-21

Takahashi H, Oyanagi K, Ohama E, Ikuta F (1992) Clarke's column in sporadic amyotrophic lateral sclerosis. *Acta Neuropathol 84*: 465-470

Tateishi J, Ikeda H, Saito A, Kuroda S, Otsuki S (1972) Myelopathy in dogs induced by iodoxyquinoline. *Neurology 22*: 702-709

Tateishi J, Kuroda S, Saito A, Otsuki S (1973) Experimental myelo-optic neuropathy induced by Clioquinol. *Acta Neuropathol 24*: 304-320

Terao S, Li M, Hashizume Y, Osano Y, Mitsuma T, Sobue G (1997) Upper motor neuron lesion in stroke patients do not induce antegrade transneuronal degeneration in spinal anteior horn cells. *Stroke 28*: 2553-2556

Terao S, Sobue G, Hashizume Y, Mitsuma T, Takahashi A (1994) Disease-specific patterns of neuronal loss in the spinal ventral horn in amyotrophic lateral sclerosis, multiple system atrophy and X-linked recessive bulbospinal neuronopathy, with special reference to the loss of small neurons in the intermediate zone. *J Neurol 241*: 196-203

Ueki K (1966) *Hemispherectomy in the human with special reference to the preservation of function*. In Tokizane T, Shade JP (eds) Progress in brain research, 21B, Correlative neuroscience, Part B: Clinical studies. Elsevier, Amsterdam, pp 285-338

Yuasa R (1970) Amyotrophic lateral sclerosis with dementia. *Clin Neurol 10*: 569-577

In: Amyotrophic Lateral Sclerosis: New Research
Editor: Christine A. Murray, pp. 197-216

ISBN 1-59454-179-5

Chapter VIII

Involvement of Neurotrophins and Their Common Receptor p75 in the Pathology of ALS

Britta Küst and Sjef Copray*

Department of Medical Physiology, University Medical Center Groningen, School for Behavioural and Cognitive Neurosciences Groningen,
University of Groningen, The Netherlands.

Abstract

For maintenance and normal functionality, spinal motoneurons depend on a continuous retrograde neurotrophic supply of muscular factors, in particular neurotrophins. Therefore, disturbances in normal neurotrophin signaling are considered to contribute - either primary or secondary - to the pathogenesis of ALS. These disturbances may not only include abnormalities in the amount and pattern of muscular neurotrophin production but also alterations in the expression of the neurotrophin receptor repertory by the motoneurons and in particularly the appearance of the neurotrophin receptor $p75^{NTR}$, an alleged 'death receptor'.

In this chapter we report on post-mortem studies performed in the past years in our lab concerning the neurotrophin production in muscles of ALS patient and the expression of the $p75^{NTR}$ neurotrophin receptor by the spinal motoneurons. Moreover, using a hSOD1 transgenic animal model that lacked the genetic information for the $p75^{NTR}$ receptor (hSOD1/$p75^{NTR-/-}$ mice) we have examined the significance of this receptor for the ALS pathogenesis process.

Our data suggest that the severe imbalances that we found in neurotrophin- and $p75^{NTR}$-levels are most likely not primary phenomena in the pathology of ALS. However, the

* Correspondence concerning this article should be addressed to Sjef Copray, Dept. of Medical Physiology, University Medical Center Groningen, A. Deusinglaan 1, 9713 AV Groningen, The Netherlands. Tel: ++31-50-363-2785; Fax: ++31-50-363-2751; e-mail: j.c.v.m.copray@med.rug.nl.

gender related differences in clinical symptom gravity and disease endpoint that we observed in the hSOD1/p75$^{NTR-/-}$ mice indicate that this neurotrophin receptor is of importance for secondary pathogenic events contributing to ALS disease progress.

Keywords: neurotrophins, p75^{NTR}, SOD1, transgenic mice, muscles, functional studies.

Introduction

The inability to fully understand the events causing the selective death of motoneurons in amyotrophic lateral sclerosis (ALS) eventuates in the most disastrous aspect of this disease: the fact that there is still no curative or even palliative treatment available.

ALS is considered a multifactorial disease since various pathogenic pathways seem to be involved. Thus, autoimmunity (Appel et al., 1994; Delbono et al., 1993; Yi et al., 2000; Smith et al., 1992), excitotoxicity (Ludolph et al., 2000), oxidative stress (Cookson and Shaw, 1999) and neurofilament abnormalities (Al Chalabi et al., 1999) may singularly or in combination account for ALS pathology. Interventions in these pathways, however, have shown only minor beneficial effects in experimental animal models and so far none of them had any inhibitory effect on disease progression in ALS patients. This indicates that the suggested pathogenic pathways for ALS as mentioned above are still disputable and that yet other mechanisms may be involved in disease etiology.

One of these alternative mechanisms may involve (a disturbance of) the continuous retrograde support of the motoneurons by neurotrophic factors produced in their targets, the muscles. Motoneurons require these neurotrophic factors not only for their development in the embryonic stage, but also for proper functional maintenance in the adult stage and for survival and regeneration in case of injury. Application of BDNF (Yan et al., 1992), neurotrophin-3 (NT-3) and neurotrophin-4/5 (NT-4/5) (Van Westerlaak et al., 2001) - three members of the neurotrophins, a prominent family of neurotrophic factors - has been shown to promote survival of adult motoneurons in various experimental injury models. Following these observations, clinical trials have been performed with the administration of several neurotrophic factors. Only one neurotrophin - BDNF - has been investigated as a potential therapeutic agent for ALS in clinical trials. Surprisingly these trials have not been preceded by a thorough examination of the actual neurotrophin levels in ALS patients to determine whether exogenous application would be meaningful or superfluous. Moreover, a few studies already have suggested that affected motoneurons presumably do not express the normal appropriate survival promoting receptor repertory (Seeburger et al., 1993; Nishio et al., 1998).

Neurotrophins mediate their biological action via two different types of transmembrane receptors: the Trk family of receptor tyrosine kinases, which have preferential binding partners (Huang and Reichardt, 2003), and the 75 kDa neurotrophin receptor p75^{NTR}, which binds all four mammalian neurotrophins with similar affinities (Chao, 2003; Hempstead, 2002; Roux and Barker, 2002). Both receptor classes are known to activate different – even opposed - downstream effector molecules. While Trk receptors seem to be mainly involved in maintenance, survival and regeneration of neurons, p75^{NTR} mediated signaling has also thought to be associated with increased cell death (Wang et al., 2001), although this receptor is best described as a mediator of cell stress responses (Dobrowsky and Carter, 2000). Motoneurons express TrkB and TrkC which specifically bind the neurotrophins BDNF and NT-4/5, and NT-3, respectively (Henderson et al., 1993; Piehl et al., 1994; Seeburger et al., 1993; Nishio et al., 1998). TrkA, the high affinity NGF-receptor, is normally not expressed in motoneurons (Nishio et al., 1998; Xu et al., 1994). In contrast, $p75^{NTR}$ is only expressed in abundance in developing motoneurons and its expression is gradually decreased to undetectable levels around the second postnatal week (Yan and Johnson, Jr., 1988). However, in the ventral spinal cord $p75^{NTR}$ is re-expressed in axotomized motoneurons (Ferri et al., 1998; Koliatsos et al., 1991) as well as in ALS-affected motoneurons (Seeburger et al., 1993; Lowry et al., 2001; Nishio et al., 1998). The question arises whether $p75^{NTR}$ signaling in spinal motoneurons could be involved in ALS related cell death? Although the cell death mechanisms in ALS affected motoneurons are not fully understood, evidence is accumulating that apoptotic pathways play a role in both human and mouse ALS pathology (Martin, 2000; Martin, 1999; Martin et al., 2000; Kostic et al., 1997; Li et al., 2000; Mu et al., 1996). Interestingly, neurotrophins are known to play a decisive role in the process of apoptosis. During embryonic development, interactions between neurotrophins and the Trk receptors prevent apoptosis through an intracellular pathway involving Bcl-2, NFκB, PI3-kinase and MAP kinases, resulting in the survival of specific neuronal populations (Al Chalabi et al., 1999; Casaccia-Bonnefil et al., 1998; Chao et al., 1998; Segal and Greenberg, 1996). On the other hand, binding of neurotrophins to $p75^{NTR}$ during embryogenesis is thought to either support the interaction between the Trk receptors and the neurotrophins, or to mediate cell death of excessive neurons. At later stages, interactions of neurotrophins with $p75^{NTR}$ activate apoptotic pathways involving Bax, ceramide, JNK kinases and caspases (Wang et al., 2001). So, it is likely that $p75^{NTR}$ functions as a 'death receptor' for ALS affected spinal motoneurons (Miller and Kaplan, 1998). In recent years, however, evidence is accumulating that the function of $p75^{NTR}$ in injured adult cells, like the ALS affected motoneurons, is presumably much more complicated. The p75 receptor is thought to play a pivotal role in determining the fate of stressed or injured cells: apoptosis or adaptation and survival (Dobrowsky and Carter, 2000; Roux and Barker, 2002).

Since aberrant neurotrophin signalling involving the p75 receptor may play a role in apoptotic events, during the last years we aimed to get more insight into the neurotrophin system in ALS related motoneuron death. Firstly we wanted to know whether ALS affected motoneurons are exposed to aberrant neurotrophin levels. To that purpose we investigated the level of expression of the neurotrophins in post-mortem muscle tissue of ALS patients. In view of the expression of $p75^{NTR}$ in affected motoneurons in ALS patients, we wanted to investigate the possible significance of $p75^{NTR}$ in ALS pathogenesis using the hSOD1 ALS mouse model. This transgenic animal model expresses one of the mutated human copper/zinc superoxide dismutase (SOD1) genes that has been demonstrated to underlie an autosomal dominant familial form of ALS (Rosen et al., 1993; Gurney et al., 1994; Hand and Rouleau, 2002; Wong and Borchelt, 1995; Bruijn et al., 1997). Reflecting the pathology of ALS in humans, these mice develop an adult-onset, progressive motoneuron degeneration ultimately resulting in muscle atrophy. They have been widely used as a model for ALS to investigate new therapeutical approaches (Gurney et al., 1996) and to study the cellular mechanisms underlying adult motoneuron death (Li et al., 2000). We examined the expression of $p75^{NTR}$ in the spinal cord of the hSOD1 mice at different stages of the disease. We then tried to establish a correlation between the expression of $p75^{NTR}$ and signs of motoneuron injury and death (apoptosis). Therefore we examined the co-expression of $p75^{NTR}$ with activating transcription factor 3 (ATF-3), a member of the ATF/CREB family of stress transcription factors and a good marker for injured motoneurons (Hai et al., 1999; Tsujino et al., 2000), and activated caspase-3, a main marker for the execution phase of apoptosis in ALS motoneurons (Li et al., 2000). To further establish the role of $p75^{NTR}$ in ALS motoneuron degeneration, we employed the original $p75^{NTR}$ knockout mouse model (Lee et al., 1992), in which disruption of exon 3 of the $p75^{NTR}$ gene inhibited extracellular neurotrophin binding without disturbing the intracellular signaling domain of the receptor. By crossing these mice with mutant hSOD1 mice we aimed to investigate the functional effects of diminished $p75^{NTR}$ signaling on the ALS pathogenic process.

Patients, Experimental Animals, Materials and Methods

Post Mortem Tissue

Samples of biceps brachii or lumbal spinal cord were obtained at autopsy (Institute for Pathology, Academic Medical Center, Amsterdam, the Netherlands) from patients who had previously given written approval for the use of their tissues, according to the guidelines of the Netherlands ALS Bank. Biceps samples were collected from 15 patients with neuropathologically confirmed sporadic ALS (age ranging from 39-75 years, disease duration varying from 7-96 months, post mortem delay between 3 and 48 hours), and from 15 control patients without evidence of neurologic diseases (age ranging from 42-69 years, post mortem delay from 3-21 h). All tissue samples were rapidly frozen in liquid nitrogen and stored at -80°C until used.

Quantification of Neurotrophin Proteins by Enzyme-Linked Immunosorbant Assay (ELISA)

Human biceps tissue was pulverized mechanically and extracted in 10 volumes of a solution containing 50 mM Tris (pH 7.4), 600 mM NaCl, 0.2% Triton-X-100, 1% BSA and 5 μl/100 mg wet weight (ww) protease inhibitor mix (P8340, Sigma), by shaking (500rpm) the mixture over night at 4°C. 2 volumes of sterile aqua bidest were added, the suspension was vortexed and centrifuged for 5 minutes at 10.000 x g, and the supernatant was collected. The total protein concentration was measured using the Pyrogallol Red test (Instruchemie, Verhildersum, the Netherlands) and expressed in albumin equivalents. The concentrations of the neurotrophin proteins were measured in the muscle extracts using a monoclonal antibody-based sandwich ELISA.

Microtitre plates (Costar, Badhoevedorp, the Netherlands) were coated overnight at room temperature (RT) on a horizontal shaker at 500 rpm in a final volume of 100 µl/well (if not mentioned otherwise, these conditions were maintained for all subsequent steps) with monoclonal NGF, BDNF, NT-3 or NT-4 antibodies (MAB256, MAB848, MAB267 or MAB 268 respectively, RandD Systems) at a dilution of 1µg/ml in 0.01 M PBS, pH 7.4 (1x PBS). Plates were then washed 3 times with a solution containing 0.025 M Tris, pH8, 0.15 M NaCl and 0.05% Tween-20 and blocked for 1 hour at RT with 2% BSA and 0.05% Tween-20 in 1xPBS. After washing, plates were incubated with the muscle lysates in duplicates at serial dilutions in incubation buffer consisting of 1xPBS, 0.2% gelatine and 0.05% Tween-20, starting with 1:1. Another washing step was followed by a one-hour incubation with secondary biotinylated antibodies (BAF256, BAM648, BAF267 and BAF268, R&D Systems) diluted to 25ng/ml in incubation buffer. Plates were washed again and incubated for 30 minutes with streptavidin conjugated to poly-horse radish peroxidase (Strepta-E^+, Centraal Laboratorium voor Bloedtransfusie, Amsterdam, the Netherlands) at a concentration of 125 ng/ml in incubation buffer. A final washing step was followed by the chromogen-reaction: 1 mg of 3'3'5'5'tetramethylbenzidin (TMB, Roth, Germany) in 0.3 ml 96% EtOH was added to 11 ml 0.1 M Na-acetate, pH6, and 0.004% H_2O_2 and plates were incubated for ca. 20 minutes with 0.1 ml of the chromogen solution until the reaction was stopped by addition of 2 N H_2SO_4. The absorbtion at 450 nm minus 570 nm was measured in a microplate reader (Labsystems, Breda, the Netherlands), the concentrations were calculated by SOFTmax PRO software (Molecular Devices, Sunnyvale, USA) and displayed as pg neurotrophin protein/ 100 mg wet weight [ww].

Experimental Animals

Wild type mice (B6SJLF1/J, Stock Nr 100012), mutant high-copy SOD1 transgenic mice (B6SJL-TgN(SOD1-G93A)1Gur, Stock Nr 002726) and $p75^{NTR}$ "knockout" mice (B6.129S4-$Ngfr^{tm1Jae}$, Stock Nr 002213) were purchased from The Jackson Laboratory (Bar Harbor, ME). Interbreeding $p75^{NTR}$ knockout mice ($p75^{-/-}$) with hSOD1 transgenic ($SOD^{1/0}$) mice generated double transgenic animals. $SOD^{1/0}/p75^{+/-}$ offsprings from the first generation were backcrossed to $p75^{-/-}$ mice to obtain $SOD^{1/0}/p75^{-/-}$ mice. All mice were housed in groups of 2-5 animals under standard conditions (12 h daylight / 12 h darkness, 21°C) in conventional translucent cages with food pellets and water ad libitum. Under these conditions, hemizygous hSOD1 transgenic mice became paralyzed in one or more limbs by 4-5 months (ca. 135 days) of age. Homozygous $p75^{NTR}$ knockout mice needed to be handled very carefully because they frequently developed ulcers and infections at their toes by 4 months of age due to decreased cutaneous innervation; the lifespan of these mice was comparable to wild type mice. More detailed information concerning the heterozygous hSOD1 transgenic mice and the homozygous $p75^{NTR}$ knockout mice can be obtained from the original publications (Gurney et al., 1994; Lee et al., 1992). All animal experiments were in accordance with National Institutional Animal Care and Use Commitee Guidelines (Dier Experimenten Commissie, DEC).

Genetic Characterisation

Mice were genotyped by collecting 0.5 cm pieces of mouse tails, subjecting them to DNA extraction (Spin tissue Mini Kit, InViTek, Berlin, Germany) and carrying out polymerase chain reaction (PCR). Heterozygous hSOD1 mice were identified by using sense (5'-CATCAGCCCTAATCCATCTGA) and antisense (5'-CGCGACTAACAATCAAAGT-GA) hSOD1 primers, annealing to exon 4 of the mutated SOD1 gene and amplifying a 236 bp product, and by using sense (5'-CTAGGCCACAGAATTGAAAGATCT) and antisense (5'-GTAGGTGGAAATTCTAGCATCATCC) Il-2 primers which amplify a product of 324 bp as an internal control. Heterozygous and homozygous $p75^{NTR}$ knockout mice were identified by using sense (5'-CTTGGGTGGAGAGGCTATTC) and antisense (5'-AGGTGAGATGACAGGAGATC) Neo-generic primers, annealing to the neo-cassette of the $p75^{NTR}$ -gene and amplifying a 280 bp product, and by using sense (5'-TGTTACGTTCTCTGACGTGGTGAG) and antisense (5'-TCAGCCCAGGGTGTGCACTC) $p75^{NTR}$ primers which amplify a 345 bp DNA fragment from the $p75^{NTR}$ wild type allele. PCR-conditions were for the hSOD1-mice:

3 min at 94°C, followed by 12 cycles of 1 min 94°C, 1 min 64°C, 1.5 min 72°C and 25 cycles of 1 min 94°C, 1 min 58°C, 1.5 min 72°C, followed by 8 min at 72°C. Amplified DNA fragments were separated by gel electrophoresis on a 2% agarose gel.

Determination of ALS-like Symptoms

The clinical signs and body weight of mice were monitored every second day over the whole experimental period. The onset of clinical signs was determined by tremor in one or both hindlimbs when mice were lifted by the tail. Disease end-points were determined by total hindlimb paralysis.

Determination of Survival

Female and male WT (n>30), $SOD^{1/0}$ (n=38), $p75^{+/-}$ (n>20), $p75^{-/-}$ (n>30), and the double transgenic $SOD^{1/0}/p75^{+/-}$ (n=69) and $SOD^{1/0}/p75^{-/-}$ (n=28) mice were followed for 160 days for survival. Mice carrying the hSOD1(G93A) mutation were sacrificed if both hindlimbs were paralysed and the animals became immobile. The maximal survival data for female and male mice were plotted into separate Kaplan-Meier survival curves, because a sex difference has been observed in ALS.

Animal Perfusion and Tissue Preparation

The mice were anaesthetised with sodium pentobarbital (60 mg/kg i.p.) and subsequently perfused transcardially with phosphate-buffered saline containing 100 units of heparin, followed by Zamboni's fixative (2% formaldehyde, 15% picric acid in 0.1 M phosphate buffer). The lumbar part of the spinal cord was removed and, after a one-night cryoprotective treatment in 25% sucrose in phosphate buffer, sections of 14 μm were cut in a cryostat. Serial sections were stained with haematoxylin-eosin or cresyl violet, for a general overview of the histological structure of the spinal cord, and by immunohistochemistry to detect various proteins as markers of the pathological process.

Histological and Immunological Characterisation of Human and Mouse Spinal Cords

Human lumbar spinal cord sections (10μm) were incubated overnight at 4°C in a primary rabbit antibody against $p75^{NTR}$ (Chemicon) diluted 1:100. Mouse lumbar spinal cord sections (14μm) were incubated overnight at 4°C in a primary rabbit antibodies against mouse/rat $p75^{NTR}$ (kindly provided by Louis F. Reichardt) diluted 1:3500; against activated caspase-3, a major apoptosis inducing caspase (Cell Signaling, #9661S) diluted 1:100; and anti-activation transcription factor-3, a stress activation factor and marker for injured motoneurons (ATF-3, Serotec) diluted 1:1000. Application of secondary antibody (goat anti-rabbit (Vector, BA1000), 1:400 for 2h) was followed by a two-step biotin-streptavidin-peroxidase procedure with diamino-benzidine as the chromogen, which allowed counting of the immuno-complex positive cells in sections of ventral spinal cords. To demonstrate specificity of the antibodies, in separate control sections the primary or secondary antibodies were omitted, which in all cases produced no signals.

Determination of Cell Numbers

For the quantification of cell numbers in lumbar spinal cord, cresyl violet-stained serial sections were used to count large motoneurons in the ventral spinal horns of wildtype and transgenic mice. In order to compare identical regions in different mice, we used a microscopy ocular with a grid-pattern covering a surface of 0.25 mm^2, which was placed over the entire ventral grey matter. The chequered square was subdivided by 100 horizontal and 100 vertical lines, the distance between which corresponded to 5 μm. Only motoneurons with cell bodies larger than 3 sections (>15μm) were counted.

Statistics

Large diameter (>15μm) motoneuron and ATF-3 or activated caspase-3 positive motoneuron cell numbers in ventral spinal cords as well as disease endpoint data are expressed as means ± standard deviations (SD) per group. Physiological data are expressed as means ± standard errors of means (SEM) per group. Statistical differences were determined by One-Way-ANOVA. $p<0.05$ was considered significant.

Results

- Expression of neurotrophin proteins in human ALS biceps
- Expression of the common neurotrophin receptor p75 in spinal motoneurons of ALS and hSOD1(G93A) transgenic mice
- Double transgenics
- Physiological tests
- Survival
- Motoneurons cell counts in ventral spinal cord, correlation to ATF-3 and caspase-3 expression

Expression of Neurotrophin Proteins in Human ALS Biceps

To determine whether motoneuron death in ALS could be due to decreased synthesis of neurotrophins in the motoneuronal targets, we investigated neurotrophin protein content in muscles of ALS patients. We performed enzyme-linked immunosorbent assays (ELISAs) using post mortem biceps brachii tissue of ALS patients and age-matched controls without neuromuscular disease. Whereas levels of NGF, BDNF or NT-4/5 were comparatively low in biceps tissue of patients without neuromuscular diseases (46 ± 5, 11 ± 3 and 28 ± 5 pg/100 mg wet weight [ww], respectively), NT-3 protein levels were notably higher (128 ± 14 pg/100 mg ww).

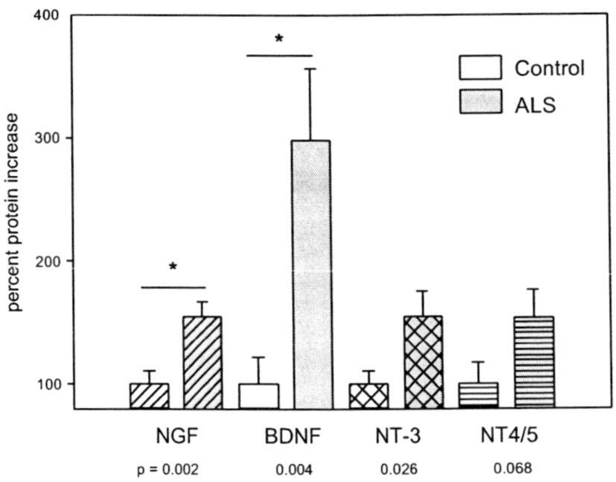

Figure 1. Neurotrophin expression in biceps brachii tissue of human controls and ALS patients. Neurotrophin levels were determined by ELISA in biceps tissue from control (n=15) and ALS patients (n=15, except for BDNF: n=14). Means of neurotrophin levels of control patients were set as 100% and correlated to mean values of ALS patients. *, $p < 0.01$ (One-Way-ANOVA).

All neurotrophin protein levels were found to be increased in biceps tissue of ALS patients. Levels of NGF and BDNF were significantly higher in diseased muscles (Fig. 1), whereas the increases of NT-3 and NT-4/5 were less pronounced. Furthermore, after separation of the ALS patients in two groups, one with a disease duration shorter than 40 months, and the other with a longer disease time course, we also found a significant elevation of NT-3 and NT-4/5 in the latter group (Kust et al., 2002). These data suggest that an elevation of neurotrophin expression is linked to disease duration. Further correlation analyses for possible associated parameters revealed that the increases of neurotrophin proteins in ALS tissue could not be correlated to the post mortem delay times, indicating a high post mortem stability of the neurotrophins. Furthermore, the expression pattern could not be correlated to patient's age or sex.

Expression of the Common Neurotrophin Receptor p75 in Spinal Motoneurons of ALS Patients and hSOD1(G93A) Transgenic Mice

To determine whether enhanced neurotrophin production could influence the motoneuronal fate, we investigated $p75^{NTR}$ expression on spinal motoneurons in ALS and the hSOD1(G93A) mouse model by immunohistochemical experiments. Confirming the data of Seeburger et al. (Seeburger et al., 1993), strong $p75^{NTR}$ immunoreactivity was observed in the membrane of lumbar spinal motoneurons in ALS tissue (Fig. 2a), while no positive staining could be observed in spinal motoneurons of healthy controls. Reminiscent of the situation in ALS, no specific $p75^{NTR}$ signals were visible in spinal motoneurons of control mice (Fig. 2b). However, a strong expression of $p75^{NTR}$ could be detected in lumbar spinal cord tissue of hSOD1(G93A) transgenic mice at the end stage of the disease (Copray et al., 2003) (Fig. 2c,d). Next to this, we observed increased $p75^{NTR}$ staining in vessels walls adjacent to the large α-motoneurons in the ventral horn of hSOD1 transgenic mice (Fig. 2c and d, arrowheads).

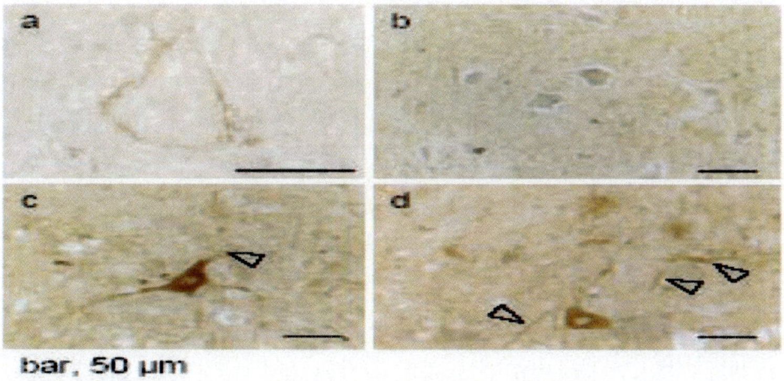

Figure 2. $p75^{NTR}$ immunoreactivity is observed in spinal motoneurons of ALS (a) and transgenic $hSOD1^{1/0}$ (c, d) tissue. **a**, human lumbar ALS motoneuron, showing $p75^{NTR}$ immunoreactivity at the cell surface. No $p75^{NTR}$ signals are observed in healthy mouse controls (**b**), while receptor protein is strongly induced in spinal motoneurons of transgenic $hSOD1^{1/0}$ mice (**c,d**). Arrowheads point to $p75^{NTR}$ positive vessels walls adjacent to the large α-motoneurons. Scale bar, 50 µm.

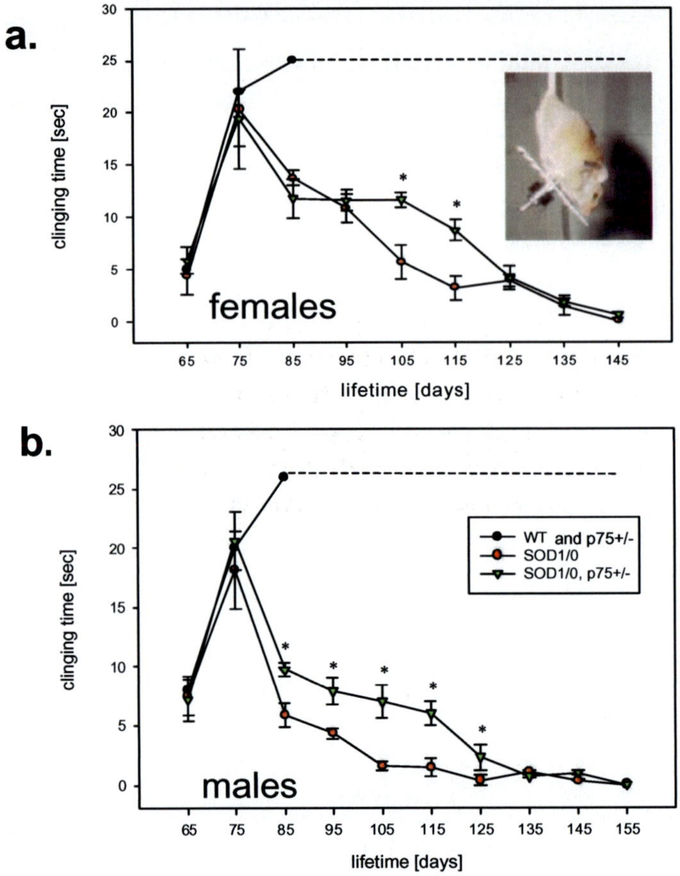

Figure 3. Grip-reflex-test to monitor motor performance of transgenic $hSOD1^{1/0}$ mice. Upon lifting, mice were allowed to cling to a 25g metal grid (Fig. 3a, insert). Female and male wildtype and $p75NTR^{+/-}$ mice (black squares) were able to cling to the grid more than 30 seconds (**a, b**). $hSOD1^{1/0}$ mice of both sexes (red circles) displayed a rapid decrease in maximal holding times from day 80 on. Female (**a**) and male (**b**) double transgenic $hSOD1^{1/0}/p75^{NTR+/-}$ mice (green triangles) could be characterized by a significant shift, a period in which these mice were able to hold the grid longer than the single transgenic $hSOD1^{1/0}$ mice. *, $p<0.01$ (One-Way-ANOVA).

Generation of $p75^{NTR}$ Deficient hSOD1 Mice

To evaluate if the observed $p75^{NTR}$ expression on motoneurons was involved in the degeneration of these cells, $p75^{NTR}$ deficient hSOD1 mice were generated. While we did not detect any apparent difference between wildtype and heterozygous $p75^{NTR+/-}$ mice over a surveillance period of two years, homozygous $p75^{NTR-/-}$ mice developed edema and ulcers on fore- and hindpaws by 4 month of age (Lee et al., 1992). Since secondary infections aggravated the ulcers, these mice had to be handled with extreme care, implying that the mice could furthermore not be monitored in one of the physiological tests mentioned below. High copy hSOD1(G93A) transgenic mice were characterized by motoneuron loss from the spinal cord, resulting in paralysis in one or more limbs and subsequent death by 4-5 month of age (120-140 days).

Double transgenic heterozygous (p75$^{NTR+/-}$) and homozygous (p75$^{NTR-/-}$) hSOD1$^{1/0}$ mice did survive into adulthood and were fertile. They furthermore developed pathological symptoms reminiscent of the single transgenic hSOD1$^{1/0}$ mice.

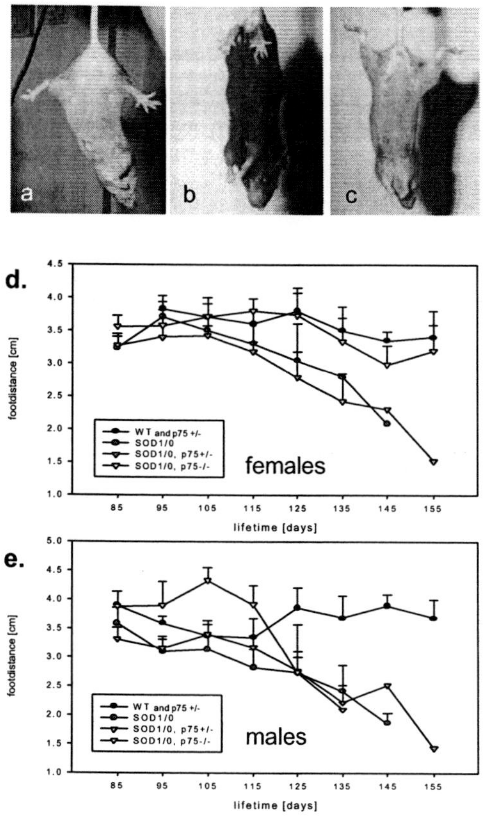

Figure 4. Monitoring of disease progression by measuring the hindlimb-stretch reflex. Upon lifting the mice at their tail their hindpaws were marked with ink. The mice were dropped from a height of 10 cm and the distance between the two footprints was measured. Female and male wildtype, p75NTR$^{+/-}$ and p75NTR$^{-/-}$ mice reacted by normal stretching of the hindlimbs upon uplifting over the whole measurement period (**a**, black squares in **d, e**). Single transgenic hSOD1$^{1/0}$ (**b,** red circles in **d, e**) and hSOD1$^{1/0}$/p75$^{NTR+/-}$ (green triangles in **d, e**) mice showed progressingly decreasing footprint distances. **c**, different posture of female and male hSOD1$^{1/0}$/p75$^{NTR-/-}$ mice, resulting in persistant (females, yellow triangles in **d**) or transient (males, yellow triangles in **e**) higher scores in the test.

Functional Screening of Single and Double Transgenic Mice

Disease progression in the mice was monitored by two different physiological tests. The first test was a grip-reflex-test (all homozygous p75$^{NTR-/-}$ mice were excluded from this test). Upon lifting the mice at their tail, they would grip and cling to any object in their surrounding, which in this test was a metal grid of circa 25g weight (Fig. 3a, insert). After a learning phase of 10 days, with measurements every second day, wildtype and p75$^{NTR+/-}$ mice were able to cling to the grid more than 30 seconds (Fig. 3). In contrast, most hSOD1$^{1/0}$ and hSOD1$^{1/0}$/p75$^{NTR+/-}$ mice were not able to hold the grid for the maximal time observed in wildtypes. Even in the presymptomatic stage (< 80 days), the maximal time was around 20 seconds, with a rapid decrease after 80 days. Female hSOD1$^{1/0}$ mice older than 95 days were not able to hold the grid longer than 10 seconds (Fig. 3a). However, double transgenic females displayed a shift between 95 and 125 days, a period in which they were able to hold the grid significantly longer than the single transgenic hSOD1$^{1/0}$ mice. A similar curve progression, e.g. learning phase, maximal strength and decline, was observed in male mice (Fig. 3 b). Like in females, double-transgenic males displayed an analogue significant shift towards later timepoints. However, compared to females, male hSOD1$^{1/0}$ mice displayed a faster reduction of the clinging time.

A second test to monitor disease progression was a hindlimb-stretch reflex test. The mice were lifted at their tail and their hindpaws were marked with ink. The mice were dropped from a height of 10 cm and the distance between the two footprints was measured. While both female and male wildtype, p75$^{NTR+/-}$ and p75$^{NTR-/-}$ mice reacted by normal stretching of the hindlimbs upon uplifting over the whole measurement period (Fig. 4a), single transgenic hSOD1$^{1/0}$ and hSOD1$^{1/0}$/p75$^{NTR+/-}$ mice could be characterized by a gradually increasing disability to stretch the hindlimbs (Fig. 4b), resulting in decreased footprint distances (Fig. 4d, e). Female and male hSOD1$^{1/0}$/p75$^{NTR-/-}$ mice, however, obviously had a different ability to move their hind extremities (Fig. 4c), which resulted in higher scores in the test. While this effect could only be observed in males up to 120 days (Fig. 4e), the greater distances between the inkmarks of hSOD1$^{1/0}$/p75$^{NTR-/-}$ mice compared to those of hSOD1$^{1/0}$ mice persisted in females over the whole measurement period.

Survival Analysis of the p75^{NTR} Deficient hSOD1 Mice

p75$^{NTR+/-}$ and p75$^{NTR-/-}$ mice did not differ from wildtype mice regarding ageing and lifetime (Lee et al., 1992), and these mice did survive longer than 200 days. High copy hSOD1(G93A) transgenic mice developed a pathology reminiscent of ALS and they died around 130 days (Table 1, and Jackson Lab protocol). Double transgenic mice, lacking one or both p75 alleles, did also develop the ALS pathology. Survival responses, however, seemed to differ from those of hSOD1$^{1/0}$ mice (Kust et al., 2003). While male SOD$^{1/0}$/p75$^{NTR+/-}$ mice displayed the same lifespan as male hSOD1$^{1/0}$ mice, survival of male SOD$^{1/0}$/p75$^{NTR-/-}$ mice seemed to be decreased by 3 days (Table 1). In contrast, but corresponding to the physiological tests, female SOD1$^{1/0}$ mice lacking one or both p75^{NTR} alleles, displayed an increased lifespan. For the female SOD$^{1/0}$/p75$^{NTR+/-}$ mice this delay in disease endpoint proved to be significant (p= 0.020).

Table 1. Quantification of mouse survival

Survival [d]	wildtype	p75$^{NTR+/-}$	p75$^{NTR -/-}$	SOD$^{1/0}$	SOD$^{1/0}$ /p75$^{+/-}$	SOD$^{1/0}$ /p75$^{-/-}$
females	> 200	> 200	> 200	131 ± 11.0	139 ± 8.6	138 ± 11.8
males	> 200	> 200	> 200	132 ± 7.7	133 ± 8.7	129 ± 5.7

Wildtype and transgenic mice were monitored for survival. Mice were sacrificed when one or both hindlimbs were paralyzed and when they were not able to reach the food any longer. Values are given as means ± standard deviations. The shaded value was found to differ significantly from the corresponding SOD$^{1/0}$ value (One-Way-ANOVA. p<0.05 was considered significant).

Table 2. Quantification of mouse motoneuron numbers in ventral lumbar spinal cords

		wildtype	p75$^{NTR -/-}$	SOD$^{1/0}$	SOD$^{1/0}$ /p75$^{+/-}$	SOD$^{1/0}$ /p75$^{-/-}$
females	Motoneuron cell number	**54.2** ± 10	**56** ± 9.2	**37.6** ± 6.6	**36** ± 9.4	29.6 ± 8.5
	ATF-3 pos. cells [%]	0	0	**11.7** ± 5.3	n.d.	**14.3** ± 6
	Caspase–3 pos. cells [%]	0	0	**5.1** ± 4.7	n.d.	**6.8** ± 4.3
males	Motoneuron cell number	**57.0** ± 4.2	**59.4** ± 6.3	**32.4** ± 8.8	**34.0** ± 6.7	**30.8** ± 5.4
	ATF-3 pos. cells [%]	0	0	**9.0** ± 2.1	n.d.	**9.5** ± 6.1
	Caspase–3 pos. cells [%]	0	0	**8.4** ± 1.2	n.d.	**7.8** ± 6.9

Perfused animals were investigated histologically and remaining large motoneurons were counted per 16 μm section of the ventral lumbar spinal cord (both horns). In the same region, motoneurons positive for the transcription factor ATF-3 or activated aspase-3 were counted. Values are given as means ± standard deviations. The shaded value was found to differ significantly from the corresponding SOD$^{1/0}$ value (One-Way-ANOVA. p<0.05 was considered significant).

Motoneurons Cell Counts in Ventral Spinal Cords

To examine whether increased physical abilities and prolonged survival in female p75^{NTR} deficient hSOD1 mice was correlated to enhanced motoneural survival, we quantified cell numbers in ventral lumbar spinal cord of wildtype and transgenic mice. In order to compare identical regions in different mice, we used a microscopy ocular with a grid-pattern covering a surface of 0.25 mm^2, which was placed over the entire ventral grey matter. The checkered square was subdivided by 100 horizontal and 100 vertical lines, the distance between which corresponded to 5 μm. Only motoneurons with cell bodies larger than 3 sections (>15μm) were counted. Comparing wildtype mice with transgenic hSOD1 mice, we observed a strong decrease of ventral horn motoneurons which was evident in females and males to a similar extent (Tabel 2). Regarding the amount of surviving motoneurons in male $p75^{NTR}$ deficient hSOD1 mice, we did not detect a significant difference between these mice and hSOD1 mice, although $SOD^{1/0}/p75^{NTR-/-}$ mice had the lowest number of remaining cells.

Surprisingly, increased survival in $p75^{NTR}$ deficient hSOD1 females was accompanied by even decreased motoneuron cell numbers: while, compared to female wildtype or $p75^{NTR-/-}$ mice, 70% of the motoneurons remained in $hSOD1^{1/0}$ mice, this reduction was exceeded in female $SOD^{1/0}/p75^{NTR-/-}$ mice, where only 55% of the motoneurons remained. Questioning whether the activation state of these motoneurons was altered in these double transgenic mice, we performed immunohistochemical experiments with antibodies against caspase-3, a major apoptosis inducing caspase, and activation transcription factor-3 (ATF-3), a stress activation factor and marker for injured motoneurons. While we did not detect a single caspase-3 or ATF-3 positive motoneuron in lumbar ventral spinal cords of wildtype or $p75^{NTR}$ deficient mice (Table 2), between 5 and 10 % of the remaining motoneurons in $hSOD1^{1/0}$ mice stained positive for one of these stress markers (Copray et al., 2003). However, we did not detect any substantial differences between staining in $hSOD1^{1/0}$ and $SOD^{1/0}/p75^{NTR-/-}$ mice, arguing against a differential execution pathway in single and double transgenic mice.

Discussion

The selective vulnerability of motoneurons to the pathogenic mechanisms that have been suggested to underlie ALS has been ascribed to their size, the large number of neurofilaments, and the continuous intensive retrograde and anterograde transport along very elaborate axons and dendrites. In addition their extraordinary metabolic activity as well as their immense excitatory input could specifically render these cells susceptible to degeneration in ALS (reviewed in Kok, 1997; Louvel et al., 1997; Rothstein, 1996). Although some motoneuron groups (e.g. oculomotor neurons and Onuf's nuclei) appear to be more resistant to ALS, which has been ascribed to the expression of protective calcium binding/buffering proteins (Ince et al., 1993; Reiner et al., 1995; Ho et al., 1996), the singular exclusive feature of motoneurons distinguishing them from other equally sized and active, but relatively ALS-resistant neurons (sensory neurons, magnocellular neurons in the brainstem, cerebellar Purkinje cells, etc.) is the fact that they innervate muscles and that there is a continuous transport of muscular proteins to the motoneurons.

Many reports have described the essential neurotrophic effects of these muscular factors, in particular the neurotrophins, on maintenance and regeneration of adult motoneurons (reviewed in Boyd and Gordon, 2003; Mendell and Arvanian, 2002). It seems obvious that (a disturbance of) this muscular dependency of motoneurons may be of importance in the selective pathogenesis of ALS. The question arises whether disruption of the muscular trophic support may be a primary event in ALS, retrogradely affecting motoneurons. Although our data on the expression of neurotrophins in post-mortem muscles from ALS patients obviously are not conclusive for that, they do demonstrate that the capacity to produce neurotrophins in ALS muscles is not affected. In contrast, the expression of all muscular neurotrophins appeared to be increased in ALS patients. This may be interpreted as a compensatory muscular response in an attempt to rescue degenerating/disconnected motoneurons. However, the pattern of increased neurotrophin expression does not correspond to the muscular responses observed in plain axotomy experiments in animal models. In general, these experiments have demonstrated that muscles upon denervation up-regulate the expression of BDNF, show no change (or a decrease) in the expression of NT-3, and down-regulate NT-4/5 (Funakoshi et al., 1993; Koliatsos et al., 1993; Griesbeck et al., 1995; Copray and Brouwer, 1997). The changes in neurotrophin expression observed in the post-mortem muscles of ALS patients in our study presumably reflect an ALS specific response. Most likely the raised levels of all neurotrophins observed here would effect the motoneurons retrogradely, if axonal transport mechanisms were not affected in the degenerating motoneurons (Collard et al., 1995). In this respect it has been demonstrated that due to alterations in the neurofilament network fast and slow axonal transport are impaired in spinal cords of hSOD1 transgenic mice (Williamson and Cleveland, 1999; Zhang et al., 1997).

Furthermore, effects of increased neurotrophic support would strongly depend on the motoneuronal pattern of expressed neurotrophin receptors. In this respect it has been shown that the expression of TrkA is altered in ALS spinal motoneurons (Nishio et al., 1998) and we and others have demonstrated that $p75^{NTR}$ mRNA and immunoreactivity is increased in spinal motoneurons of ALS patients and hSOD1 transgenic mice (Lowry et al., 2001; Copray et al., 2003).

Originally, activation of the p75 neurotrophin receptor expressed by affected spinal motoneurons was thought to induce apoptosis pathways (Miller and Kaplan, 1998; Lowry et al., 2001). However, our data on motoneuron cell counts obtained from the transgenic animal model could not reveal an involvement of $p75^{NTR}$ in the occurrence of motoneuron death via apoptosis. In contrast, absence of $p75^{NTR}$ in female hSOD mice seemed to result in even a greater reduction of spinal motoneuron numbers. The paradox of a reduction of spinal motoneurons in female hSOD1/$p75^{NTR-/-}$ mice concomitant with a delay in disease progress may be explained by the occurrence of a less intense astrogliosis in these mice (Kust et al., 2003). Albeit speculative, the decreased toxic influence of these astrocytes on the few surviving motoneurons might have compensated for the loss of the degenerated motoneurons. In the past 5 years, it has become obvious that $p75^{NTR}$ is not just an assistant receptor of the Trk receptors during embryogenesis nor merely a death receptor. It is a receptor expressed in stressed cells and it plays a key role in determining the fate of stressed or injured cells: apoptosis or adaptation and survival (Dobrowsky and Carter, 2000). Activation of $p75^{NTR}$ may be involved, possibly via the stress transcription factor ATF3, in the production and release of the distress signals (e.g. cytokines, chemokines) known to be produced by injured neurons. These distress signals are thought to recruit astrocytes and microglia either for neurotrophic rescue or for fast apoptotic removal depending on the gravity of the injury. Our observations on the altered astrogliosis in female hSOD1/$p75^{NTR-/-}$ seem to be in accordance with studies that have shown a relationship between sex hormones and modulation of astrocytic properties, although the mechanisms underlying this regulation are still obscure (Garcia-Segura et al., 1999).

Our original hypothesis that re-expressed p75^{NTR} on ALS motoneurons induces their degeneration (in response to higher neurotrophin amounts from the muscles), did not prove to be universally valid. It has become conceivable that the severe imbalances that we found in neurotrophin- and p75^{NTR}-levels are not primary phenomena in the pathology of ALS. Furthermore, regarding the sexual difference between the double transgenic mice, p75^{NTR} seems not to be directly involved in motoneuronal death, since p75^{NTR} deficient hSOD1 mice did not display enhanced cell survival.

However, the milder clinical symptom gravity and the shift of disease endpoints that we observed in female hSOD1/p75$^{NTR-/-}$ mice indicate that this neurotrophin receptor is of importance for the pathology of ALS. Most likely this enigmatic neurotrophin receptor is indirectly influencing neuronal (and presumably also glial) properties and thereby is contributing to secondary pathogenic events in ALS.

References

[1] Al Chalabi A, Andersen PM, Nilsson P, Chioza B, Andersson JL, Russ C, Shaw CE, Powell JF, Leigh PN (1999) Deletions of the heavy neurofilament subunit tail in amyotrophic lateral sclerosis. *Hum Mol Genet 8*: 157-164.

[2] Appel SH, Smith RG, Engelhardt JI, Stefani E (1994) Evidence for autoimmunity in amyotrophic lateral sclerosis. *J Neurol Sci 124* Suppl:14-9.: 14-19.

[3] Boyd JG, Gordon T (2003) Neurotrophic factors and their receptors in axonal regeneration and functional recovery after peripheral nerve injury. *Mol Neurobiol 27*: 277-324.

[4] Bruijn LI, Becher MW, Lee MK, Anderson KL, Jenkins NA, Copeland NG, Sisodia SS, Rothstein JD, Borchelt DR, Price DL, Cleveland DW (1997) ALS-linked SOD1 mutant G85R mediates damage to astrocytes and promotes rapidly progressive disease with SOD1-containing inclusions. *Neuron 18*: 327-338.

[5] Casaccia-Bonnefil P, Kong H, Chao MV (1998) Neurotrophins: the biological paradox of survival factors eliciting apoptosis. *Cell Death Differ 5*: 357-364.

[6] Chao M, Casaccia-Bonnefil P, Carter B, Chittka A, Kong H, Yoon SO (1998) Neurotrophin receptors: mediators of life and death. *Brain Res Brain Res Rev 26*: 295-301.

[7] Chao MV (2003) Neurotrophins and their receptors: a convergence point for many signalling pathways. *Nat Rev Neurosci 4*: 299-309.

[8] Collard JF, Cote F, Julien JP (1995) Defective axonal transport in a transgenic mouse model of amyotrophic lateral sclerosis. *Nature 375*: 61-64.

[9] Cookson MR, Shaw PJ (1999) Oxidative stress and motor neurone disease. *Brain Pathol 9*: 165-186.

[10] Copray JC, Brouwer N (1997) Neurotrophin-3 mRNA expression in rat intrafusal muscle fibres after denervation and reinnervation. *Neurosci Lett 236*: 41-44.

[11] Copray JC, Jaarsma D, Kust BM, Bruggeman RW, Mantingh I, Brouwer N, Boddeke HW (2003) Expression of the low affinity neurotrophin receptor p75 in spinal

motoneurons in a transgenic mouse model for amyotrophic lateral sclerosis. *Neuroscience 116*: 685-694.

[12] Delbono O, Magnelli V, Sawada T, Smith RG, Appel SH, Stefani E (1993) Fab fragments from amyotrophic lateral sclerosis IgG affect calcium channels of skeletal muscle. *Am J Physiol 264*: C537-C543.

[13] Dobrowsky RT, Carter BD (2000) p75 neurotrophin receptor signaling: mechanisms for neurotrophic modulation of cell stress? *J Neurosci Res 61*: 237-243.

[14] Ferri CC, Moore FA, Bisby MA (1998) Effects of facial nerve injury on mouse motoneurons lacking the p75 low-affinity neurotrophin receptor. *J Neurobiol 34*: 1-9.

[15] Funakoshi H, Frisen J, Barbany G, Timmusk T, Zachrisson O, Verge VM, Persson H (1993) Differential expression of mRNAs for neurotrophins and their receptors after axotomy of the sciatic nerve. *J Cell Biol 123*: 455-465.

[16] Garcia-Segura LM, Naftolin F, Hutchison JB, Azcoitia I, Chowen JA (1999) Role of astroglia in estrogen regulation of synaptic plasticity and brain repair. *J Neurobiol 40*: 574-584.

[17] Griesbeck O, Parsadanian AS, Sendtner M, Thoenen H (1995) Expression of neurotrophins in skeletal muscle: quantitative comparison and significance for motoneuron survival and maintenance of function. *J Neurosci Res 42*: 21-33.

[18] Gurney ME, Cutting FB, Zhai P, Andrus PK, Hall ED (1996) Pathogenic mechanisms in familial amyotrophic lateral sclerosis due to mutation of Cu, Zn superoxide dismutase. *Pathol Biol (Paris) 44*: 51-56.

[19] Gurney ME, Pu H, Chiu AY, Dal Canto MC, Polchow CY, Alexander DD, Caliendo J, Hentati A, Kwon YW, Deng HX, Chen WZPSRL&ST (1994) Motor neuron degeneration in mice that express a human Cu,Zn superoxide dismutase mutation. *Science 264:* 1772-1775.

[20] Hand CK, Rouleau GA (2002) Familial amyotrophic lateral sclerosis. *Muscle Nerve 25*: 135-159.

[21] Hempstead BL (2002) The many faces of p75NTR. *Curr Opin Neurobiol 12*: 260-267.

[22] Henderson CE, Camu W, Mettling C, Gouin A, Poulsen K, Karihaloo M, Rullamas J, Evans T, McMahon SB, Armanini MP, Berkemeier L, Phillips HS, Rosenthal A (1993) Neurotrophins promote motor neuron survival and are present in embryonic limb bud. *Nature 363*: 266-270.

[23] Ho BK, Alexianu ME, Colom LV, Mohamed AH, Serrano F, Appel SH (1996) Expression of calbindin-D28K in motoneuron hybrid cells after retroviral infection with calbindin-D28K cDNA prevents amyotrophic lateral sclerosis IgG-mediated cytotoxicity. *Proc Natl Acad Sci U S A 93*: 6796-6801.

[24] Huang EJ, Reichardt LF (2003) Trk receptors: roles in neuronal signal transduction. *Annu Rev Biochem 72*:609-42.: 609-642.

[25] Ince P, Stout N, Shaw P, Slade J, Hunziker W, Heizmann CW, Baimbridge KG (1993) Parvalbumin and calbindin D-28k in the human motor system and in motor neuron disease. *Neuropathol Appl Neurobiol 19*: 291-299.

[26] Kok AB (1997) Ascorbate availability and neurodegeneration in amyotrophic lateral sclerosis. *Med Hypotheses 48*: 281-296.

[27] Koliatsos VE, Clatterbuck RE, Winslow JW, Cayouette MH, Price DL (1993) Evidence that brain-derived neurotrophic factor is a trophic factor for motor neurons in vivo. *Neuron 10*: 359-367.

[28] Koliatsos VE, Crawford TO, Price DL (1991) Axotomy induces nerve growth factor receptor immunoreactivity in spinal motor neurons. *Brain Res 549*: 297-304.

[29] Kostic V, Jackson-Lewis V, de Bilbao F, Dubois-Dauphin M, Przedborski S (1997) Bcl-2: prolonging life in a transgenic mouse model of familial amyotrophic lateral sclerosis. *Science 277*: 559-562.

[30] Kust BM, Brouwer N, Mantingh IJ, Boddeke HW, Copray JC (2003) Reduced p75NTR expression delays disease onset only in female mice of a transgenic model of familial amyotrophic lateral sclerosis. *Amyotroph Lateral Scler Other Motor Neuron Disord 4*: 100-105.

[31] Kust BM, Copray JC, Brouwer N, Troost D, Boddeke HW (2002) Elevated levels of neurotrophins in human biceps brachii tissue of amyotrophic lateral sclerosis. *Exp Neurol 177*: 419-427.

[32] Lee KF, Li E, Huber LJ, Landis SC, Sharpe AH, Chao MV, Jaenisch R (1992) Targeted mutation of the gene encoding the low affinity NGF receptor p75 leads to deficits in the peripheral sensory nervous system. *Cell 69*: 737-749.

[33] Li M, Ona VO, Guegan C, Chen M, Jackson-Lewis V, Andrews LJ, Olszewski AJ, Stieg PE, Lee JP, Przedborski S, Friedlander RM (2000) Functional role of caspase-1 and caspase-3 in an ALS transgenic mouse model. *Science 288*: 335-339.

[34] Louvel E, Hugon J, Doble A (1997) Therapeutic advances in amyotrophic lateral sclerosis. *Trends Pharmacol Sci 18*: 196-203.

[35] Lowry KS, Murray SS, McLean CA, Talman P, Mathers S, Lopes EC, Cheema SS (2001) A potential role for the p75 low-affinity neurotrophin receptor in spinal motor neuron degeneration in murine and human amyotrophic lateral sclerosis. *Amyotroph Lateral Scler Other Motor Neuron Disord 2*: 127-134.

[36] Ludolph AC, Meyer T, Riepe MW (2000) The role of excitotoxicity in ALS--what is the evidence? *J Neurol 247 Suppl 1*:I7-16.: I7-16.

[37] Martin LJ (1999) Neuronal death in amyotrophic lateral sclerosis is apoptosis: possible contribution of a programmed cell death mechanism. *J Neuropathol Exp Neurol 58*: 459-471.

[38] Martin LJ (2000) p53 is abnormally elevated and active in the CNS of patients with amyotrophic lateral sclerosis. *Neurobiol Dis 7*: 613-622.

[39] Martin LJ, Price AC, Kaiser A, Shaikh AY, Liu Z (2000) Mechanisms for neuronal degeneration in amyotrophic lateral sclerosis and in models of motor neuron death (Review). *Int J Mol Med 5*: 3-13.

[40] Mendell LM, Arvanian VL (2002) Diversity of neurotrophin action in the postnatal spinal cord. *Brain Res Brain Res Rev 40*: 230-239.

[41] Miller FD, Kaplan DR (1998) Life and death decisions: a biological role for the p75 neurotrophin receptor. *Cell Death Differ 5:* 343-345.

[42] Mu X, He J, Anderson DW, Trojanowski JQ, Springer JE (1996) Altered expression of bcl-2 and bax mRNA in amyotrophic lateral sclerosis spinal cord motor neurons. *Ann Neurol 40*: 379-386.

[43] Nishio T, Sunohara N, Furukawa S (1998) Neutrophin switching in spinal motoneurons of amyotrophic lateral sclerosis. *Neuroreport 9*: 1661-1665.

[44] Piehl F, Frisen J, Risling M, Hokfelt T, Cullheim S (1994) Increased trkB mRNA expression by axotomized motoneurones. *Neuroreport 5*: 697-700.

[45] Reiner A, Medina L, Figueredo-Cardenas G, Anfinson S (1995) Brainstem motoneuron pools that are selectively resistant in amyotrophic lateral sclerosis are preferentially enriched in parvalbumin: evidence from monkey brainstem for a calcium-mediated mechanism in sporadic ALS. *Exp Neurol 131*: 239-250.

[46] Rosen DR, Siddique T, Patterson D, Figlewicz DA, Sapp P, Hentati A, Donaldson D, Goto J, O'Regan JP, Deng HX, Rahmani Z, Krizus A, McKenna-Yasek D, Cayabyab A, Gaston SM, Berger R, Tanzi RE, Halperin JJ, Herzfeld B, Van den Bergh R, Hung W-Y, Bird T, Deng G, Mulder DW, Smyth C, Laing NG, Soriano E, Pericak-Vance MA, Haines J, Rouleau GA, Gusella JS, Horvitz HR, Brown Jr RH (1993) Mutations in Cu/Zn superoxide dismutase gene are associated with familial amyotrophic lateral sclerosis. *Nature 362*: 59-62.

[47] Rothstein JD (1996) Therapeutic horizons for amyotrophic lateral sclerosis. *Curr Opin Neurobiol 6*: 679-687.

[48] Roux PP, Barker PA (2002) Neurotrophin signaling through the p75 neurotrophin receptor. *Prog Neurobiol 67*: 203-233.

[49] Seeburger JL, Tarras S, Natter H, Springer JE (1993) Spinal cord motoneurons express p75NGFR and p145trkB mRNA in amyotrophic lateral sclerosis. *Brain Res 621*: 111-115.

[50] Segal RA, Greenberg ME (1996) Intracellular signaling pathways activated by neurotrophic factors. *Annu Rev Neurosci 19*:463-89.: 463-489.

[51] Smith RG, Hamilton S, Hofmann F, Schneider T, Nastainczyk W, Birnbaumer L, Stefani E, Appel SH (1992) Serum antibodies to L-type calcium channels in patients with amyotrophic lateral sclerosis. *N Engl J Med 327*: 1721-1728.

[52] Van Westerlaak MG, Bar PR, Cools AR, Joosten EA (2001) Malonate-induced cortico-motoneuron death is attenuated by NT-4, but not by BDNF or NT-3. *Neuroreport 12*: 1355-1358.

[53] Wang X, Bauer JH, Li Y, Shao Z, Zetoune FS, Cattaneo E, Vincenz C (2001) Characterization of a p75(NTR) apoptotic signaling pathway using a novel cellular model. *J Biol Chem 276*: 33812-33820.

[54] Williamson TL, Cleveland DW (1999) Slowing of axonal transport is a very early event in the toxicity of ALS-linked SOD1 mutants to motor neurons. *Nat Neurosci 2*: 50-56.

[55] Wong PC, Borchelt DR (1995) Motor neuron disease caused by mutations in superoxide dismutase 1. *Curr Opin Neurol 8*: 294-301.

[56] Xu H, Federoff H, Maragos J, Parada LF, Kessler JA (1994) Viral transduction of trkA into cultured nodose and spinal motor neurons conveys NGF responsiveness. *Dev Biol 163*: 152-161.

[57] Yan Q, Elliott J, Snider WD (1992) Brain-derived neurotrophic factor rescues spinal motor neurons from axotomy-induced cell death. *Nature 360*: 753-755.

[58] Yan Q, Johnson EM, Jr. (1988) An immunohistochemical study of the nerve growth factor receptor in developing rats. *J Neurosci 8*: 3481-3498.

[59] Yi FH, Lautrette C, Vermot-Desroches C, Bordessoule D, Couratier P, Wijdenes J, Preud'homme JL, Jauberteau MO (2000) In vitro induction of neuronal apoptosis by anti-Fas antibody-containing sera from amyotrophic lateral sclerosis patients. *J Neuroimmunol 109*: 211-220.

[60] Zhang B, Tu P, Abtahian F, Trojanowski JQ, Lee VM (1997) Neurofilaments and orthograde transport are reduced in ventral root axons of transgenic mice that express human SOD1 with a G93A mutation. *J Cell Biol 139*: 1307-1315.

In: Amyotrophic Lateral Sclerosis: New Research
Editor: Christine A. Murray, pp. 217-243

ISBN 1-59454-179-5

Chapter IX

The Use of Acoustic Speech Analysis and Dysarthria Profile Tests in Detecting Early Speech Disturbances in Patients with Amyotrophic Lateral Sclerosis

B. Tomik[1,*] , W. Wszołek[2], A. Pichór[1] and A. Szczudlik[1]
[1]Department of Neurology, Jagiellonian University, Krakow
[2]Academy of Mining and Metallurgy, Krakow, Poland.

Abstract

Background

A diagnosis of definite amyotrophic lateral sclerosis (ALS) requires the presence of motor neuron degeneration signs on at least three spinal levels or two spinal and bulbar levels. In the initial stage of the disease there is a group of patients in whom only limbs involvement is apparent. EMG studies of bulbar region muscles are of limited value. There is a need for development of new diagnostic tools facilitating the early detection of bulbar involvement in ALS patients.

Objective

To evaluate the usefulness of acoustic speech analysis (ASA) and dysarthria profile tests (DPT) in the early detection of speech disturbances in ALS.

* Correspondence concerning this article should be addressed to: Barbara Tomik MD, PhD; Department of Neurology, Medical College Jagiellonian University; 3 Botaniczna St, 31-503 Krakow, Poland; Tel. + 48 12 424 86 00 ,fax +48 12 424 86 26; E-mail:tomik@neuro.cm-uj.krakow.pl

Methods

We studied 56 sporadic, definite and probable ALS subjects. Te disease severity was scored on the Norris scale. The evidence of dysarthria was measured using two independent, quantitative and semiquantitative methods such as ASA, which is based on the sounds test and DPT including tests of the respiration, phonation, articulation, speech intelligibility, prosody, face movements, diadochokinesis and reflexes, respectively. Firstly, DPT and ASA were carried out in ALS subjects and 67 healthy age-matched controls. Secondly, limb and bulbar onset ALS subjects were compared separately in three consecutive examinations.

Results

The mean sound distances from the pattern of all the sounds measured by ASA were greater both in bulbar and limb onset ALS subjects as compared to the controls ($p<0.001$). The mean sound distances from the pattern for 4 out of 5 sounds measured were greater in the bulbar than in limb onset ALS patients: "W" ($p<0.001$), "I" ($p<0.05$), "O" ($p<0.05$), "B" ($p<0.05$). The mean score of DPT in the whole ALS group was significantly lower as compared to the controls ($p<0.001$). A comparison between bulbar and limb onset ALS subjects, as well as between the limb onset group and healthy controls revealed in each case the significant difference in the mean DPT score ($p<0.01$).

Conclusion

Our results confirm the usefulness of ASA and DPT in the early detection of bulbar pathology in limb onset ALS patients.

Keywords: ALS, early speech disturbances, detection

Introduction

Amyotrophic lateral sclerosis (ALS) is a progressive disorder in which degeneration of upper and lower motor neurones leads to the subsequent weakness of the bulbar, limb, thoracic and abdominal muscles with relative sparing of oculomotor muscles and the sphincter function. The neurodegenerative process of cortical, brainstem and spinal cord motoneurones is of unknown origin [1,2]. Most often the signs of motoneurones' degeneration occur first in the limbs. Early bulbar symptoms i.e., dysarthria (i.e., the voice deterioration, slurred speech), dysphagia (choking, swallowing difficulties) and sometimes pathological emotional lability [3], are less frequent and appear in 25% of patients. Death from ventilatory failure ensues usually within 5 years from the onset. Patients with bulbar signs deteriorate more rapidly, usually 1 or 2 years after the diagnosis [1,2]. The mechanism underlying these differences at a rate of disease progression is unknown. The prevalence and measurement of the cranial motor neurone involvement in ALS is of particular interest, because the loss of bulbar function contributes to the communication disability requiring speech therapy and is responsible for the increased mortality rate.

Dysarthria is a neurogenic motor speech impairment characterised by abnormalities in the facial movement rate, phonation, articulation, and intelligibility of speech [1] The speech disturbance of ALS patients is typically classified as a mixed dysarthria due to the presence of both the upper and lower motor neuron involvement. The relative contribution of flaccidity and spasticity in the impairment of speech intelligibility varies among individuals [1,3]. The dysarthria resulting from the disease can be rapidly progressive and have an impact on the whole speech system [3]. The ALS patients with the limb onset of ALS lose their speaking communication relatively later as compared with bulbar onset ALS subjects.

Dysarthria in ALS is characterised by the grossly defective articulation, short phrases, inappropriate pauses, imprecise consonants, extremely slow laborious speech, marked hypernasality and severe harshness [1,3,4]. In addition to the strained/strangled voice there is almost a complete disruption of prosody. In regards to the phonatory system, perceptual features can include: harshness, strain-strangled voice, breathiness, tremor, and pitch abnormalities [1,3].

Better understanding of the nature and course of dysarthria in ALS is certainly an important topic. The identification of initial speech changes without a strong evidence of bulbar dysfunction would assist with an early speech therapist intervention and clinical trials. Ball et al [5] showed that the strongest early predictors of bulbar speech dysfunction included altered voice quality (laryngeal control), speaking rate, and communication effectiveness.

Although different approaches have been tried so far, currently there are no objective methods available to assess early symptoms of speech dysfunction due to ALS. Until now voice assessment in ALS patients has been done mainly by perceptual analysis [6]. Only a few detailed reports have been published on the nature of speech and voice changes during the course of ALS. Dysarthria has been studied by the application of the physiological (electromyographic and kinematic) and computerised acoustic methods [7-22], aerodynamics method [6] but still there is no a standardized, easy and commonly used objective method to detect and follow the progression of dysarthria due to ALS.

The purpose of this study was to evaluate the usefulness of two different methods i.e., up-to-date, detailed, quantitative assessment of the speech disturbances by using the acoustic speech analysis (ASA) and the semiquantitative, traditional method by using the dysarthria profile tests (DPT) for detection of the early speech disturbances in ALS patients and clarified if they could be useful in clinics for assessment of speech dysfunction.

For the detailed assessment by ASA we used the Euclidian principle for analyses of sequences of sound formants and the mean sound distances from the pattern /Δf=125 Hz, ΔT=9ms, Δs=0,5dB/. The attempt to define the specific profile of dysarthric speech, by the acoustic computer analysis based on the Euclidian principle, has never been previously undertaken in ALS patients.

Study Design

We studied 56 sporadic, definite and probable ALS subjects. The disease severity was scored on the Norris scale. The evidence of early signs of dysarthria was measured using two independent, quantitative and semiquantitative methods as ASA, which is based on the measure of the sounds distances as compared to pattern and the DPT including test of the respiration, phonation, articulation, speech intelligibility, prosody, face movements, diadochokinesis and reflexes, respectively. Three out of 56 patients included in the study withdrew their consent for the examination during the first analysis, so they were excluded from the study. Firstly, ASA and DPT were carried out in the total number of 53 ALS subjects and 67 healthy age-matched controls. Secondly, limb and bulbar onset ALS subjects were compared separately in groups containing different numbers of patients which was the result of excluding some patients from particular stages of the examination or was due to the aggravation of symptoms of the disease, inability to be present in three consecutive examinations of ASA and DPT. In ASA examinations we included 53 out of 56 ALS patients and divided this group into the bulbar and limb patients based on neurological examination and the occurrence of the speech disturbances. The results obtained from this group were compared with 30 healthy volunteers (controls). In DPT examinations we included 43 out of 56 ALS patients and divided this group into nondysarthric (n=28) and dysarthric (n=15) patients based on the dysarthria features in the history of the patient's disease and perceptual changes of the speech. The results obtained from this group were compared with 37 healthy volunteers (controls). The main aim of both of the performed examinations was to evaluate the early speech changes in ALS subjects.

Patients for the Acoustic Speech Analysis (ASA)

In the ALS group there were 53 patients (21 females, 32 males), mean age of 53.66± 10.30 (29-76 yrs). Subjects with only sporadic ALS were studied and classified as definite (n=27) or probable (n=26) ALS based on El Escorial WFN criteria [23].All of them were treated in MND Centre in Krakow in 1996-1999 yr. The duration of ALS symptoms ranged from a few months to 2 years. Each patient was visited every 10-12 weeks, by the same neurologist. To evaluate disease severity Norris scale (maximum - 120 point) [26] and ALSFRS (maximum - 40 point) were used [24]. Bulbar examination included assessment of difficulties in chewing food, swallowing, speech, breathing, presence of cough, evidence of labile emotions, jaw jerk, muscle wasting or fasciculations. Patients were categorised into two groups of ALS: 15 bulbar patients (with presence of dysarthria and bulbar or pseudobulbar signs in the neurological examination) and 38 limb patients (no clinical evidence bulbar or corticobulbar involvement). The control group consisted of 30, aged and sex -matched healthy subjects (19 females, 11 males), aged 46.87± 6.24 (24-78 yrs) with no prior history of neurological disease, speech, hearing, voice, or language disorders. The control group provided the basic pattern for the computerised acoustic analysis. A written consent for this study was obtained from all patients as well as from controls.

Procedure of Acoustic Speech Analysis

Each patient (47 out of 53) underwent the series of acoustic and computer-based speech sounds and voice articulation testing. They were recorded during three test sessions every 10-12 weeks. Only two patients died before the third acoustic test and three patients were excluded because their state deteriorated quickly (due to anarthria) prior to the third acoustic examination. One patient did not appear for the third test. Two speech tasks were performed by each subject (ALS and control group). First, each subject read and repeated a test sound three times. In the second task, each subject read and repeated three times a standard sentence. The tasks were tape-recorded. The following consonants and vowels were analysed: R, L, D, T, M, W, P, B, G, K , H, Q , O, U, I. They were analysed separately and then in the standard Polish sentence: *W CALYM KRAJU DZIS JEST LADNA POGODA (The weather is nice in the whole country today.).* The sounds and the standard sentence were written on flashcards and presented to the subjects, who were instructed to read the sounds and the test sentence. The examinations were done by the same engineer in all cases. The acoustic signal of speech was transduced by a microphone (Bruel&Kjaer), placed approximately 10 cm from the subject's mouth, and then recorded on a low-noise tape (NAGRA IV SJ, Kudelski SA). All the sessions for all the subjects were recorded in a sound-proof room. The sound measurements, including articulation time and pause duration, were made using a sonograph (Bruel&Kjaer, 3348) set to a wideband filter (FF-2425, Bruel&Kjaer) of 25 Hz and a frequency range from 0 to 7000 Hz. The tape-recorded speech samples of the separate sounds and the standard sentence were studied with spectrograms prepared by a spectrograph and then with a microcomputer speech analysis program (computer PC 486). This programme allows to measure the mean sound distances between chosen consonants and vowels in ALS patients and to compare them with the basic pattern in the control group. The change of sound articulation was measured using the time-frequency computer analyses, (Δf=125 Hz, Δ T=9ms, Δs=0,5dB). The Euclidian principle *(see Appendix)* was applied to assess the sound mean distances from the pattern in the matrix (characteristic attribute: M0, M1, M2, WS1, WS2, WS3, WS4). Finally this prompted the selection of the most discriminatory sounds. Acoustic analyses were done by measuring the mean distances between the sound and the pattern in the three subsequent acoustic tests, every 12 weeks for the detailed observation of the speech changes as the disease progressed. The Norris scales obtained from patients during the time of ASA examinations were also monitored.

Statistical Data

For statistical analyses t-Student tests were used to compare demographic data between ALS and control subjects, and mean sound distances between bulbar, limb and control groups. ANOVA was used to test the difference between the mean value of mean sound distances in both ALS groups and mean sound distances of the pattern (control subjects) at first and third acoustic analyses.

Patients for Dysarthria Profile Tests (DPT) Analysis

Forty-three out of 56 ALS patients were included in the DPT study. These 43 ALS sporadic patients (19 females, 24 males), aged from 45 to 69 years (mean age: 54.1±10.2 yr.), were treated in MND Centre in Krakow in 1996-1999 yr. They were classified as definite (n=17) or probable (n=26) ALS according to El Escorial WFN Criteria [23]. The duration of ALS symptoms ranged from 5 months to 33 months. Each patient was examined every 12 weeks by the same neurologist and scored using the Norris scale [24]. The neurological examination included a detailed evaluation of the bulbar function i.e., difficulties in chewing food, swallowing, speech, breathing, presence of cough, evidence of emotional lability, presence of a jaw jerk and gag reflexes, and muscle and tongue wasting or fasciculations. The lack of evidence of dysarthria in the neurological examination and perceptual assessment was used to select ALS "nondysarthric" subjects (n=28) from the whole group of ALS patients examined during this time (n=43). The used term: "nondysarthric" did not exclude the occurrence of some not very aggravated bulbar sings in ALS subjects but excluded the patients with any speech changes. Nine (definite ALS according to El Escorial Criteria) out of 28 nondysarthric patients were presented with some bulbar signs in the neurological examination i.e., brisk jaw jerk, lack of gag reflexes, brisk gag reflexes. None of them noticed any changes of speech. None of them was presented with wasting or fasciculations of face's muscles and the tongue. None of them was presented with any swallowing or breathing problems (there were no changes in FVC examinations done obligatorily by spirometry). There were 15 ALS patients with dysarthria (dysarthric) who declared the occurrence of the progressive speech difficulties and presented bulbar and pseudobulbar signs in the neurological examinations as well as the perceptual changes of speech (i.e., defective articulation, short phrases, imprecise consonants, slowness of speech, hypernasality).There were 37 age, sex -matched healthy control subjects (22 females, 15 males), aged from 24 to 78 years (mean: 52.3 ± 12.8 yr.) without a previous history of neurological disease, speech, hearing, voice, or language disorders. A written consent for this study was obtained from all the patients as well as from the controls.

Procedure of Dysarthria Profile Tests Analysis

Dysarthria profile tests (DPT) [18] were used to assess the occurrence of early speech disturbances and observe them during the disease progression in "nondysarthric" ALS subjects. All DPT examinations were done by the same speech therapist. The study was performed in two independent stages. First, during the recruitment to the study, DPTs were carried out in 28 "nondysarthric" ALS subjects (see demographic data in table I) and the results were compared to the 15 ALS dysarthric patients and separately to the 37 age, sex - matched healthy controls. Secondly, 28 "nondysarthric" ALS subjects were included in the study of three subsequent examinations of DPT and the Norris scale, every 12 weeks for analysis of the speech disturbances and disease progression. Only 25 out of 28 ALS patients underwent all three examinations of DPT and the Norris scale. Three patients did not take part in the third test.

Dysarthria profile tests (DPT) [18] (*see Appendix*) are a semiquantitative method assessing different functional elements of the productive speech organs by tests of: respiration, phonation, articulation, and intelligibility of speech, prosody and movements of face and tongue, diadochokinesis and face reflexes. Each out of 8 tests is composed of different numbers of tasks evaluated according to 5-point rating scales (4-normal, 3-good, 2-fair, 1-poor, 0-nil). The mean scores ($\bar{x} \pm SD$) of DPT were compared separately for each test between the control and the ALS subjects (stage I) and then among the whole ALS group of patients in three subsequent DPT examinations (stage II). Finally, the correlation between the mean scores ($\bar{x} \pm SD$) of each DPT and the mean value ($\bar{x} \pm SD$) of the Norris scale in ALS subjects, in each out of three subsequent examinations was calculated (step II).

Table 1. The mean values of the Norris score in the ALS subjects,the bulbar ALS group and the limb ALS group (test I-III) (ANOVA- A1-A3 and t-Student test, independent- A3-B3)

Group	Test I Norris score X±SD	Test II Norris score X±SD	Test III Norris score X±SD
ALS subjects	92.13 ± 19.96	83.32 ± 25.45	77.71 ± 30.10
Bulbar group (**A**)	81.33 ± 18.93	65.61 ± 21.84	*** 54.84 ± 16.05
Limb group (**B**)	92.13 ± 20.72	83.32 ± 25.46	* 77.71 ± 30.10

*** - $p < 0.001$ for A1 – A3 * - $p < 0.05$ for A3 – B3

Statistical Data

For statistical analyses a Student t- independent test was used to compare demographic data between ALS and the control subjects and the mean scores in each dysarthria profile test between ALS and the control groups. ANOVA was used to test differences between the mean scores in DPT test in ALS group studied in three subsequent examinations and to calculate the correlation between the mean scores of each DPT and the mean value of the Norris scale in ALS subjects, in each out of three subsequent examinations.

Results

Acoustic Speech Analysis (ASA)

Disease progression was measured using the Norris scale. In our study it was clear that the initial mean Norris scores in the two ALS groups were different (bulbar ALS group 81.33 ±18.93, limb group 92.13 ± 20.72). Over the course of the disease, the mean Norris scores decreased significantly in both groups ($p<0.05$) (Figure 1a-b), but the bulbar group mean

Norris score deteriorated significantly quicker (Norris score- bulbar group: 54.84 ±16.05, limb group 77.71 ± 30.10) ($p<0.001$). Table 1 and figures 1a-c show the Norris scores for each ALS group in the first and third examination.

Based on the initial analyses the following sounds were chosen for further studies: "B","I","O","W","T". Acoustic analyses were done by measuring the mean distances between the sound and the pattern in the three acoustic tests. In the control group the maximum mean sounds distance was $\bar{x} = 0.12$, and in all ALS group $\bar{x} = 0.62$. The differences between the mean distances for each sound in both ALS groups were significant ($p < 0.001$). Table 2 and figure 2 demonstrate the mean sounds distances in the ALS and control subjects in the first examination.

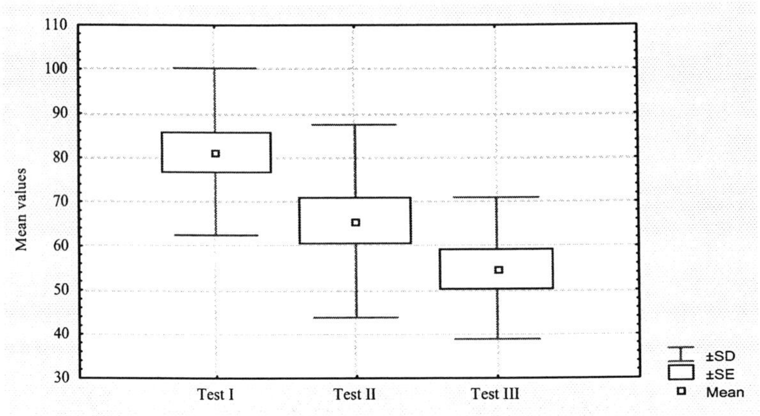

Figure 1a. The mean values of the Norris score in the bulbar ALS group (test I-III).

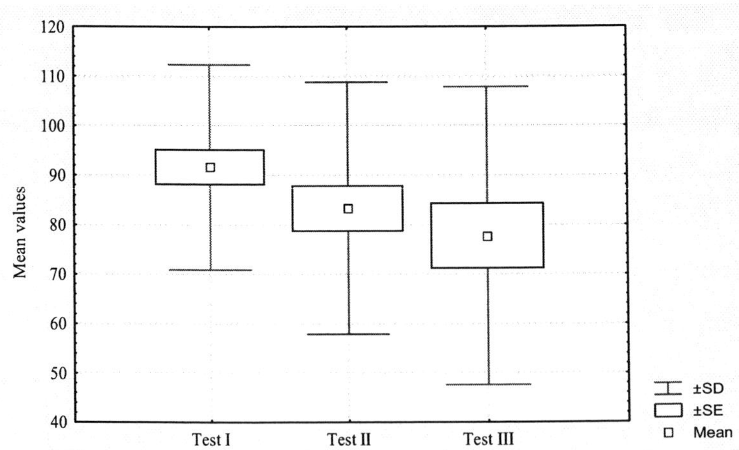

Figure 1b. The mean values of the Norris score in the limb ALS group (test I-III).

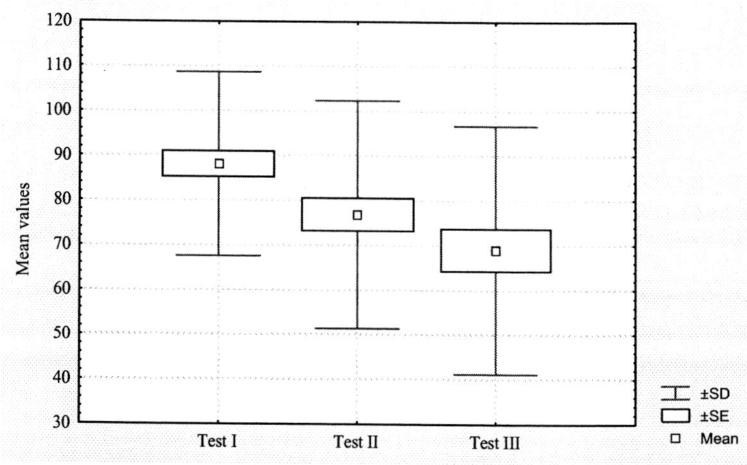

Figure 1c. The mean values of the Norris score in all ALS patients (test I-III).

Table 2. The comparison of mean sounds distances in all ALS patients as compared to the control subjects (t- Student, independent test)

Sounds	Control group N = 30		ALS group N = 47		Value *P*
	$\bar{X} \pm SD$	[range] min – max	$\bar{X} \pm SD$	[range] min – max	
I	0.08 ± 0.03	0.04 – 0.13	0.50 ± 0.23	0.20 – 1.36	*< 0.001*
T	0.11 ± 0.03	0.05 – 0.18	0.59 ± 0.18	0.27 – 0.94	*< 0.001*
W	0.08 ± 0.03	0.02 – 0.15	0.57 ± 0.25	0.24 – 1.30	*< 0.001*
O	0.10 ± 0.04	0.05 – 0.20	0.46 ± 0.19	0.10 – 1.11	*< 0.001*
B	0.12 ± 0.05	0.04 – 0.22	0.62 ± 0.25	0.20 – 1.47	*< 0.001*

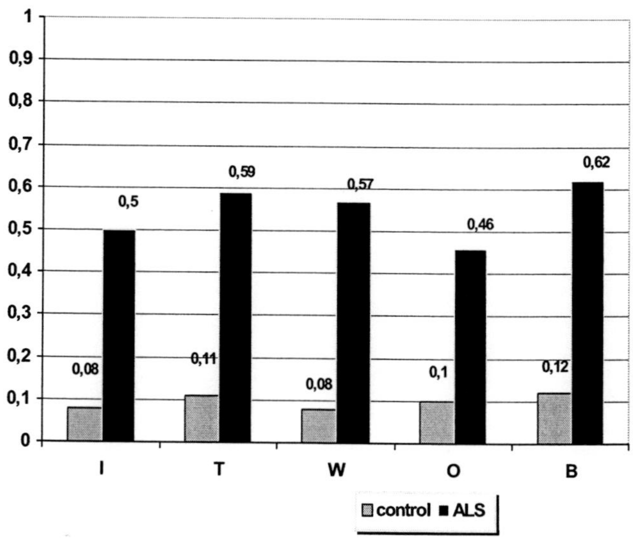

Figure 2. The comparison of mean sounds distances in all ALS patients as compared to the control subjects (t- Student, independent test).

When comparing the mean sound distance to the control group (pattern) we noted a significant increase over the time of study of the mean distances for all chosen sounds in both ALS groups, ($p<0.001$) (Table 3, Figure 3,4). These results proved the progression of pathological changes (i.e. slowness of the speech) for all examined sounds in both ALS groups. We draw attention to the significant increase of the mean distances for chosen sounds over the three acoustic tests of all examined sounds, in the nondysarthric limb ALS group (Table 3). To characterise the apparent specific dysarthria profile of ALS, the patients underwent the third speech acoustic test which compared the mean sound distances to those of the controls, and in which the Euclidian principle was applied. The significant increase in mean distances for the chosen sounds obtained between the first and third test was compared to the controls (Table 3).

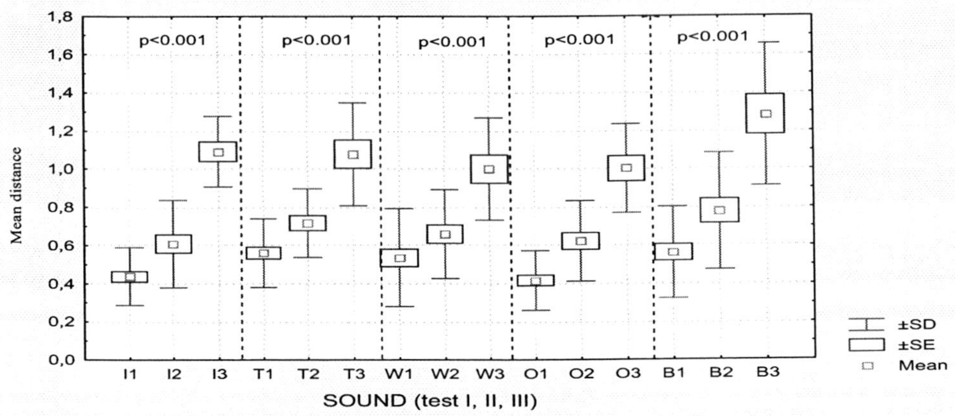

Figure 3. The comparison of mean distances of the chosen sounds in the bulbar group as compared to the control pattern. Acoustic computer analyses, test I-III.(*ANOVA test*).

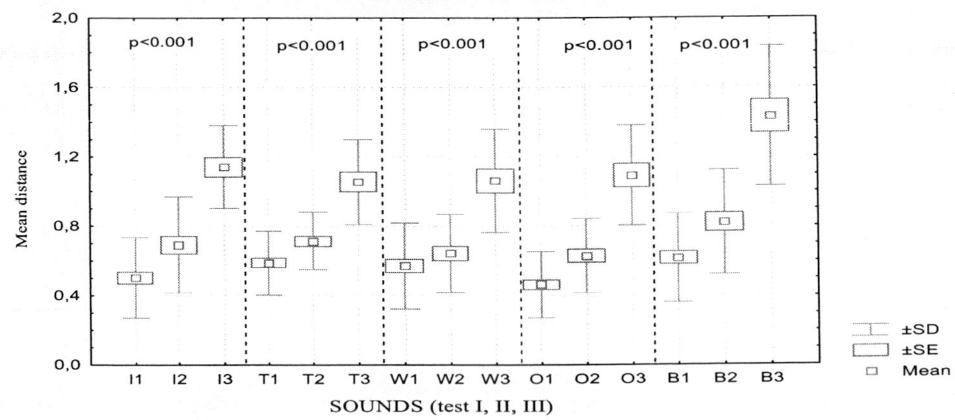

Figure 4.The comparison of mean distances of the chosen sounds in the limb group as compared to the control pattern. Acoustic computer analyses, test I-III.(*ANOVA test*).

Table 3. The comparison of mean distances of the chosen soundsin all ALS patientsas compared to the control group. Acoustic computer analyses, test I-III (*ANOVA test)*

	The mean sounds distances as compared to the control pattern. Acoustic computer- analyses, test I-III				
		ANOVA			
Group	**Sounds**	**Test I**	**Test II**	**Test III**	**Value p**
		$\bar{X} \pm SD$	$\bar{X} \pm SD$	$\bar{X} \pm SD$	
All ALS patients	I	0.44 ± 0.23	0.66 ± 0.27	1.14 ± 0.24	*< 0.001*
	T	0.50 ± 0.18	0.68 ± 0.16	1.05 ± 0.24	*< 0.001*
	W	0.44 ± 0.25	0.57 ± 0.22	1.06 ± 0.29	*< 0.001*
	O	0.39 ± 0.19	0.59 ± 0.21	1.09 ± 0.28	*< 0.001*
	B	0.49 ± 0.25	0.76 ± 0.30	1.43 ± 0.40	*< 0.001*
Bulbar Group	I	0.56 ± 0.31	0.88 ± 0.27	1.27 ± 0.32	*< 0.001*
	T	0.56 ± 0.18	0.67 ± 0.11	0.99 ± 0.18	*< 0.001*
	W	0.48 ± 0.21	0.50 ± 0.21	1.22 ± 0.35	*< 0.001*
	O	0.47 ± 0.22	0.62 ± 0.24	1.30 ± 0.32	*< 0.001*
	B	0.60 ± 0.25	0.91 ± 0.26	1.82 ± 0.11	*< 0.001*
Limb Group	I	0.40 ± 0.15	0.58 ± 0.23	1.09 ± 0.18	*< 0.001*
	T	0.48 ± 0.18	0.63 ± 0.18	1.08 ± 0.27	*< 0.001*
	W	0.42 ± 0.26	0.59 ± 0.23	1.00 ± 0.27	*< 0.001*
	O	0.37 ± 0.16	0.58 ± 0.21	1.00 ± 0.23	*< 0.001*
	B	0.45 ± 0.24	0.71 ± 0.31	1.28 ± 0.37	*< 0.001*

In the bulbar group, consonant “T” distance increase was the smallest (0.99- absolute value based on Euclidian principle) while consonant ”B” distance increase was the most significant (1.82) (Table 4).

Table 4. The comparison of mean distances of the chosen sounds in the bulbar group as compared to the control pattern. Acoustic computer analyses, test I-III . *Euclidian principle*

EUCLIDIAN PRINCIPLE	Test I	Test II	test III
Sound “B”	*0.56*	*0.88*	*1.82*
Sound “O”	*0.47*	*0.62*	*1.3*
Sound “W”	*0.48*	*0.5*	*1.22*
Sound “T”	*0.56*	*0.67*	*0.99*
Sound “I”	*0.56*	*0.88*	*1.27*

In the limb group, the increase of the distances for sounds “O”, “W”(both at 1.00) was the smallest, and consonant “B” was the most significant (1.28) (Table 5).

Table 5. The comparison of mean distances of the chosen sounds in the limb group as compared to the control pattern. Acoustic computer analyses, test I-III . *Euclidian principle*

EUCLIDIAN PRINCIPLE	test I	Test II	test III
Sound "B"	0.45	0.71	1.28
Sound "O"	0.37	0.58	1.00
Sound "W"	0.42	0.59	1.00
Sound "T"	0.48	0.63	1.08
Sound "I"	0.40	0.58	1.09

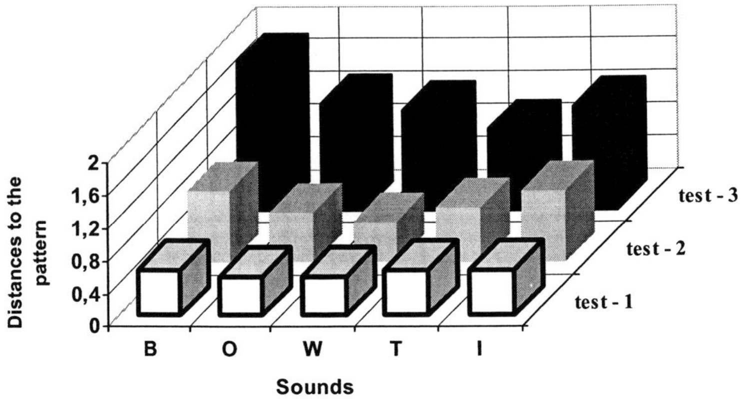

Figure 5. The comparison of mean distances of the chosen sounds in the bulbar group as compared to the control pattern. Acoustic computer analyses, test I-III . *Euclidian principle.*

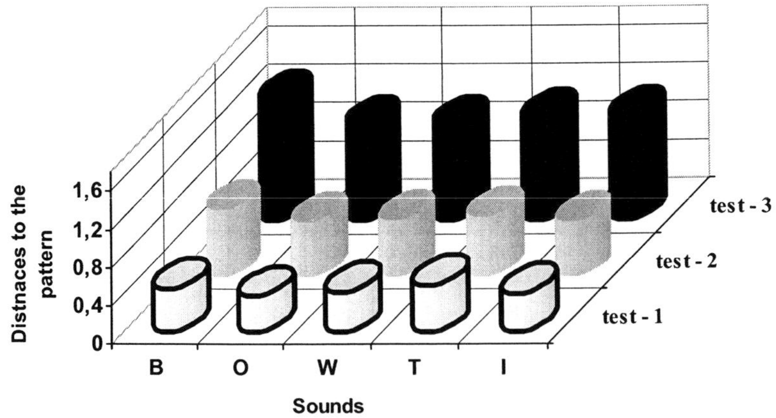

Figure 6 . The comparison of mean distances of the chosen sounds in the limb group as compared to the control pattern. Acoustic computer analyses, test I-III . Euclidian principle.

Our results indicate that the limb and bulbar ALS groups differ in that each demonstrates its smallest deterioration of the sound distance for different consonants. On the basis of this, we designed a specific dysarthria profile for each ALS group. In the bulbar group it would be: "B","O","I","W","T" (Figure 5) while in the limb group: "B","I","T","W","O" (Figure 6) (for both first sounds displayed the biggest mean distance increase to the control pattern).

Results of the Dysarthria Profile Tests (DPT)

The mean scores in each DPT achieved by subjects from the control group were close to maximum values but the mean scores in each DPT test achieved by "nondysarthric" ALS subjects were abnormal i.e.: the mean score of respiration in controls was 19.11 ±1.01 vs 13.61±5.03 in ALS subjects, phonation:46.03±3.27 vs 37.64±9.31,facial musculature 79.24±1.4 vs 76.32±3.17, daiadochkinesis 43.00±1.55 vs 37.43±5.09, reflexes 27.62±1.07 vs 25.93±2.81, articulation 19.97±0.16 vs 19.18±1.12, intelligibility of speech 24.00±0.01 vs 22.50±2.35, prosody/rate 20.00±0.01 vs.18.11±3.65, respectively. The mean scores of each DPT in "nondysarthric" ALS subjects were significantly lower ($p<0.01$) as compared to the control group (Table 6).

Table 6. The comparison of results of dysarthria profile tests between the nondysarthric ALS and the control subjects *(Student t-, independent test)*

Dysarthria profile tests	The maximum score	Control group N = 37 $\bar{X} \pm SD$	Nondysarthrics ALS N=28 $\bar{X} \pm SD$	t	value p
Respiratory	20	19.11 ± 1.01	13.61 ± 5.03	*6.49*	*p = 0.000000*
Phonation	48	46.03 ± 3.27	37.64 ± 9.31	*5.08*	*p = 0.000004*
Facial musculature	80	79.24 ± 1.4	76.32 ± 3.17	*4.97*	*p = 0.000005*
Diadochokinesis	44	43.00 ± 1.55	37.43 ± 5.09	*6.29*	*p = 0.000000*
Reflexes	28	27.62 ± 1.07	25.93 ± 2.81	*3.35*	*p = 0.001371*
Articulation	20	19.97 ± 0.16	19.18 ± 1.12	*4.25*	*p = 0.000072*
Intelligibility of speech	24	24.00 ± 0.01	22.50 ± 2.35	*3.89*	*p = 0.000241*
Prosody/rate	20	20.00± 0.01	18.11 ± 3.65	*3.16*	*p = 0.002437*

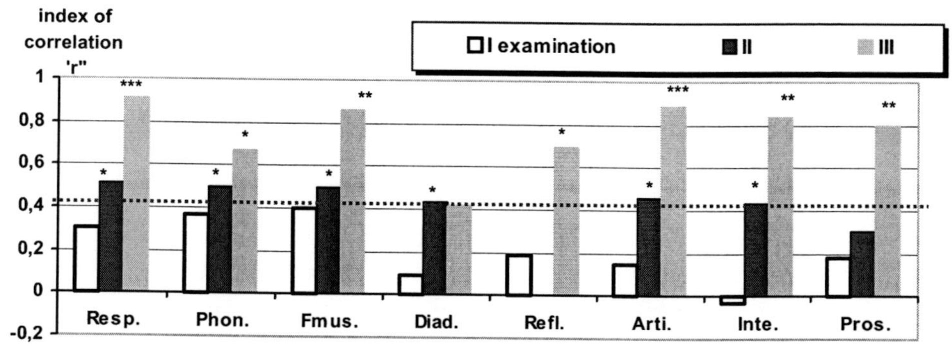

Figure7. The correlation between the mean results of Norris scale and the mean results of each DPT test. * - $p < 0,05$; ** - $p < 0,01$; *** - $p < 0,001$, Resp.=Respiration,Phon.= Phonation, Fmus.=Facial musculature, Diad.= Diadochokinesis, Refl.= Reflexes, Arti.= Articulation, Inte.= Intelligibility of speech, Pros.= Prosody/rate.

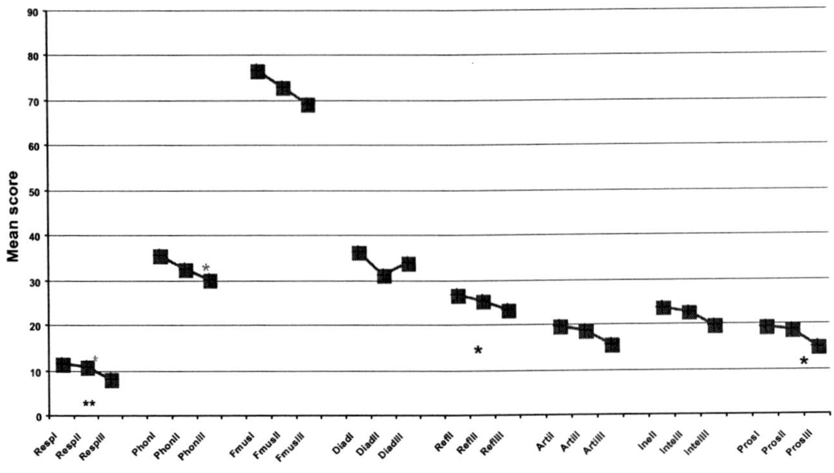

Figure 8. The comparison between the mean scores of each DPT in three subsequent examinations. * - p < 0,05; ** - p < 0,01.

Resp I-III.=Respiration in three subsequent examinations , Phon I-III= Phonation, Fmus. I-III=Facial musculature, Diad.I-III= Diadochokinesis, Refl I-III.= Reflexes, Arti . I-III= Articulation Inte.I-III= Intelligibility of speech, Pros. I-III= Prosody/rate; respectively

With the progression of the disease during the time of our observation (examination I-II-III every 12 weeks, in summer 36 weeks), the comparison of results of each DPT in ALS subjects demonstrated that all of these tests were changed pathologically (towards the lower value; excluding the changes of the diadochokinesis test between the second and third examination) in the three subsequent examinations i.e., the mean score of respiration test in examination I was 11.66±4.75 vs 10.83±5.23 in examination II vs 8.16±4.78 in examination III; phonation: 35.8±10.38 vs 32.6±11.24 vs 30.3±10.18; facial musculature: 76.8±3.47 vs 73.16±10.64 vs 69.16±13.09; diadochokinesis: 36.8±5.21 vs 31.16±7.62 vs 34.0±7.97; refelxes: 26.83±3.35 vs 25.56 ± 4.81 vs 23.33±4.02; articulation: 19.66±1.4 vs 18.83±2.58 vs 15.66±4.83; intelligibility of speech: 23.66±2.29 vs 22.66±3.18 vs 19.66±5.41: prosody/rate: 19.33±4.47 vs 18.66±3.03 vs 15.0±5.0; respectively. Differences between the mean scores were significantly lower for the tests of respiration ($p<0.05$) and phonation ($p<0.05$) in three subsequent examinations (Table 7, Figure 8). The mean value of the Norris scale was 92.13±20.72 during the first DPT examination, 83.32±25.46 during the second DPT examination and 77.71±30.10 during the last DPT examination. A decrease of the mean value of the Norris scale was statistically significant 92.13 ±20.72 vs. 77.71±30.10, $p<0.05$ with the progression of the disease (respectively, from the first to the third examination). There were no correlations between the mean value of the Norris scale and the mean scores of each dysarthria test during the first DPT examination, during the second - we noted the correlation between: Norris scale vs. respiratory test ($r=0.50$, $p<0.05$), Norris scale vs. phonation test ($r=0.50$, $p<0.05$), Norris scale vs. movements of face and tongue test ($r=0.50$, $p<0.05$, Norris scale vs. diadochokinesis test ($r= 0.43$, $p<0.05$), Norris scale vs. articulation ($r=0.46$, $p<0.05$),

Norris scale vs. intelligibility of speech. During the tird examination we observed : Norris scale vs. respiratory test ($r=0.91$, $p<0.001$), Norris scale vs. phonation test ($r=0.67$, $p<0.05$), Norris scale vs. movements of face and tongue test ($r=0.86$, $p<0.01$), Norris scale vs. reflexes ($r=0.70$, $p<0.05$), Norris scale vs. articulation ($r=0.90$, $p<0.001$), Norris vs. intelligibility of speech ($r=0.84$, $p<0.01$) and Norris scale vs. prosody ($r=0.80$, $p<0.01$), respectively. These results are shown in Figure 7.

Table 7. The comparison of results of dysarthria profile tests between the whole ALS group and the dysarthric and the nondysarthric ALS subjects in three subsequent examinations *(ANOVA)*

Group	Dysarthria profile tests	ANOVA			
		Examination I	**Examination II**	**Examination III**	value p
		$\bar{X} \pm SD$	$\bar{X} \pm SD$	$\bar{X} \pm SD$	
The whole ALS group	**Respiratoion**	10.16 ± 5.76	9.42 ± 5.51	7.25 ± 5.12	*< 0.001*
	Phonation	31.42 ± 12.89	29.25 ± 12.66	25.67 ± 12.89	*< 0.01*
	Facial musculature	67.5 ± 17.16	65.16 ± 16.27	59.42 ± 17.17	NS
	Diadochokinesis	32.75 ± 10.29	29.83 ± 9.53	28.48 ± 10.29	NS
	Reflexes	23.17 ± 7.02	22.75 ± 6.74	18.5 ± 7.03	*< 0.01*
	Articulation	17.5 ± 4.89	16.83 ± 4.86	13.91 ± 4.90	*< 0.01*
	Intelligibility of speech	19.5 ± 6.40	20.17 ± 5.96	16.75 ± 6.40	NS
	Prosody/rate	16.0 ± 5.94	16.41 ± 5.50	12.5 ± 5.94	*< 0.05*
Dysarthric ALS subjects	Respiration	8.70 ± 4.88	8.0 ± 4.87	6.33 ± 5.06	*< 0.01*
	Phonation	27.00 ± 13.3	25.80 ± 11.99	21.0 ± 17.84	NS
	Facial musculature	58.16 ± 19.9	57.16 ± 20.08	49.66 ± 21.96	NS
	Diadochokinesis	28.66 ± 12.4	28.5 ± 11.21	22.8 ± 12.84	NS
	Reflexes	10.50 ± 8.9	20.0 ± 8.25	13.66 ± 8.38	*< 0.05*
	Articulation	15.30 ± 6.5	14.8 ± 6.39	12.16 ± 6.53	NS
	Intelligibility of speech	15.30 ± 6.9	17.66 ± 8.04	13.8 ± 8.52	NS
	Prosody/rate	12.66 ± 6.38	14.16 ± 7.30	16.1 ± 7.25	*< 0.05*
Nondysarthric ALS subjects	Respiration	11.66 ± 4.75	10.83 ± 5.23	8.16 ± 4.78	*< 0.05*
	Phonation	35.8 ± 10.38	32.6 ± 11.24	30.3 ± 10.18	*< 0.05*
	Facial musculature	76.8 ± 3.47	73.16 ± 10.64	69.16 ± 13.09	NS
	Diadochokinesis	36.8 ± 5.21	31.16 ± 7.62	34.0 ± 7.97	NS
	Reflexes	26.83 ± 3.35	25.56 ± 4.81	23.33 ± 4.02	NS
	Articulation	19.66 ± 1.4	18.83 ± 2.58	15.66 ± 4.83	NS
	Intelligibility of speech	23.66 ± 2.29	22.66 ± 3.18	19.66 ± 5.41	NS
	Prosody/rate	19.33 ± 4.47	18.66 ± 3.03	15.0 ± 5.0	NS

NS – no statistical significance

The Comparison of the Results of Dysarthria Profile Tests Between ALS and the Control Group

The mean scores in each dysarthria profile test achieved by the subjects from the control group were close to the maximum values, but the mean scores in each dysarthria profile test achieved by ALS subjects were evidently abnormal. Differences between the mean scores of each dysarthria profile test in ALS subjects were significantly lower ($p<0.001$) as compared to the control subjects. We noted that the mean scores of each dysarthria profile test in the dysarthric ALS subjects were significantly lower ($p<0.001$) as compared to the nondysarthric ALS subjects (table 8).

Also the mean scores of each dysarthria profile test in the nondysarthric ALS subjects were significantly lower ($p<0.01$) as compared to the control group (table 6).

Table 8.The comparison of results of dysarthria profile tests between the dysarthric and the nondysarthric ALS subjects (Student t-, independent test)

Dysarthria profile tests	The maximum score	ALS subjects		t	value p
		Dysarthric N = 15 $\bar{x} \pm SD$	Nondysarthric N = 28 $\bar{x} \pm SD$		
Respiration	20	7.40 ± 4.88	13.61 ± 5.03	*3.90*	*p=0.00035*
Phonation	48	22.73 ±13.27	37.64 ± 9.31	*4.30*	*p=0.000102*
Facial musculature	80	50.0 ± 19.90	76.32 ± 3.19	*6.80*	*p = 0.000000*
Diadochokinesis	44	24.60 ±12.39	37.42 ± 5.09	*4.81*	*p = 0.000021*
Reflexes	28	17.13 ± 8.89	25.93 ± 2.81	*4.85*	*p = 0.000018*
Articulation	20	13.00 ± 6.55	19.18 ± 1.12	*4.91*	*p = 0.000015*
Intelligibility of speech	24	12.87 ± 6.92	22.50 ± 2.35	*6.74*	*p = 0.000000*
Prosody/rate	20	10.60 ± 6.39	18.11 ± 3.65	*4.92*	*p = 0.000014*

The Comparison of Results of Dysarthria Profile Tests Between the Whole ALS Group and the Dysarthric and the Nondysarthric ALS Subjects in three Subsequent Examinations

The comparison of results of each dysarthria profile test in ALS subjects demonstrated that all of these tests were changed pathologically (towards the lower value) in the three subsequent examinations. Differences between the mean scores in each dysarthria profile test in all ALS groups were significantly lower in the tests of respiration ($p<0.001$), phonation ($p<0.01$), reflexes ($p<0.01$), articulation ($p<0.01$) and prosody ($p<0.05$) in three subsequent examinations (Table 7). Our results indicate that dysarthric and nondysarthric ALS subjects differ. Differences between the mean scores in each dysarthria profile test were significantly lower in the dysarthric ALS subjects in the tests of respiration ($p<0.01$), reflexes ($p<0.05$) and prosody ($p<0.05$) and in the nondysarthric ALS in the tests of respiration ($p<0.05$) and phonation ($p<0.05$) in three subsequent examinations (Table 7, Figure 8). We noted that only the mean scores of the respiratory test were significantly lower in all ALS groups assessed in three subsequent examinations of dysarthria profile tests. We draw attention to the mean scores in some of dysarthria profile tests i.e. respiration and phonation in the nondysarthric

ALS subjects which were significantly lower in three subsequent examinations of dysarthria profile tests.

Summary of DPT Results

1. When comparing the results of mean scores in each dysarthria profile test between ALS and the control groups we noted significantly lower values in ALS subjects than when comparing the ALS nondysarthrics to the controls, separately.
2. With the progression of the disease during the time of our observation (36 weeks) the results of each dysarthria profile test deteriorated in all the ALS subjects studied. These results also proved the progression of some pathological changes in dysarthria profile tests, which were specific (because of statistical significance) for different ALS subjects in three subsequent examinations of dysarthria profile tests.
3. Comparing the results among all three examinations of dysarthria profile tests in all ALS subjects we demonstrated significant decreases in the tests of respiration, phonation, reflexes, articulation, and prosody.
4. This deterioration of results among all three examinations of dysarthria profile tests occurred in the dysarthric ALS subjects (in the tests of respiration, reflexes and prosody) as well as in the nondysarthric ALS subjects (in the tests of respiration and phonation).

Discussion

Acoustic Speech Analysis (ASA)

Although dysarthria in ALS patients has been studied by the application of the perceptual, physiological and acoustic methods [7-22], there are still not many widely known methods assessing the changes and the nature of speech due to ALS. Presented computer-based acoustic analysis relying on the Euclidian principle is a sensitive method for the detecting and measurement of dysarthria. To the best of our knowledge, the presented acoustic method has not been used previously to assess dysarthria in ALS patients. This study demonstrated that when ALS progresses over the time there is a significant deterioration of speech and individual sound production as assessed by computer-based acoustic analyses. Sounds were affected by disease in both studied groups of patients, i.e., with bulbar (dysarthric) or limb (nonbulbar and nondysarthric) signs. Bulbar group deterioration was significantly more rapid. We have identified and characterised a specific dysarthria profile for each ALS group. We have also shown a deterioration in the speech quality as measured by the sounds distance increase from the basic control pattern. This may allow earlier identification of imminent bulbar involvement. Improved understanding of the dysarthria pathophysiology in ALS will help us both to assess the speech disorder in greater depth and to better anticipate and manage patients with the loss of speech. Detection and measurement of dysarthria can be of great importance to the language pathologist. It facilitates an individualised program possible for the patient.

Some of acoustic aberrations have been noted in the dysarthric populations and affected the perception of the fast speaking rate. Kent et al., [25-27] studied the speech and voice in

ALS patients with a number of techniques with a particular emphasis on placebo intelligibility. The measurement of intelligibility was accomplished by a multiple-choice, single-word identification test. Kent et al. [25] studied the relationship between acoustic parameters of speech and intelligibility. Phonatory instability in ALS has been observed with the use of acoustic measures by Ramig et al[16] and Ramig et al [28]. Weismer et al. [29] showed that the changes and slowing of articulation may constitute a general index of the severity of speech disturbance.

From more recent studies Kent and Kim et al. mentioned [30] that acoustic methods have progressed to the point where an acoustic typology of the motor speech disorders can be constructed from a parametric assessment of the speech subsystems (e.g., phonation, nasal resonance, vowel articulation, consonant articulation, intelligibility and rhythm). The results obtained from a speech acoustic analysis can be interpreted with respect to global functions in speech (e.g., voice quality, intelligibility, and prosody). Typically acoustic analyses of the voice have revealed deviant fundamental frequency (Fo), amplitude and frequency, perturbation (e.g., shimmer, jitter), voice range, vocal quality and phonatory instability [3,14].

Acoustic analyses of our speech tests showed that it is possible to measure an articulatory dysfunction in ALS patients with acoustic methods, as well as the form of a characteristic "acoustic signatures", based on the Euclidian principle. Our results, based on the measurement of the mean distances in the chosen sounds, show a significant increase of these distances to the pattern. It helps to demonstrate the occurrence of a specific dysarthria profile, which is different for both examined ALS groups as well as to allow us to estimate the profiles' degree of abnormality. It revealed that the specific dysarthria profile for ALS patients, as specified by the chosen mean sound distances, may have its origin in functional and structural changes reflecting the motor neurone dysfunction in ALS as well as the orofacial diadochokinesis in the speech production system (tongue, lips, soft palate, larynx). We have suggested that the changes in the mean sound distances may constitute a functional indicator of structural degeneration. This may be particularly important as far as the tongue function (relative to jaw and lips) is concerned. Most of the sounds are produced with the use of the tongue and lips, and palatal function is required. The vocalisation of consonants like "P","T","K" which are formed by a firm contact between the lips, tongue and hard palate are particularly important to be tested, as well as vocalisation of the vowels, like "I", formed by the tongue, lips, and the lower jaw. The abnormalities shown in this study are consistent with the previous reports which showed disturbances of lingual, velopharyngeal and laryngeal articulations [9,10,31-34]. These authors defined three functional regions: articulatory (lips, tongue, mandible), velopharyngeal (palate, pharynx), and phonatory (larynx) for studying myometric characteristics of the orofacial structures in both normal subjects and dysarthric patients. Langrmore et al [7] described that bulbar ALS patients were generally more severely affected than the corticobulbar or spinal ALS patients, and the tongue was generally the most affected structure in all ALS groups.

Our study demonstrated also that the refined bending adjustments needed for lingual consonants are affected more than the gross positioning of the tongue body which is required to produce vowels. A possible explanation is that the motoneurones of the intrinsic tongue musculature are lost [35]. It is expected that intrinsic fibres are particularly important in producing bending movements of the tongue [34].

Our hypothesis of disproportion of tongue weakness is supported by earlier clinical [36] and neuropathologic observations [37]. They showed that in ALS dysarthria, hypoglossal motor neurones were affected differently from facial or masticatory motor neurones. More recent research characterising the motor deficits in the orofacial system in ALS patients, has confirmed the selective vulnerability of cranial motor neurones. Although earlier reports demonstrated significant impairments of lingual strength in ALS patients [9,33,38] other studies indicated a greater weakness of the tongue as compared to the jaw and lower lip, even among ALS patients without bulbar signs and/or symptoms [34]. Quantitative measurements of lip, mandible, and tongue function performed by DePaul et al [34] in 25 men with ALS revealed that the greatest dysfunction occurred in hypoglossal motor neurons. The tongue weakness was detected not only in the patients with involved bulbar ALS, but also in those with affected limb muscles and no dysarthria. A magnetic resonance study of 16 patients with ALS by Cha and Pattern [39] also revealed some tongue abnormalities. The tongues of all the patients were 30% smaller, more rectangular, and situated more posteriorly and ventrally in the oral cavity. The internal structure of the tongue showed an abnormal loss of the radial and curvilinear bands of the intrinsic tongue muscles.

In our study we have also found that the limb ALS group who was not dysarthric, and had no clinical signs of bulbar or corticobulbar involvement as well as any perceptual disturbances of speech, also demonstrated some changes disturbances in the mean sound distances in the following: "B","I", "T","W","O". The sounds could therefore be used as an early indication of a preclinical dysarthria in those patients. The occurrence of speech changes in apparently free of bulbar symptoms ALS patients has been described in the literature, but the authors have used different methods [34, 40]. Darley et al [32] described also the presence of silent physiologic parameters in both flaccid and spastic dysartrhia in ALS patients. They identified muscle weakness as a key factor of lower motor neurone involvement with slowness of movement and variable weakness as a feature of upper motor neurone dysarthria.

Severity of dysarthria was more highly correlated with the measures of the repeated contraction rate than with the measures of strength, suggesting that more severe dysarthria may be largely due to the slower movement of the orofacial structures until the substantial muscle strength has been lost. [7]. Acoustic-perceptual patterns have been developed in the Kent and colleagues' studies [25,30] and also Weismer et al [11,21,29], Turner and Tjaden [22] studies. They focused on creating the patterns of speech performance at different levels of speech intelligibility among individuals with ALS without being concerned with the underlying pathophysiology. DePaul, Langmore and Carpenter [34,7, 36] studied physiologic patterns that characterised aspects of the disease. These studies were more concerned with underlined pathophysilogic mechanisms of dysarthria. It was shown that differential impairment which occurred in the cranial systems with the tongue and larynx more impaired than the facial and mandibular motor systems is a significant contribution to the understanding how ALS affects the speech and swallowing musculature. The subtle changes can be detected without any apparent functional speech change. The recent study done by Weismer at al [21] in ALS dysarthric subjects assessed the acoustic and perceptual effects of speaking rate. The ALS patients showed the bigger compression of the acoustic vowel space and the ability to increase their speaking rate but significantly slower as compare to controls, neurologically normal subjects.

Also Turner and Tjaden [22] analysed the acoustic characteristics of speech produced for explanation of the intelligibility deficits in ALS patients with mild to moderate dysarthria with comparison to controls. Both groups were acoustically distinguished /i/ /ae/, /u/ and /a/ in content and function words. The duration of vowels was also measured. The authors showed that in ALS speakers the vowel space area was different as compared to healthy controls, but the results were not statistically significant, however, there was a tendency for the difference in vowel space area for content and function words to be smaller for ALS speakers.

Our study showed that the differences in the mean sound distance in patients with and without dysarthria may be a good marker of the severity and progression of bulbar motoneurones dysfunction. We have also found that the nondysarthric limb ALS group with no clinical signs of bulbar or corticobulbar involvement, also demonstrated some changes in the mean sound distances in the following: ”B”,”I”, ”T”,”W”,”O”. The sounds could therefore be used as an early indication of a preclinical dysarthria in those patients. These hypotheses were confirmed by Robert et al [6], who demonstrated that acoustic parameters are more sensitive than aerodynamics parameters for early detection of bulbar involvement in ALS patients and also Silbergleit et al [14], who compared the acoustic analysis and perceptual assessment in dysarthric ALS patients. Their results showed that acoustic analysis can detect the early signs affecting the laryngeal system and may be useful in ALS patients for evaluation of early speech changes before the occurrence of perceptual aberrant vocal characteristics.

In conclusion, let us state that improving communicative abilities in ALS has a significant impact on the overall disease management, patient comfort and quality of life.

Dysarthria Profile Tests (DPT) Analysis

The analysis of DPT study allows us to suggest that it is possible to measure some changes in different functional elements of speech due to ALS by means of dysarthria profile tests. Using this method we have shown the early occurrence of some speech disturbances in the nondysarthric ALS subjects, which were significant when compared to the controls, as well as while comparing the deterioration of changes in dysarthria profile tests between dysarthric and nondysarthric ALS subjects over the time of the study. With the progression of the disease different changes in the dysarthria profile tests occurred characteristically in different ALS subjects. It seems that assessing only 5 out of 8 dysarthria profile tests i.e., respiration, phonation, reflexes, articulation, and prosody is sufficient enough to characterise dysarthria in all ALS subjects. Some of them may be used to select the dysarthrics and the nondysarthrics from the whole ALS group and also to detect dysarthria in the limb onset ALS subjects. Of all the dysarthria profile tests we have identified the tests of respiratory, reflexes and prosody as specific for dysarthria in the dysarthric ALS subjects and the tests of respiration and phonation as specific for the early stage of dysarthria in the nondysarthric ALS subjects in three subsequent examinations.

We have not found the information in the literature about systematic studies using dysarthria profile tests to assess dysarthria in ALS subjects. The method assessing dysarthria, especially measuring motor speech function, as Frenchay Dysarthria Assessment [41], closest to the dysarthria profile tests used in our study, was used by Riddel et al [8]. It also provides the scale assessment of speech disturbances in the analyses of reflexes, respiration, muscular function of speech of facial organs, diadochokinesis and also phonetic factors. The authors examined 29 ALS subjects, 14 of whom were dysarthrics but without the comparison with the control group. They detected the occurrence of early phonetic disturbances of speech in all the ALS subjects studied, notwithstanding the high intelligibility of their speech. These disturbances were most advanced in the dysarthrics. Using the dysarthria profile tests we also have discovered the occurrence of dysarthria in all ALS studied subjects, as well as the deterioration of dysarthric process in the dysarthrics. In Langmore and Lehman's study [7] the authors analysed several parameters of dysarthria in ALS subjects i.e., facial musculature, diadochokinesis, intelligibility of speech, articulation and changes in facial reflexes, and demonstrated the occurrence of pathological changes in diadochokinesis and facial musculature in all ALS subjects. However, statistically significant changes occurred only in the dysarthric (bulbar) subjects. On the contrary, we have shown that abnormalities of phonation and respiratory functions significantly occur in the nondysarthric ALS subjects. Other authors studied single aspects of dysarthria due to ALS. Wiesmer et al. [11] observed the intensification of respiratory and articulation dysfunction and also changes in the quality of voice i.e. hoarseness and lower pitch of voice, but only in the dysarthric ALS subjects. Kent et al. [25] examined phonetic parameters in 25 ALS men and noted that the analysis of intelligibility of speech and phonation was vital to the assessment of dysarthria in ALS patients. DePaul and Brooks [42] using physiological measures have found some disturbances in oral motor functioning even among ALS patients with high levels of speech intelligibility. In addition, in the studies in which acoustic methods have been used, early changes have been documented in the speech of highly intelligible individuals with ALS [11,13,16,17,20,22, 25,27,29].

Theodoros et al [43] described also the use of Assessment of Intelligibility of Dysarthric Speech (ASSIDS), which gives the percentage of word and sentences intelligibility, words per minute and a rating of communication efficiency for the assessment of motor speech disorders. But the results obtained from this study are not comparable with our results because of different protocols.

The direct comparison between others studies' results and ours is difficult because of considerable methodological differences in these analyses. We are quite aware that DPT used by us to the assessment of dysarthria is not an up-to-date research tool and poses a certain limitation in the analysis and the comparison of results with the studies using newer, noninstrumental methods of the speech disturbance assessment. However, our aim was the assessment of speech disturbances in ALS patients with the use of up-to-date, instrumental, objective research tool ASA and the comparison of results with simple- to- perform (also by the neurologist) logopedic test DPT. It seems that the results obtained by us confirm the rightness of using these methods for the assessment of dysarthria in ALS patients.

In spite of this, most of the results indicate the occurrence of early speech disturbances in the nondysarthric ALS subjects. This allows us to suggest that the neurodegeneration process due to ALS affects both corticospinal and bulbar motorneurones nearly simultaneously but it is still difficult to find a precise method to assess the dysarthric signs preclinically. The value of the assessment of dysarthria profile tests and their role in characterising the orofacial involvement in the early stages of ALS bulbar impairment will certainly be discussed.

Conclusions and Future Directions

Computer-based acoustic analysis relying on the Euclidian principle is a sensitive method of measurement of dysarthria in bulbar and limb onset ALS patients on the grounds of the acoustic analysis (ASA) of only several sounds. Abnormalities detected in different dysarthria profiles in the two ALS subject groups may appear prior to any clinical symptoms of these disturbances. The semiquantitative assessment of speech disturbances based on dysarthria profile tests (DPT) might be also useful in the clinical practice of detection of the early dysarthric processes occurring among the clinically nondysarthric ALS subjects. Additionally, DPT is a very easy and cheap method, which can be performed not only by a speech therapist but also by the neurologist. On the basis of our findings we suggest that the examination of DPT, used for observing the deterioration of speech disturbances due to disease progression, especially a test of respiration and phonation, may be an indicator of the occurrence of early speech changes in primary, clinically nondysarthric ALS patients. It can be a good point for starting an early speech therapy and the orofacial voluntary rehabilitation.

On the grounds of our study we start using the bedside short examination of DPT and continuing the acoustic analysis of the occurrence of early speech disturbances in ALS patients without dysarthria.

Appendix

I. The Euclidian Principle (The Mathematical Method)

Acoustic analysis of speech requires a scalar measure of acoustic signals' similarity. The word "scalar" is used here to emphasise the necessity of a single, synthetic indicator but not a multidimensional assessment of signals' divergence in the time, frequency or spatial configuration (or any other). The basic assumption is as follows: we look for a principle or method of measurement of the similarity by creating an appropriate configuration of acoustic signals' description (a space in which one can describe this signal-acoustic wave) and measure this space by applying one of the methods measuring the distance.

Principles:

1. Hammings' principle
2. **Euclidian principle**

3. Camberrs' principle
4. Bray and Curtis principle
5. Clark's principle
6. Jeffreys-Mutusist principle.

II. Dysarthria profile tests [18]

Dysarthria profile tests	Task	Normal	Good	Fair	Poor	Nil
1. Respiration	1. Sustain /s/ on exhalation					
	2."Crescendo" on /s/					
	3. "Diminuendo" on /s/					
	4. Repeat series of /s/					
	5. Synchronise respiration / phonation					
2. Phonation	1. Initiate /a:/					
	2. Sustain /a:/					
	3. Say /a:/ loudly					
	4. " Crescendo" on /a:/					
	5. "Diminuendo" on /a:/					
	6. Repeat series of /a:/					
	7. Raise pitch on /a:/					
	8. Lower pitch on /a:/					
	9. Glide up scale on /a:/					
	10. Glide down scale on /a:/					
	11. Maintain adequate volume in speech					
	12.Quality of voice					
3. Facial musculature	1. Symmetry of face at rest					
	2. Change expression to smile					
	3.Purse lips					
	4. Stretch lips					
	5. Maintain lip closure at rest					
	6. Achieve lip closure during speech					
	7. Open/ close month					
	8. Move mandible to right					
	9. Move mandible to left					
	10. Protrude tongue					
	11. Retract tongue					
	12. Move tongue to right					
	13. Move tongue to left					
	14. Pass tongue over teeth					
	15. Move tongue tip into right cheek					
	16. Move tongue tip into left cheek					
	17. Raise tongue tip in mouth					
	18. Raise tongue tip outside mouth					
	19. Elevate soft palate on / a:/					
	20. Elevate soft palate on series of /a:/					

II. Dysarthria profile tests [18] Continued

Dysarthria profile tests	Task	Normal	Good	Fair	Poor	Nil
4. Diadochokinesis	1. Open/close mouth rapidly					
	2. Protrude/Retract lips rapidly					
	3. Protrude /Retract tongue rapidly					
	4. Elevate/Lower tongue tip rapidly					
	5. Move tongue side/side rapidly					
	6. Repeat "oo-ee" rapidly					
	7. Repeat "pa..."rapidly					
	8. Repeat "ta..."rapidly					
	9. Repeat "ka...: rapidly					
	10. Repeat 'kala...' rapidly					
	11. Repeat "p.t.k...' rapidly					
5. Reflexes	1. Chewing					
	2. Swallow solid food					
	3. Swallow liquids					
	4. Prevent drooling at rest					
	5. Prevent drooling during eating					
	6. Prevent drooling during speech					
	7. Cough/clear throat					
6.Articulation	1. Repeat initial consonant					
	2. Accuracy of vowel sounds					
	3. Repeat consonant clusters					
	4. Repeat polysyllabic words					
	5. Repeat phrase					
7. Intelligibility	1. Intelligibility of reading to therapist					
	2. Intelligibility of reading to rel/friend					
	3. Intelligibility of reading to stranger					
	4. Intelligibility of speech to therapist					
	5. Intelligibility of speech to rel/friend					
	6. Intelligibility of speech to stranger					
8. Prosody/rate	1. Maintain appropriate rate					
	2. Increase rate					
	3. Maintain appropriate rhythm					
	4. Use appropriate rhythm					
	5. Imitate different stress patterns					

References

[1] Mitsumoto H., Chad D.A., Pioro E.P.: Speech and communication management, chapter 23. In: Amyotrophic lateral sclerosis, ed. *F.A., Davis Company* – Philadelphia, 1998,p 405-419.

[2] Leigh N.: Amyotrophic lateral sclerosis and other motor neurone diseases. *Current Opinion in Neurol Neurosur* 1991, 4, 586-596.

[3] Watts CR, Vanryckeghem M. Laryngeal dysfunction in Amyotrophic Lateral Sclerosis: a review and case report. *BMC Ear Nose Throat Disord.* 2001;1(1):1. Epub 2001 Nov 13.

[4] Yorkston K, Strand E, Miller R, Hillel A, et al. Speech deterioration in Amyotrophic lateral sclerosis; Implications for the timing of intervention. *J Med Speech-Lang Pathol* 1993;1: 35-46.

[5] Ball LJ, Willis A, Beukelman DR, Pattee GL.A protocol for identification of early bulbar signs in amyotrophic lateral sclerosis. *J Neurol Sci.* 2001 Oct 15;191(1-2):43-53.

[6] Robert D, Pouget J, Giovanni A, Azulay JP, Triglia JM.Quantitative voice analysis in the assessment of bulbar involvement in amyotrophic lateral sclerosis. *Acta Otolaryngol.* 1999;119(6):724-31.

[7] Langmore SE, Lehman ME. Physiologic deficits in the orofacial system underlying dysarthria in amyotrophic lateral sclerosis. *J Speech Hear Res* 1994; 37: 28-37.

[8] Riddel J, McCauley RJ, Mulligan M, Tandan R.,1995 Intelligibility and phonetic contrast errors in highly intelligible speakers with amyotrophic lateral sclerosis. *J Speech Hear Res.*; 38: 304-314.

[9] Dworkin,J.P.,1980a. Tongue strenght measurement in patients with amyotrophic lateral sclerosis: Qualitative vs quantitative procedures. *Arch Phys Med Rehab*, 61,422-424

[10] Carrow,E.,Rivera,V.,Maudlin,M., Shamblin,L.,1974.Deviant speech characteristic in motor neuron disease. *Arch Otolaryngol Head Neck Surg*, 100, 212-218.

[11] Weismer G, Kent RD, Hodge M, Martin R. The acoustic signature for intelligibility test words. *J Acoust Soc Am.* 1988; 84: 1281-91.

[12] Kent,R.D.,Sufit,R.L.,Rosenbek,J.C.,Kent,J.F.,Weismer,G.,Martin,R.E.,Brooks,B.R., 1991. Speech deterioration in amyotrophic lateral sclerosis: a cases study, *J Speech Hear Res,* 34, 1269-1275.

[13] Kent,J.F.,Kent,R.D.,Rosenbek,J.C.,Weismer,G.,Martin,R.,Sufit R., Brooks B.R.,1992. Quantative description of dysarthria in women with amyotrophic lateral sclerosis. *J Speech Hear Res,* 35, 723-733.

[14] Silbergleit AK, Johnson AF, Jacobson BH.Acoustic analysis of voice in individuals with amyotrophic lateral sclerosis and perceptually normal vocal quality. *J Voice.* 1997 Jun;11(2):222-31.

[15] Turner GS, Tjaden K, Weismer G. The influence of speaking rate on vowel space and speech intelligibility for individuals with amyotrophic lateral sclerosis. *J Speech Hear Res.* 1995; 38: 1001-1013.

[16] Ramig L, Scherer R, Klasner E, Titz, Horii Yl. Acoustic analysis of voice in amyotrophic lateral sclerosis: A longitudinal case study. *J Speech Hear Disord.* 1990;55: 2-14

[17] Mulligan M, Carpenter J, Riddel J, Delaney MK, Badger G, Krusinski P, et al. Intelligibility and the acoustic characteristics of speech in amyotrophic lateral sclerosis. *J Speech Hear Res* 1994; 37: 496-503

[18] Robertson SJ, Thomson F (1986): Working with dysarthric clients. Tucson, AZ: *Communication Skill Builders.*

[19] Tomik B, Glodzik-Sobanska L, Lechwacka A, Bala-Slodowska M, Kolasa M, Szczudlik A. The application of dysarthria profile tests in ALS patients for the detection of speech disturbances. *Neurol Neurochir Pol.* 2000 Mar-Apr;34(2):269-79.

[20] Tomik B, Krupinski J, Glodzik-Sobanska L, Bala-Slodowska M, Wszolek W, Kusiak M, Lechwacka A. 1999Acoustic analysis of dysarthria profile in ALS patients.

Acoustic analysis of dysarthria profile in ALS patients. *J Neurol Sci.* Oct 31;169(1-2):35-42.

[21] Weismer G, Laures JS, Jeng JY, Kent RD, Kent JF.Effect of speaking rate manipulations on acoustic and perceptual aspects of the dysarthria in amyotrophic lateral sclerosis. *Folia Phoniatr Logop.* 2000 Sep-Oct;52(5):201-19.

[22] Turner GS, Tjaden K. Acoustic differences between content and function words in amyotrophic lateral sclerosis. *J Speech Lang Hear Res.* 2000 Jun;43(3):769-81.

[23] Brooks BR, Hormigo A, Larumbe R, et al. El Escorial World Federation of Neurology criteria for the diagnosis of amyotrophic lateral sclerosis. *J Neurol Sci* 1994;124(suppl):96-107.

[24] Norris FH Jr, U KS, Sachais B, Carey M. Trial of baclofen in amyotrophic lateral sclerosis. *Arch Neurol.* 1979 Nov;36(11):715-6.

[25] Kent,R.D.,Kent,J.F.,Weismer,G.,Martin,R.E.,Sufit,R.L.,Rosenbek,J.C.,Brooks,B.R., 1989a., Relationships between speech intelligibility and the slope of second-formant transitions in dysarthric subjects. *Clin Linguist Phon*, 3, 347-358.

[26] Kent,R.D.,Weismer,G.,Kent,J.F.,Rosenbek,J.C,1989b.Towards phonetic intelligibility testing in dysarthria. *J Speech Hear Res*, 54, 482-499.

[27] Kent RD, Kent JF, Weismer G, Sufit RL, Rosenbeck JC, Martin RE, et al. Impairment of speech intelligibility in men with amyotrophic lateral sclerosis. *J Speech Hear Res* 1990; 5: 721-728.

[28] Ramig,L.O.,Titze,I.R.,Scherer,R.C., Ringel, S.P.,1988. Acoustic analysis of voices of patients with neurologic disease: Rationale and preliminary data. *Ann Otol Rhinol Laryngol*, 97(2),164-172

[29] Weismer G, Jeng JY, Laures JS, Kent RD, Kent JF. Acoustic and intelligibility characteristics of sentence production in neurogenic speech disorders. *Folia Phoniatr Logop.* 2001 Jan-Feb;53(1):1-18.

[30] Kent RD, Kim YJ. Toward an acoustic typology of motor speech disorders. *Clin Linguist Phon.* 2003 Sep;17(6):427-45.

[31] Darley,F.,Aronson,A.,Brown,J., 1969a. Clusters of deviant speech dimensions in the dysarthrias. *J Speech Hear Res* , 12, 462-496.

[32] Darley,F.,Aronson,A., Brown,J., 1969b. Differential diagnostic patterns of dysarthria. *J Speech Hear Res* , 12, 246-269.

[33] Dworkin,J.,Aronson,A.,Mulder,D.,1980b. Tongue force in normals and in dysarthric patients with amyotrphic lateral sclerosis. *J Appl Speech Hear Res.* 23, 828-837.

[34] DePaul, R.,Abbs,J. H.,Caligiuri,M., et al., 1988. Hypoglossal, trigeminal, and facial motorneurone involvement in amyotrophic lateral sclerosis. *Neurology.*, 38, 281-283.

[35] Shawker TH, Sonies BC, Stone M.Soft tissue anatomy of the tongue and floor of the mouth: an ultrasound demonstration. *Brain Lang.* 1984 Mar;21(2):335-50.

[36] Carpenter,R.J.,McDonald, T.J., Howard, F.M., 1978,The otolaryngologic presentation of amyotrophic lateral sclerosis. *J Otol Rhinol Laryngol*, 86, 479-484.

[37] Lawyer,T.,Netsky, M.G.,1953.Amyotrophic lateral sclerosis: A clinicoanatomic study of fifty-three cases. *AMA Arch Neurol Psychiatry.* , 69, 171-192.

[38] Dworkin,J.P., Hartman,D.E.,1979. Progressive speech deterioration and dysphagia in amyotrophic lateral sclerosis. Case report. *Arch Phys Med Rehab,* 60:423-425.

[39] Cha,C.H.,Pattern,B.M.,1989. Amyotrophic lateral sclerosis: Abnormalities of the tongue on magnetic resonance imaging. *Ann Neurol,* 25, 468-472.

[40] Dworkin,J.P.,Aronson,A.E.,1986. Tongue strength and alternate mation rates in normal and dysarthric subjects. *J Commun Disor*, 19, 115-132

[41] Enderby P., 1988. The assessment of dysarthria: A challenge to more than the ears. *Clin Rehab* 2(4), 267-273.

[42] DePaul R, Brooks BR.: Multiple orofacial indices in amyotrophic lateral sclerosis. *J Speech Hear Res*. 1993; 36: 1158-1167.

[43] Theodoros D, Russell TG, Hill A, Cahill L, Clark K. Assessment of motor speech disorders online: a pilot study. *J Telemed Telecare*. 2003;9 Suppl 2:S66-8.

In: Amyotrophic Lateral Sclerosis: New Research
Editor: Christine A. Murray, pp. 245-262
ISBN 1-59454-179-5

Chapter X

Evaluation of Oesophageal Peristalsis in Amyotrophic Lateral Sclerosis' Patients with Dysphagia (Early Report)

B. Tomik[1,*], K. Lorens[2], A. Pichor[1], A. Szczudlik and W. Pawlik[2]

[1]Department of Neurology and [2]Department of Physiology,
Medical College Jagiellonian University, Krakow, Poland.

ABSTRACT

Background

There are currently only few techniques available to reliably assess the stages of swallowing dysfunction due to ALS, including mainly videofluoroscopy and different clinical scales which are based on symptomatology only. The occurrence of the oropharyngeal phases of swallowing in ALS patients has been well documented.
We suggest that the oesophageal manometry (OM) can be useful in determining the degree of dysphagia even on the level of the oesophageal body.

Objective

To evaluate the use of oesophageal manometry as the diagnostic procedure in amyotrophic lateral sclerosis' (ALS) patients with dysphagia.

* Correspondence concerning this article should be addressed to Barbara Tomik MD, PhD; Department of Neurology, Medical College Jagiellonian University; 3 Botaniczna St, 31-503 Krakow, Poland; Tel. + 48 12 424 86 00 ,fax +48 12 424 86 26; E-mail:tomik@neuro.cm-uj.krakow.pl

Material and Methods

The study was carried out in 20 bulbar onset ALS patients with dysphagia, fulfilling WFN criteria (aged from 36 to 74 yr.) and 20 sex- and age matched healthy volunteers. The standard transnasal oesophageal manometry was performed in all subjects using a flexible catheter with the solid state transducers (Synectics, Sweden). The proximal part of oesophageal body was evaluated by locating the proximal transducer 3 cm below the distal border of the upper oesophageal sphincter (UOS). Five ml of water (wet swallows) and saliva (dry swallows) were given at 30-sec intervals.

Results

The comparison of mean oesophageal contractile amplitude, mean oesophageal contractile duration and mean oesophageal contractile velocity during the wet swallows between ALS and control subjects were: 99± 58 vs. 60±22mmHg ($p=0.009$), 3.91±1.4 vs. 2.7±0.7 sec ($p=0.001$), 4.6±1.8 vs. 2.8±0.4 cm/sec ($p<0.001$), respectively and during the dry swallows were: 96 ±59 vs. 44±25 mm Hg ($p<0.001$), 4.8±1.9 vs. 2.5±1.7 sec($p<0.001$), 5.4±2.0 vs. 3.9±0.5 cm/sec ($p=0.002$), respectively. The differences of the results of these parameters during wet vs. dry swallows in the studied groups were statistically significant only for the amplitude and the velocity in controls ($p<0.001$) but not in ALS subjects.

Conclusion

The most remarkable result of the study is the evidence that all ALS patients with dysphagia showed significant abnormalities in all parameters measured by oesophageal manometry as compared to controls. Our study showed the presence of oesophageal dysmotility in all ALS patients with dysphagia, which had not been systematically studied before.

Keywords: ALS, dysphagia, oesophageal manometry.

Introduction

A neurogenic mechanism of dysphagia, which may have either sensory or motor components, or both, can result from a disorder of the oral, pharyngeal, or oesophageal phase of swallowing. They may arise from the involvement of the cortical areas concerned with swallowing, their efferent pathway, the brain stem motor and sensory nuclei, the lower cranial nerves in their distal course, their neuromuscular junctions, or the striated muscle components of the swallow pathway [1].

It is well known that symptoms of bulbar dysfunction due to ALS represent the first manifestations in about 30% of patients, and about 90% of patients usually develop bulbar symptoms by the time of death. Dysphagia is not uncommon as an initial symptom in ALS, but it appears typically several months after the onset of the symptoms [2,3]. Swallowing disorders of ALS patients are usually the major handicaps to the quality of life and an addition to the increasing risk of aspiration pneumonia and impaired nutritional status as well as dehydratation. [3-5]. All of them are independent prognostic factors for worsened survival [6]. In patients with progressing bulbar neurodegeneration signs also dysphagia dramatically progressed and limited food and fluid consumption [7]. ALS dysphagic patients are presented with a slowed ability to eat a meal, retention of solid food in the pharynx, delayed food passage, loss of salivary control with drooling, episodic coughing, choking and nasal regurgitation, wet voice as well as aspiration and asphyxia due to a solid bolus obstructing the airway [8,9].

Dysphagia in ALS patients is difficult to assess objectively. Bedside examination and clinical evaluation of swallowing cannot be accurate because the clinical scales of swallowing are mainly based on symptomatology. There are currently a few techniques available to reliably assess the swallowing dysfunction due to ALS. Videofluoroscopy (VFES, also called cineradiography) visualised the bolus path and related structures from the mouth to the stomach [10-13]. VEFS combining with various food textures, postural changes and specific swallowing manoeuvres can show more information regarding the disturbances of the swallowing mechanism [14-18]. The presence of dysphagia in ALS cases can be diagnosed by videofluoroscopic/manometric methods even before the bulbar symptoms or swallowing difficulty appear clinically [11,13,15]. The combination of videofluoroscopy and manometry conducted simultaneously (videomanoflourometry) has measured the changes in intraluminal pressure precisely correlated with the movement of the bolus and different structures [15,16]. The fibreoptic endoscipic examination [19] and ultrasound (detecting the movements of the tongue and pharyngeal wall) can also be used [20]. The objective measurment of oropharyngeal voluntarily initiated swallowing can be made by the electrophysiological studies [2].

According to the literature it is known that the combination of bulbar spasticity and flaccid muscular weakness and wasting in ALS patients provide for abnormalities mainly in the oropharyngeal phases of swallowing, which have been well documented [4,11,21-24]. The occurrence and the mechanism of disturbances of the oesophageal phase of swallowing in ALS patients have not been systematically studied. Detection and measurement of the oesophageal stage of swallowing can be of great importance for improving the full understanding of dysphagia pathophysiology due to the disease, and maybe a good opportunity for the future rehabilitation (biofeedback) of swallowing disturbances in ALS patients.

In this study, we investigated the disturbances of oesophageal peristalsis due to swallowing abnormalities in ALS patients by using the oesophageal manometry (OM) method. OM can detect and characterise the disturbances of oesophageal motility during the swallowing disorders.

Material and Methods

Subjects

The study was carried out in 20 bulbar onset sporadic ALS patients with the clinical evidence of dysphagia, and 20 sex- and age matched healthy volunteers. All ALS patients were diagnosed according to El Escorial WFN Criteria (1994) [25] based on the information from the database of Krakow MND Centre of the Department of Neurology of Jagiellonian University. ALS group consisted of 12 women and 8 men , aged: 36-74 yr. (mean: 56.8±11.4 yr.). At the time of the investigation, additional signs of the lower motor neurone (LMN) involvement in the limbs were prominent in 13 patients, while the signs of the upper motor (UMN) neurone involvement in the limbs predominated in 7 patients. These 7 patients (35%) fulfilled WFN ALS definite criteria and remaining 13 patients (65%) were diagnosed as having probable ALS. Disease duration calculated from the first bulbar symptoms' onset was from 5 to 72 months, (mean 16.5±14.9 months). To evaluate disease severity Norris scale (maximum - 120 point) [26] and ALSFRS (maximum - 40 point) were used [27]. Bulbar and pseudobulbar signs other than dysphagia occurred in all of the investigated patients e.g. emotional liability, an increase of brainstem reflexes and a loss of the lingual motor function as well as the fasciculation and atrophy of the tongue muscles and the decrease of brainstem reflexes. Dysphagia was the first symptom only in 3 out of 20 investigated ALS patients with bulbar onset. In the remaining patients the first clinical bulbar presentation showed signs of

Table 1. ALS swallowing scores form Hillel et al, 1989 (27)

Normal eating habit

10. Normal swallowing: Patient denies any difficulty chewing or swallowing

9. Nominal abnormality: Only patient notices slight indicators such as food lodging in the recesses of the mouth or sticking in the throat

Early eating problems

8. Minor swallowing problems: Complains of some swallowing difficulties

7. Prolonged time/smaller bite size: Meal time has significantly increased and smaller bite sizes are necessary

Dietary consistency changes

6. Soft diet: Diet is limited primarily to soft foods

5. Liquefied diet: Nutrition is limited primarily to liquefied diet

Needs tube feeding

4. Supplemental tube feedings: Patient uses or needs a tube to supplement intake; patient continues to take significant (greater than 50%) nutrition orally

3. ube feeding with occasional oral nutrition: Primary nutrition and hydration accomplished by tube; receives less than 50% nutrition orally

No oral feeding

2. Secretions managed with aspirator and/or medications

1. Aspiration of secretion: Secretion cannot be managed noninvasively

dysarthria, however, difficulties with swallowing occurred in all of them during the later stage of progression of the disease. Early, predominant symptoms of dysphagia noticed by the patients were: accumulation of saliva in the mouth, coughing during swallowing and difficulty with liquid swallowing. Our patients were presented with dysphagia in varying degrees. However, at the time of the investigation and recruitment to the oesophageal manometry procedure no patient required nutrition through a nasogastric tube or gastrostomy (PEG), all of them were able to ingest orally but most of them preferred taking semisolid food. To evaluate dysphagia severity 10-point clinical scale of swallowing (table 1) was used, in which 10 points mean the normal swallowing and 1 point means the aspiration. (from Hillel et al., 1989 [27]. The inclusion criteria to the study if ALS patients were: [1] bulbar evidence in the clinical examination, [2] clinical evidence of dysphagia in the swallowing severity scale ≤ 7 point (means the prolonged time of swallowing, small pieces of food), but >5 point (means: liquid diet), [3] forced vital capacity -FVC >50% (done obligatorily by the standard spirometry, examined in the sitting position), [4] written informed consent. In the control group (healthy adult volunteers who declared no swallowing problems) there were 9 women and 11 men, aged: 35-65 yr. (mean :48.7±12.3 yr.). Each subject gave a written informed consent after being fully informed about the aim of the study and the freedom to withdraw from the trial. The study protocol was approved by the Ethics Committee of the Jagiellonian University Medical School in Krakow. The subjects with the past medical history of the major surgery of the neck, local radiotherapy and with additional conditions that could effect the oesophageal function e.g. previous stroke, parkinsonism, diabetes mellitus, thyroid disease and lymphadenopathy were excluded from the study. No patient studied was on any drug that could affect oesophageal motility (eg. calicum antagonists, beta blockers, nitrates, prokinetics, antidopaminergics, sedatives) [28]. One patient who withdrew his written consent during the OM procedure was also excluded from the study.

Oesophageal Manometry Procedure

A manometric study of the oesophageal body was used to assess the strength, duration and propagation of the muscular contractions and to detect the motility and abnormalities of the peristaltic waves [14,29-31]. The standard transnasal oesophageal manometry (OM) was performed in all subjects in the Manometry Laboratory of the Department of Physiology of the Jagiellonian University, Krakow, in which more than 10 000 OM examinations were performed without any clinical complications (except a few cases with epistaxis, which was stopped after catheter insertion*)*. Three peristaltic parameters were assessed: amplitude, duration and velocity. Amplitude is a measure of the strength of the peristaltic contraction and is expressed in millimetres of mercury (mmHg). Duration of the contraction is expressed in seconds (s). Velocity is the rate of progression of the contraction down the oesophagus and is expressed in centimeters per second (cm/s) [28,31].

Organic diseases of the upper gastrointestinal tract (UGT)) were excluded before examination after endoscopy. OM was performed in each patient by the same examiner in the morning, after a 12-hour fast. The study was carried out in the same position, using the same technique in all subjects. OM was performed using computerised Synectics' System

(Sweden) consisting of Polygraph VIII, solid state catheter Königsberg Instruments, Pasadena, USA, number P 33-4200 DM60, and software Polygram Upper GI Edition, version 5.06 (Synectics). The manometric tracings were analysed using Synectics' software. Oesophageal pressures values were estimated directly by the solid state transducers in the catheter [31,32]. Four manometric transducers were located in the distal part of the catheter with a distance between each one 3,2,5 cm, respectively. The proximal part of the oesophagus was evaluated by locating the first transducer 3 cm below the distal border of the upper oesophageal sphincter (UOS). Before insertion of the catheter each patient was in the comfortable sitting position just in front of the computer screen. After the local anaesthesia the flexible catheter was passed via the nose into the oesophagus (without the helpful swallowing to exclude the possibility of aspiration in patients with more severe dysphagia). After catheter insertion the patient had a 5 minutes' rest for habituation and the better acceptance of the catheter presence. During this period of time the patients were observing their manometric changes occurring in real time during the swallowing of saliva, cough and breathing without the examiner's assistance.

Each diagnostic procedure of OM consists of 10 wet and 10 dry successful swallows, respectively. All patients with dysphagia presented an individual rhythm of successful, primary swallowing and that fact determined the total time of the examination. Wet swallowing means swallowing of 5 ml of room temperature water (all subjects were able to hold the beaker of water close to their own mouth) and dry swallowing means swallowing of saliva. The manometric profile of wet swallowing was reproducible but not for dry swallowing because sialorrhea excluded the standardisation of this procedure.

After collecting the manometric data in the computer system dry and wet swallowings were analysed. According to the problems with standardisation of dry swallowing only the wet swallows' rhythm was reliable. The mean time of diagnostic procedure was 20 minutes.

During OM procedure the primary wet and dry swallows (primary peristaltic waves) and secondary waves (oesophageal clearing) and tertiary peristaltic waves were analysed, respectively. Primary oesophageal peristalsis during wet and dry swallows was established after the voluntary oropharyngeal manoeuvre. During the analysis: the individual frequency of primary peristalsis (a number of successful primary swallows/minute), the presence of secondary peristalsis, the basal oesophageal body pressure, the mean and maximum pressure of wet and dry contractions, velocity (cm/sec) of wet and dry contractions and a number of tertiary peristalsis were studied in detail. Most of the patients excellently tolerated the procedure of the examination excluding only two patients with the brisk jaw jerk and the involuntary spastic closure of the mouth (due to the severe lesion of pseudobulbar innervation*)* who had to be additionally passed out from the study.

Statistical analysis: Chi-square, Student t-independent test, non-parametric Mann-Whitney-Wilcoxon and Pearson's correlation tests were done by using STATA . A p *value* ≤ 0.01 was accepted as statistically significant.

Results

There were no significant differences between the age and sex in the studied group. The mean value of Norris scale was 72.7 ± 27.2 point (range: 46-101). The mean value of ALSFRS was 22.9 ± 8.5 point (range: 16-37). The mean value of clinical scale of swallowing was 6.2±1.6 point (range:5-7 point). The mean time of dysphagia duration was 8.6±6.4 months (range:1-26). The demographic data are shown in table 2.

Table 2. Characteristics of the studied groups

	Age	Sex	WFN Criteria	Duration of the disease (months)	Duration of dysphagia (months)	Swallowing scale (point)	Norris scale (point)	ALSFRS (point)
ALS bulbar onset subjects	36-74 yr. 56.8±11.4	Females n=12 Males n=8	Definite ALS n=7 (35%) Probable ALS n=13 (65%)	5-72 16.5±14.9	1-26 8.6±6.4	5-7 6.2±1.6	46-101 72.7±27.2	16-37 22.9±8.5
Control subjects	35-65 yr. 48±12.3	Females n=9 Males n=11						

Table 3. The comparison of values of the mean oesophageal contractile amplitude, the mean oesophageal contractile duration and the mean oesophageal contractile velocity during the wet swallows between ALS and control subjects

Oesophageal body: 3cm below the UES	ALS	Control group	p value
Mean oesophageal contractile amplitude	99±58	60±22	p=0.009
Mean oesophageal contractile duration	3.91±1.4	2.7±0.7	p=0.001
Mean oesophageal contractile velocity	4.6±1.8	2.8±0.4	p<0.001

Table 4. The comparison of values of the mean oesophageal contractile amplitude, the mean oesophageal contractile duration and the mean oesophageal contractile velocity during the dry swallows between ALS and control subjects

Oesophageal body: 3cm below the UES	ALS	Control group	p value
Mean oesophageal contractile amplitude	96±59	44±25	p<0.001
Mean oesophageal contractile duration	4.8±1.9	2.5±1.7	p<0.001
Mean oesophageal contractile velocity	5.4±2.0	3.9±0.5	p=0.002

The comparison of the mean oesophageal contractile amplitude, the mean oesophageal contractile duration and the mean oesophageal contractile velocity during the wet swallows between ALS and control subjects were: 99±58 vs. 60±22mmHg (p=0.009), 3.91±1.4 vs. 2.7±0.7 sec (p=0.001), 4.6±1.8 vs. 2.8±0.4 cm/sec (p<0.001), respectively (table 3). The comparison of the mean oesophageal contractile amplitude, the mean oesophageal contractile duration and the mean oesophageal contractile velocity during the dry swallows between ALS and control subjects were 96 ±59 vs. 44±25 mm Hg (p<0.001), 4.8±1.9 vs. 2.5±1.7 sec(p<0.001), 5.4±2.0 vs. 3.9±0.5 cm/sec (p=0.002), respectively (table 4). The results are shown also on the graphs [1-3]. The differences of the results of these parameters during wet vs. dry swallows in the studied groups were statistically significant only for the amplitude and the velocity in controls (p<0.001) but not in ALS subjects. The tracings obtained during the OM procedure from control and ALS subjects are shown in following figures [1-3]. There was no statistical dependence between the values of the mean oesophageal contractile amplitude, duration and velocity of peristaltic contractions and the mean values of the clinical scale of swallowing, Norris scale and ALSFRS during the dry and wet swallows, respectively.

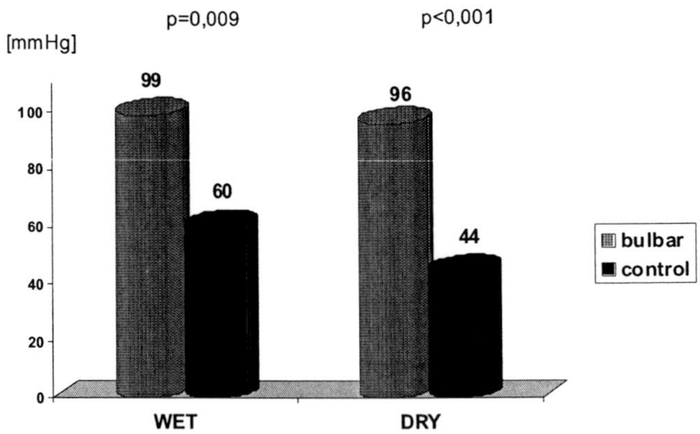

Graph 1. The comparison of the mean upper oesophageal contractile amplitude during the wet and dry swallows between ALS and control subjects.

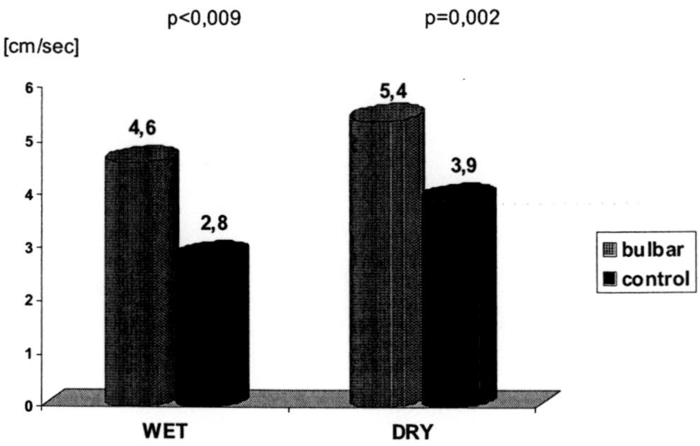

Graph 2. The comparison of the mean upper oesophageal contractile velocity during the wet and dry swallows between ALS and control subjects.

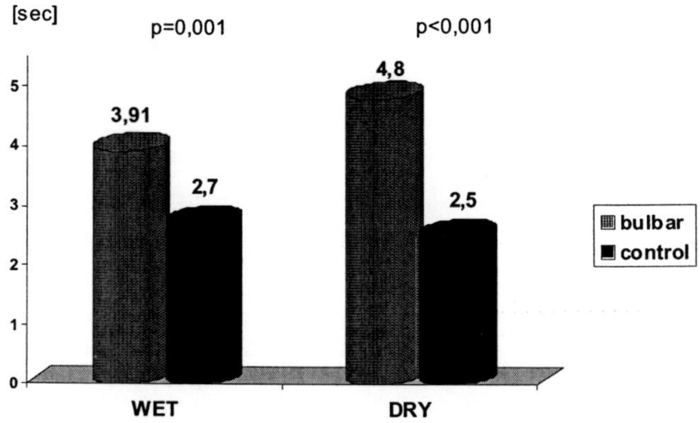

Graph 3. The comparison of the mean upper oesophageal contractile duration during the wet and dry swallows between ALS and control subjects.

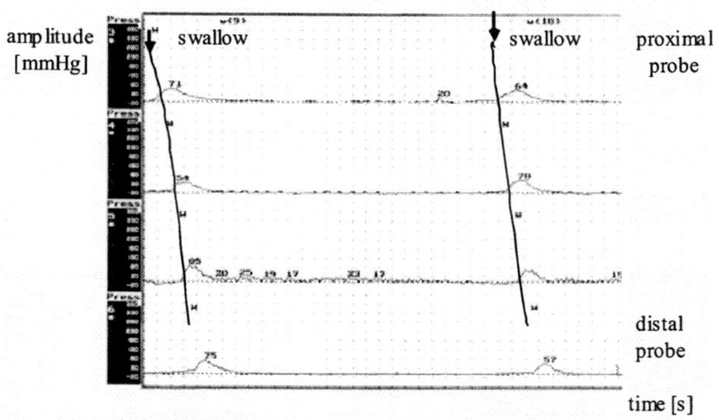

Figure 1. Normal oesophageal peristalsis. In this tracing, four transducers are positioned in the oesophagus, with the proximal one 3 cm below the UOS. At the initiation of swallowing, a peristaltic wave sweeps the length of the oesophagus, sealing the lumen behind the bolus.The maximum pressures are shown for each wave.

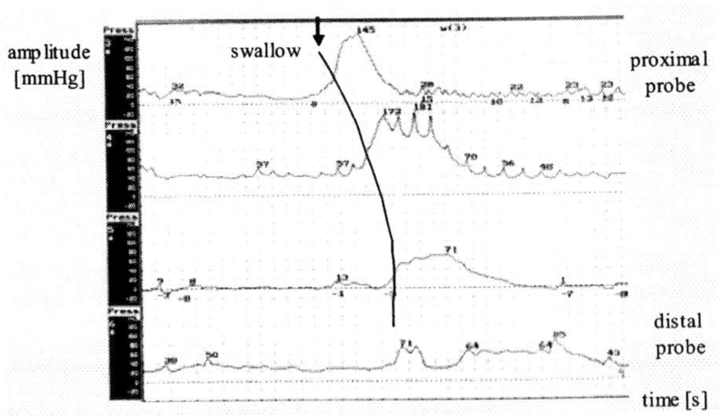

Figure 2. Disturbed oesophageal peristalsis in pseudobulbar syndrome (ALS). In this tracing four transducers are positioned in the oesophagus, with the proximal one 3 cm below the UOS. The maximum pressures are shown for each wave. The maximal pressures in the proximal oesophagus (the striated muscles) are increased, velocity of propagation is decreased and progression of waves in the distal oesophagus is disrupted.

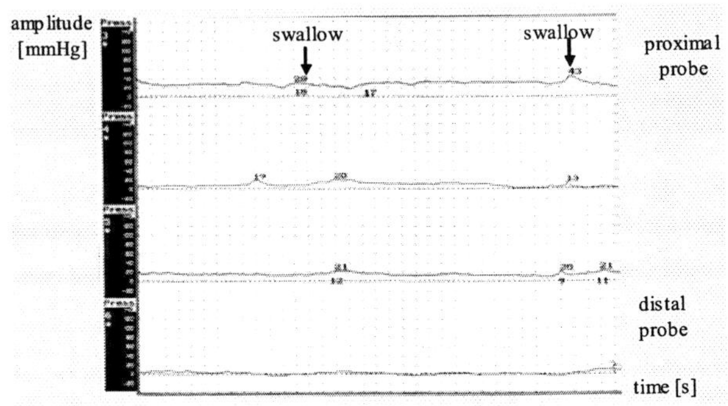

Fig 3. Oesophageal hypomotility in the patient with severe dysphagia (ALS). In this tracing, four transducers are positioned in the oesophagus, with the proximal one 3 cm below the UOS. There is no evidence of propulsive peristalsis despite the oral phase stimuli and thepositive intraoesophageal pressure.

Discussion

Swallowing is usually subdivided into three phases; an initial oral phase, a pharyngeal phase and an oesophageal phase [2]. The oral phase is under voluntary control and highly variable in many respects. The pharyngeal phase encompasses several closely co-ordinated actions that involve the bolus transport from the oropharynx into the oesophagus without aspiration. The oesophageal phase is completely involuntary and automatic. In the normal swallowing process the cranial nerve involvement in the bolus preparation (V-motor and sensory and VII), the bolus propulsion (X and XII), and the palatal elevation (X) is well appreciated[2,3,33]. The airway is protected by apposition of the true and false vocal cords and of the arytenoids against the base of the epiglottis (the sphincteric action of the larynx); the epiglottis inhibits the direct contact of the bolus with the laryngeal vestibule (all X) [33,34]. Upward and forward movement of the hyoid and larynx (V, VII, C1-3) enhances airway protection and pulls open the relaxed upper oesophageal sphincter. Breathing is centrally inhibited during the swallow (deglutition apnoea) and after it the structures return to their original position passively or aided by the infrahyoid muscles [34]. The mechanisms controlling the tongue, pharynx and UOS are associated with a wide variety of local, neurological and muscular disorders, and can also occur after surgery in the area and in response to the gastro-oesophageal reflux (GOR) [28,31].

It is well known that dysphagia in ALS is caused by degeneration of the motor nuclei of the IXth, Xth, and XIIth cranial nerves of the brain stem, and bulbar palsy is the principal feature. Hughes and Wiles [35] reported that in the motor neurone disease patients with a brisk rather than depressed pharyngeal response are associated with more impaired swallowing. Also Hughs and Wiles [35] presented that a loss of corticobulbar pyramidal fibres may lead to brisker palatopharyngheal reflex responses because of a reduction in descending inhibition, and therefore probably produces the swallowing disorders due to ALS. Marked degeneration of the motor nucleus of the XIIth cranial nerve resulting in atrophy and a loss of fine movements of the tongue causes apparent disorders at the oral phase of swallowing [36]. It is also reported that dysphagia in ALS is aggravated by disturbances at the pharyngeal phase of swallowing, including disorders of the laryngeal elevation, the soft palate elevation, and a decrease in the swallowing pressure due to the decreased pharyngeal contraction [36,37]. Patients with oropharyngeal dysphagia are usually presented with difficulty in initiating swallowing and associated coughing, choking or nasal regurgitation and hypernosality of the speech. The dominant mechanism causing neurogenic dysphagia (ALS patients) may differ in two patients with the same disease and can clearly change over time.

In cases of bulbar ALS, dysphagia can result from the involvement of the trigeminal, facial, hypoglossal, glossopharyngeal, or vagus cranial nerves [38]. Hillel and Miller [4] described a temporal progressive pattern of affected musculature due to the course of bulbar ALS. These authors suggested that the tongue and lips were affected first (resulting in possible oral stage swallowing difficulties). The group of muscles affected secondly included the palatal, jaw, and pharyngeal muscles. The facial, upper trunk, and laryngeal muscles formed the third group of affected muscles followed by the last group consisting of extra-ocular muscles. Swallowing difficulties can be one of the earliest complaints of bulbar onset ALS patients. Early swallowing problems include managing foods with tough texture, foods that fragment easily, thin liquids, and saliva control as well as increasing eating time [38,39]. More severe swallowing disturbances in ALS patients included reduced nutritional intake, severe problems controlling liquids during the swallow, and increased saliva control problems [38].

Ertekin et al [3] suggested that two pathophysiological mechanisms operate dysphagia in ALS cases i.e.(a) the triggering of the swallowing reflex for the voluntarily initiated swallows is delayed, disordered and eventually absent while the spontaneous reflexive swallows are preserved until the preterminal stage of ALS and (b) the cricopharyngeal sphincter muscle of pharyngo-oesophageal segment becomes hyperreflexive and hypertonic, resulting in the loss of coordination of voluntarily initiated oropharyngeal swallowing by the laryngeal protective system. These authors claim that the described above pathophysiological changes due to dysphagia in ALS patients are primarily associated with the progressive degeneration of the excitatory and inhibitory corticobulbar pyramidal fibres. Perkin et al [1] described also the abnormal oral phase of swallowing encompassing both a prolonged oral transit time and repetitive lingual pumping, probably reflecting reduced lingual force. The ALS patients usually employ changing head postures to facilitate swallowing. A prolonged delay time (duration from arrival of the bolus at the midpoint of the velum until the initiation of maximal hyoid excursion) is strikingly apparent in the bulbar group, whereas the pharyngeal response time (from the initiation of maximal hyoid excursion to hyoid return to rest) shows no differences between the patients with the bulbar and nonbulbar form of the disease. Laryngeal aspiration can occur before, during, or after the pharyngeal phase of swallowing. However, there are also some bases for involving the oesophageal phase of swallowing in ALS patients with bulbar signs because of the degeneration of Xth nerve, especially nucleus ambiguus from which the nervous fibres go down and innervate the striated muscle of the upper part of the oesophagus. Additionally, oesophageal disturbances are commonly manifested by pharyngeal or even oropharyngeal symptoms. This underscores the fact that the whole swallowing process should be examined [40].

The use of oesophageal manometry procedure for detecting the occurrence of disturbances in the oesophageal phase of swallowing in ALS patients is a new concept, however, oesophageal manometry has been used as a diagnostic test in oesophageal diseases for over 40 years. It provides both qualitative and quantitative assessment of oesophageal pressures, coordination and motility [28,31]. Gambitta et al [41] reported that OM can detect the abnormalities of oesophageal motility in 90% of the patients with dysphagia. Manometric examination of the oesophagus frequently reveals dysmotility whose cause in unknown and whose physiological importance in not clear. Although manometric abnormalities are frequent, authorities disagree on how to interpret and classify the aberrant oesophageal motility patterns [28,31,42-44]. This is caused by several factors. Firstly, the cause of dysmotility is not known and next, a number of manometric abnormalities has no apparent physiological consequences. There is also no clear consensus on the ideal technique for performing oesophageal manometry resulting in the lack of the widely accepted system for classifying the abnormal oesophageal motility patterns, and the lack of uniform diagnostic criteria for the putative disorders [44]. Contraindications of OM are limited to: pharyngeal or upper oesophageal obstructions, oesophageal bullous disorder, cardiac conditions in which vagal stimuli cannot be tolerated, severe coagulopathy and patient non-compliance [45].

In the present study, oesophageal peristalsis was estimated in 20 ALS patients with mild or moderate dysphagia using oesophageal manometry and the results were compared with results obtained from the control subjects. We found a strong evidence of the occurrence of disturbances of the oesophageal phases of swallowing in ALS patients, which previously had not been well documented in the literature. We presented a detailed analysis of changing the parameters by describing the upper oesophageal peristalsis e.g. the mean oesophageal contractile amplitude, the mean oesophageal contractile duration and the mean oesophageal contractile velocity, which significantly differed during the wet and also dry swallows in ALS patients as compared to the controls. Also the result differences between the parameters obtained during the wet and dry swallowings in the studied groups were statistically significant only for the amplitude and the velocity in controls ($p<0.001$) but not in ALS subjects. However, we also obtained no statistical dependence between the values of the mean oesophageal contractile amplitude, duration and velocity during the wet and also dry swallowings (compared separately) and the mean values of clinical scales assessing the disease severity (Norris scale, ALSFRS) as well as the mean values of the clinical scale of swallowing. Our data suggest that the neurodegeneration of cortical and bulbar motoneurones in ALS patients is parallel to the observed oesophageal motility abnormalities. The process of denervation leads to disruption of neural reflexes controlling the swallowing and limits the possibility of effective oesophageal primary peristalsis. The number of primary swallows was lower in all ALS patients than in controls. Central denervation and limitation of mechanical stimulation of the striated muscle in the oesophageal wall leads to atrophic changes which aggravate dysphagia. We observed no significant differences between wet and dry swallows in ALS patients. This phenomenon demonstrates the absence of specific swallowing reflexes induced by saliva or water. Dry swallows in ALS patients with a long duration of contraction (4.8±1.9 s) and higher velocity (5.4±2.0 cm/s) explain the difficulties in saliva swallowing reported by the patients. Of course these symptoms may be also caused by oropharyngeal dysmotility and sialorrhea.

The limitation of our study is the restriction of the measurement of only the upper oesophageal swallowing parameters by OM, which is connected with the anatomical structure and the innervation of the oesophagus. Extrinsic innervation of the oesophagus is via the vagus nerve. Fibres innervating the striated muscle originate from the cell bodies in the nucleus ambiguus, whereas the innervation of the smooth muscle is provided by the dorsal motor nucleus of vagus [46,47]. A complete manometric evaluation of oesophageal peristalsis should include measurements of both the smooth muscle of the distal oesophagus and the striated muscle of the proximal oesophagus and usually begins with the lower oesophageal sphincter (LOS) [31]. However, the choice of the evaluation of only the upper oesophageal peristalsis in ALS patients was intended and is explained by the characteristic type of neurodegeneration due to ALS in which the smooth muscles (lower oesophagus) are not damaged by the disease.

The estimation of the use of this method for detection of the disturbances of the oesophageal peristalsis in ALS patients due to dysphagia is also difficult because of the lack of comparable studies. The pharyngooesophageal manometry was used in ALS patients by Mac Dougall et al [12]. This study was conducted on a small group which consisted of 13 ALS patients and 13 controls. The authors showed the lack of significant difference between ALS patients and control subjects in the distal oesophageal motility or the lower oesophageal sphincter (LOS) motility and no pressure parameter of the pharyngooesophageal motility. The significant reduction of the postcontraction amplitude of UOS during wet and solid swallows was noticed only in 7 (out of 13) ALS patients with severe dysphagia as compared to the controls. Contrary to the listed results our study demonstrated significant abnormalities of all measured parameters of the upper oesophageal peristalsis in all dysphagic ALS patients as compared to controls. Kawai et al [48] using also the pharyngooseophageal manometry in 11 ALS patients showed that manometric studies were almost normal in all cases except one but the authors studied ALS patients with the early stage of dysphagia. They concluded that in the early stage of dysphagia in ALS patients only the oral phase of swallowing was changed because the transport of the bolus by the tongue was impaired. The above-mentioned authors suggest also that the principal feature of the relatively early stage of dysphagia in ALS occurs at the oral phase, in which a limitation in the lingual movement and atrophy of the tongue are dominant features. Thus, the ability of holding the bolus appears to be the most important in the determination of the severity of the relatively early stage of dysphagia in ALS. In 2002 Higo et al [16] published the results of the time-course changes of the swallowing function in 21 ALS cases (divided into five groups according to the type of disease and according to the length of time following the appearance of bulbar symptoms) by using videomanofluorometry which is a videofluoroscopic and manometric study conducted simultaneously. The authors showed that in ALS patients the decrease of swallowing pressure first appeared in the oropharynx, after that in the hypopharynx. Oropharyngeal swallowing pressure was decreased to approximately 50 mm Hg within 6 months after the presentation of bulbar symptoms whereas hypopharyngeal swallowing pressure was relatively maintained until 1 year after the onset of bulbar symptoms. Most of the patients with ALS maintained the normal upper esophageal sphincter relaxation, and the upper esophageal sphincter spasm was also seen in some patients with ALS. Higo et al [16] concluded that both videofluoroscopic and manometric evaluations are necessary to assess the swallowing disturbances due to ALS and they are quite useful for the follow-up of the swallowing function in patients with ALS and dysphagia. We did not find any data showing the use of oesophageal manometry for evaluation and characterizing the oesophageal peristalsis in ALS patients. The authors of the three papers mentioned above did not use the manometric method for the assessment of the oesophageal phase of swallowing, they focused on the oropharyngeal changing of swallowing in ALS subjects. Also the protocols of their studies differ as compared to ours. The manometric method was successfully used in the primary muscle disease as the myotonic dystrophy and showed the weakness affecting the pharynx, cricopharyngeal sphincter and the oesophagus [1]. Also defective peristalsis of the upper oesophagus was described in the inflammatory muscle disease as polymyositis and dermatomyositis. The incomplete relaxation of the upper oesophageal sphincter and abnormal peristaltic activity of the oesophageus are also described in oculopharyngeal muscular dystrophy [1].

Taking into consideration the literature data survey it is difficult to predict what practical, clinical significance our results may have. The study was conducted on the selected group of patients with slight or moderately advanced dysphagia. The assumption was necessary for the patients' convenience and the safety of performed examinations. On account of the uncommon occurrence of the disease and the selection of patients for the study (according to the strictly definite and described criteria of our study), the possibility of verification of the initial, presented results and the development of investigations is time-limited. The study will be still continued all the more that the initial results of using the method of oesophageal striated muscle rehabilitation (i.e., biofeedback training, BT) with OM indicate the swallowing function improvement in patients and body mass index (BMI) stabilization. The psychological aspect of introducing the set of drills teaching to improve swallowing functions also seems to be extremely essential.

Conclusions and Future Directions

To the best of our knowledge it is the first study to explore the influence of neurodegeneration on the oesophageal phase of swallowing in ALS patients with dysphagia. We showed that all dysphagic ALS patients studied by us showed significant abnormalities in all the parameters measured by oesophageal manometry as compared to controls. Based on these conclusions we suggest the existence of disturbances of swallowing in ALS patients with dysphagia not only in the well described oropharyngeal phase but also in the oesophageal phase. We have to mention that the results presented have to be recognised as preliminary and that they support the reports which concern the mechanisms of dysphagia in ALS.

On the basis of the demonstrated results we start the biofeedback training (BT) with visualisation of oesophageal manometric changes during wet and dry swallows in most of our dysphagic ALS patients to improve their swallowing. We hope that the continuation of the presented study and the use of OM as the diagnostic method for evaluation of oesophageal disturbances in ALS patients can allow us to describe the "pattern" of oeosphageal peristaltic parameter changes specific for the predominant bulbar and psuedobulbar presentation according to the criteria described by Spechler and Castel. This can be helpful in evaluating the occurence of life-threatening aspiration. We also plan to use this method for the follow – up of the assessment of presented disturbances of oesophageal peristalsis due to disturbances of swallowing in ALS patients. OM can be an easy, objective method for recording the time-course changes of swallowing function in amyotrophic lateral sclerosis The results will be reported.

References

[1] Perkin GD, Murray-Lyon I. Neurology and the gastrointestinal system. *Neurol Neurosurg Psychiatry.* 1998 Sep;65(3):291-300.

[2] Ertekin C, Aydogdu I, Yuceyar N, Tarlaci S, Kiylioglu N, Pehlivan M, Celebi G. Electrodiagnostic methods for neurogenic dysphagia. *Electroencephalogr Clin Neurophysiol.* 1998 Aug;109(4):331-40.

[3] Ertekin C, Aydogdu I, Yuceyar N, Kiylioglu N, Tarlaci S, Uludag B. Pathophysiological mechanisms of oropharyngeal dysphagia in amyotrophic lateral sclerosis. *Brain.* 2000 Jan;123 (Pt 1):125-40.

[4] Hillel AD, Miller R. Bulbar amyotrophic lateral sclerosis: patterns of progression and clinical management. *Head Neck.* 1989 Jan-Feb;11(1):51-9.

[5] Strand EA, Miller RM, Yorkston KM, Hillel AD. Management of oral-pharyngeal dysphagia symptoms in amyotrophic lateral sclerosis. *Dysphagia.* 1996 Spring;11(2):129-39.

[6] Desport JC, Preux PM, Magy L, Boirie Y, Vallat JM, Beaufrere B, Couratier P. Factors correlated with hypermetabolism in patients with amyotrophic lateral sclerosis. *Am J Clin Nutr.* 2001 Sep;74(3):328-34.

[7] Silani V, Kasarskis EJ, Yanagisawa N.Nutritional management in amyotrophic lateral sclerosis: a worldwide perspective. *J Neurol.* 1998 Aug;245 Suppl 2:S13-9; discussion S29.

[8] Belsh JM, Schiffman PL. Rehabilitation Management of the ALS Patient, chapter 13 In: Amyotrophic Lateral sclerosis:Diagnosis and management for the clinician. Armonk, NY: *Futura Publishing Company*, 1996:327-331.

[9] Hughes TA, Wiles CM. Neurogenic dysphagia: the role of the neurologist. *J Neurol Neurosurg Psychiatry.* 1998 May;64(5):569-72.

[10] Robbins J.: Swallowing in ALS and motor neuron diosrders. *Neurol Clin.* 1987; 5, 213-229.

[11] Leighton SE, Burton MJ, Lund WS, Cochrane GM. Swallowing in motor neurone disease. *J R Soc Med.* 1994 Dec;87(12):801-5.

[12] Mac Dougal G, Wilson J.A,Pryde A and Grant R.:Analysis of the pharyngoesophageal pressure profile in amytrophic lateral sclerosis.Otolaryngol *Head Neck Surg* 1995;112:258-61

[13] Briani C, Marcon M, Ermani M, Costantini M, Bottin R, Iurilli V, Zaninotto G, Primon D, Feltrin G, Angelini C. Radiological evidence of subclinical dysphagia in motor neuron disease. *Neurol.* 1998 Apr;245(4):211-6.

[14] Parkman H.P., Maurer A.H., Caroline D.F., Miller D.L., Krevsky B., Fisher R.S.: Optimal evaluation of patients with nonobstructive oesophageal dysphagia. Manometry, scintigraphy, or videoesophagography ? *Dig Dis - Sci.* 1996; 41, 1355-1368.

[15] Castell JA, Olsson R, Castell DO, *et al.* Simultaneous video radiography and manometry in dysphagia with normal barium swallow. *Am J Gastroenterol* 1993;88:1483.

[16] Higo R, Tayama N, Watanabe T, Nito T. Videomanofluorometric study in amyotrophic lateral sclerosis. *Laryngoscope.* 2002 May;112(5):911-7.

[17] Chen MY, Peele VN, Donati D, Ott DJ, Donofrio PD, Gelfand DW. Clinical and videofluoroscopic evaluation of swallowing in 41 patients with neurologic disease. *Gastrointest Radiol.* 1992 Spring;17(2):95-8.

[18] Wilcox F., Liss J., Siegel G.: Interjudge agreement on videofluoroscopic studies of swallowing. *J Speech Hear Res.* 1996; 39, 144-152

[19] Kidney D, Harney M, Alexander M, Patil N, Walsh P, Hardiman O. Assessing dysphasia in motor neurone disease. Abstracts from 14th International Symposium on ALS/MND, Milan, Italy 17-19 November, *Amyotrophic Lateral Sclerosis and other Motor Neuron Disorders,* vol 4, suppl, December 2003, p. 51.

[20] Miller JL, Watkin KL. Lateral wall pharyngeal motion during swallowing using real time ultrasound. *Dysphagia* 1997;12:125-132.

[21] Mitsumoto H, Chad D, Pioro E.P. Nutritional Management, chapter 24. In : Amyotrophic Lateral sclerosis,, F.A. *Davids Co*, Philadelphia 1998;421-436.

[22] Roller NW, Garfunkel A, Nichols C, Ship II. Amyotrophic lateral sclerosis. *Oral Surg Oral Med Oral Pathol.* 1974 Jan;37(1):46-52.

[23] Carpenter RJ 3rd, McDonald TJ, Howard FM Jr. The otolaryngologic presentation of amyotrophic lateral sclerosis. *Otolaryngology.* 1978 May-Jun;86(3 Pt 1):ORL479-84.

[24] McGuirt WF, Blalock D. The otolaryngologist's role in the diagnosis and treatment of amyotrophic lateral sclerosis. *Laryngoscope.* 1980 Sep;90(9):1496-501.

[25] Brooks BR, Hormigo A, Larumbe R, et al. El Escorial World Federation of Neurology criteria for the diagnosis of amyotrophic lateral sclerosis. *J Neurol Sci* 1994;124(suppl):96-107.

[26] Norris FH Jr, U KS, Sachais B, Carey M. Trial of baclofen in amyotrophic lateral sclerosis. *Arch Neurol.* 1979 Nov;36(11):715-6.

[27] Hillel AD, Miller RM, Yorkston K, McDonald E, Norris FH, Konikow N. Amyotrophic lateral sclerosis severity scale. *Neuroepidemiology.* 1989;8(3):142-50.

[28] Castell DO. Clinical applications of esophageal manometry. *Dig Dis Sci.* 1982 Sep;27(9):769-71.

[29] Mujica V.R., Conklin J.: When it is hard to swallow. What to look for patients with dysphagia. *Postgrad Med J.* 1999; 105, 131-145.

[30] Di Marino A.J. Jr., Allen M.L., Lynn R.B., Zamani S.: Clinical value of oesophageal motility testing. *Dig Dis.* 1998; 16, 198-204.

[31] Castell JA, Gideon M, Castell D.O Esophagus. Chapter 9.In: Atlas of Gastrointestinal motility in health and disease, Schuster M.M ; *Williams & Wilkins Co*, 1993;134-157.

[32] Feussner H., Kauer W., Siewert J.R.: The place of oesophageal manometry in the diagnosis of dysphagia. *Dysphagia.* 1993; 8, 98-104.

[33] Logemann JA. Swallowing physiology and pathophysiology. *Otolaryngol Clin North Am.* 1988 Nov;21(4):613-23.

[34] Hughes TA, Wiles CM. Clinical measurement of swallowing in health and in neurogenic dysphagia. *QJM.* 1996 Feb;89(2):109-16.

[35] Hughes TA, Wiles CM. Palatal and pharyngeal reflexes in health and in motor neuron disease. Neuro*l Neurosurg Psychiatry.* 1996 Jul;61(1):96-8.

[36] Ohkubo, H (1980). Dysphagia in amyotrophic lateral sclerosis — electromyographic and, radiological investigations. *Otol Fukuoka* 26: 44-78.

[37] Okamura, H, Mori, T, Inaki, S (1991). Dysphagia due to neuromuscular diseases.*J Jpn Bronchoesophagol Soc* 42: 400-406.

[38] Watts CR, Vanryckeghem M. Laryngeal dysfunction in Amyotrophic Lateral Sclerosis: a review and case report. *BMC Ear Nose Throat Disord.* 2001;1(1):1. Epub 2001 Nov 13.

[39] Hillel A, Dray T, Miller R, Yorkston K, Konikow N, Strande E, Browne J. Presentation of ALS to the otolaryngologist/head and neck surgeon: getting to the neurologist. *Neurology.* 1999;53(8 Suppl 5):S22-5; discussion S35-6.

[40] Jones B, Donner MW. How I do it: examination of the patient with dysphagia. *Dysphagia.* 1989;4(3):162-72.

[41] Gambitta P, Indriolo A, Grosso C, Pirone Z, Colombo P, Arcidiacono R. Role of oesophageal manometry in clinical practice. *Dis Esophagus.* 1999;12(1):41-6.

[42] Ragunath K, Williams JG.A review of oesophageal manometry testing in a district general hospital. *Postgrad Med J.* 2002 Jan;78(915):34-6.

[43] Spieker MR. Evaluating dysphagia. *Am Fam Physician.* 2000 Jun 15;61(12):3639-48.

[44] Spechler SJ, Castell DO. Classification of oesophageal motility abnormalities. *Gut.* 2001 Jul;49(1):145-51.

[45] Passaretti S, Zaninotto G, Di Martino N, Leo P, Costantini M, Baldi F. Standards for oesophageal manometry. A position statement from the Gruppo Italiano di Studio Motilita Apparato Digerente (GISMAD). *Dig Liver Dis.* 2000 Jan-Feb;32(1):46-55.

[46] Higgs B, Kerr FW, Ellis FH Jr. The experimental production of esophageal achalasia by electrolytic lesions in the medulla. *J Thorac Cardiovasc Surg.* 1965 Nov;50(5):613-25.

[47] Kahrilas PJ, Clouse RE, Hogan WJ. American Gastroenterological Association technical review on the clinical use of esophageal manometry. *Gastroenterology.* 1994 Dec;107(6):1865-84.

[48] Kawai S, Tsukuda M, Mochimatsu I, Enomoto H, Kagesato Y, Hirose H, Kuroiwa Y, Suzuki Y. A study of the early stage of Dysphagia in amyotrophic lateral sclerosis. *Dysphagia.* 2003 Winter;18(1):1-8.

In: Amyotrophic Lateral Sclerosis: New Research
Editor: Christine A. Murray, pp. 263-277
ISBN 1-59454-179-5

Chapter XI

Assessment of Deficient Motor Function of the Hand in Amyotrophic Lateral Sclerosis

Dennis A. Nowak [*]
Department of Neurology and Clinical Neurophysiology,
Academic Hospital Bogenhausen of the Technical University of Munich

Abstract

We analyzed the coordination between grip and load force profiles in patients with ALS performing vertical point-to-point arm movements with a hand-held instrumented object. This task necessitates a complex temporal coupling of motor activity in the proximal arm and shoulder muscles responsible for transporting the object and in the fingers used to grasp it. In healthy subjects, the precise regulation of grasping forces is reflected in (a) modulation of the grip force profile in parallel with the movement-induced fluctuations in load and (b) scaling of grip force in such a way that grip force is only a small amount greater than load at all phases of the movement. The grip force control of ALS patients exhibits two major pathologies: (a) they apply inefficiently high grip forces against a hand-held object and (b) there is a desynchronisation of the temporo-spatial coupling between grip and load force profiles. Current rehabilitation concepts commonly focus on the measurement of maximum grip force to objectively evaluate the progress in rehabilitation. Based on our theory that an overflow in grip force contributes significantly to the disability in patients with ALS, it seems fruitful to define the reduction of unnecessarily high finger forces as the preferential goal in hand motor rehabilitation. A potential treatment scheme these patients should include the measurement of grip force during natural unencumbered arm movements with a hand-held load. The finding of

[*] Correspondence concerning this article should be addressed to Dr. Dennis A. Nowak, Department of Psychiatry III, University of Ulm, Leimgrubenweg 12, D-89075 Ulm, Germany; Tel.: 0049 (0)731 500 41275; Fax: 0049 (0)731 500 41065; E-mail: Dennis.Nowak@uni-ulm.de.

uneconomically high grip force should motivate an individual training program to decrease the amount of force overshoot, facilitating fine finger movements and prevent early fatigue of affected hand muscles.

Keywords: Grasping forces; predictive force control; motor neuron disease;

1. Introduction

The numerous skeletal and muscular degrees of freedom of the human hand, orchestrated by highly developed neural control systems, provide an enormous dexterity that allows a highly precise manipulation of objects. The human hand can take on a huge variety of shapes and functions, serving as a hammer at one time or a delicate pair of forceps at another. The universal utility of hand movements are even more enhanced by our ability to amplify the function of the hand by using tools. To understand and appreciate how the central nervous system controls the movements of the hand, it is important to investigate the healthy motor behavior of the hand and its dysfunction during everyday manipulative tasks. Over the past decade, the analysis of finger force control during object manipulation has evolved as a useful tool for the objective evaluation of impaired hand movements. This chapter provides a brief review of the physiological aspects of manipulative finger force control and gives a detailed description of the specific impairments in amyotrophic lateral sclerosis (ALS).

2. Physiological Aspects of Manipulative Finger Force Control

True opposition between the thumb and index finger is only observed in humans, the great apes and Old World monkeys. The human thumb is much longer, relative to the index finger, than the thumb of other primates [33]. This allows humans to grasp and manipulate small objects between the tips of the thumb and index finger [23,24]. Humans have more individuated muscles and tendons with which to control the digits [33]. Primates have evolved extensive cortical systems for controlling the hand and the corticospinal pathways have taken on an increasing dominant role in controlling movements[4,14,25,29,48]. In humans the corticospinal tracts include direct connections between neurons in cortical motor areas and spinal motoneurons [4,29]. Through these cortico-motoneuronal connections, the cerebral cortex possesses monosynaptic control over motoneurons whose axons directly connect with the hand muscles. There is a strong linkage between the amount of cortico-motoneuronal connections and manual dexterity in terms of performing manipulative tasks that require individual finger movements. Through cortical motor structures the hand is under rapid access from most other cortical areas and from subcortical structures, e.g. the cerebellum and basal ganglia, directly involved in motor control. Although there are many advantages of cortical involvement in hand movements, the reliance on cortical control comes at a cost. Pyramidal tract section in monkeys results in impairments of independent finger movements and causes an increase of the grip force built up times [17]. Lesions of the motor cortex or corticospinal pathways can be particularly devastating in humans resulting in severe impairments of prehensile finger force control [7,16,18,45].

When we grasp and transport an object the applied grip force (normal to the grip surfaces) and the load force (tangential to the grip surfaces) are the result of a complex interplay of sensory feedback signals and muscle activity in the hand and arm [12,22,54,55]. Grip forces should be large enough to prevent the hand-held object from slipping, but on the other hand too large grip forces should be avoided as they may hamper fine object manipulation or even crush fragile objects. Hence, a stable grasp entails prevention of accidental slips as well as excessive grip forces. Consequently, successful manipulation requires the selection of motor commands according to the manipulative intend and the relevant physical object properties. In healthy subjects, grip force is efficiently scaled in such a way that it is always a small amount higher than the minimum force required to obtain a stable grasp. Object properties, such as weight, slipperiness, shape, and weight distribution impose constraints on the finger forces, including their magnitude, direction and points of application. Visual information about the physical object properties may help to roughly select appropriate grip force levels [12,22]. However, sensory information from the grasping fingers, mainly provided by cutaneous mechanoreceptors, is the most useful feedback to adjust grip force accurately to the constraints of weight and surface friction [22,23,24]. The hand area of the motor cortex receives proprioceptive and cutaneous afferent input from the hand and arm [53] and interruption of the spinal dorsal columns or disconnection between the first somatosensory and motor cortices result in deficits of the refined control of the hand and fingers similar to those induced by pyramidal tract lesions [1]. The weight and surface friction of a hand-held object are well represented in the discharge of cortical motor neurons and cutaneous afferent information significantly modulates motor cortical activity [48]. Indeed, individuals with impaired manual sensibility have great difficulties when manipulating small objects [37,38,40,41,43]. In particular, they often drop objects and experience problems during fine manipulative tasks, such as writing or using a tool. A peculiar feature of grip force control in subjects with reduced sensibility of the grasping digits is an uneconomically high force level [37,38,40,43].

Skilled grip force behavior involves different modes of control which rely on prediction and sensory feedback to different extents. When holding an object between the fingertips, sufficient grip force must be generated to prevent slip due to load force exerted by the object. When the object's behavior is unpredictable – like holding a dog's leash – sensory feedback provides the most useful signal for estimating the load [12,24,36,39]. In this situation, grip force is modified reactively in response to sensory feedback from the fingers, with the consequence that grip tends to lag some 100 ms behind load due to nerve conduction and central processing delays. In contrast, when we manipulate objects in the environment that exhibit stable properties, predictive control mechanisms can be effectively exploited. For example, when the load of a hand-held object is increased by a self generated action, such as moving the arm, the grip force increases in parallel with load force without an obvious time delay [13,39,54]. Sensory detection of the change in load force is too slow to account for the in time change in grip force which relies on predictive processes. Such a predictive or anticipatory force control is essential for the rapid movements usually observed in dexterous behavior.

When a hand-held object is moved in a point-to-point fashion, it is first accelerated from rest and then decelerated to be held stationary again at the desired end position. In this situation, grip force has to overcome acceleration induced inertial loads of the grasped object. During vertical point-to-point movements with a hand-held object, load force fluctuates, reaching a maximum early in upward and late in downward movements. The acceleration (ACC) and load force traces during upward and downward point-to-point movements are illustrated in the bottom and mid panels of Figure 1. In healthy adults, grip force starts to increase in parallel with load force during the acceleratory phase of an upward movement and during the deceleratory phase of downward movement [13,54]. A grip force maximum coincides with maximum load force early in upward and late in downward movements. These characteristic features of physiological grip force behavior during vertical point-to-point movements can be obtained from the grip force profile illustrated in the top panel of Figure 1.

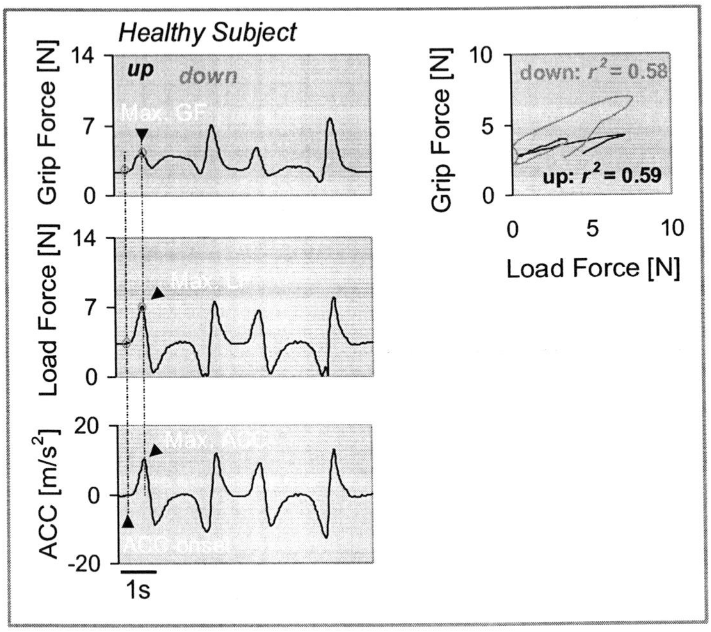

Figure 1. Acceleration (ACC), load force and grip force profiles for consecutive point-to-point upward and downward movements with the grasped object performed by a healthy subject. Vertical lines indicate the movement onset and the maximum of kinematic acceleration for a single upward movement. Right hand to the grip force panel, grip force is plotted against load force for single upward and downward movements. The r^2 correlation coefficients of the least square regression lines are given. ACC onset = movement onset; Max. ACC = maximum of kinematic acceleration; Max. LF = maximum load force; Max. GF = maximum grip force.

When the object is held in the air at rest in between single movements, only its weight has to be counteracted by adequate grip force. At all phases of the transport movement grip force is modulated in parallel with the movement-induced fluctuations in load force without an obvious time delay. The absence of a temporal delay between grip and load force profiles implies that the central nervous system is able to precisely predict the load variations before the intended manipulation takes place and consequently regulates grip force in anticipation [12,54]. In other words, when we move a hand-held object we rely more on a predictive force control policy in which grip force control parameters are derived from internal neural representations of the task and relevant physical object properties, rather than from sensory feedback information from the grasping fingers that would result in large time lags between grip and load force profiles [14,31,54,55]. Investigating grip force control during the combined holding-moving task described here is a sensitive method to demonstrate healthy grip force behavior and its dysfunction. For example, we demonstrated an impaired coordination between grip and load forces during point-to-point movements with a hand-held load in Parkinson's disease [35], stroke [45], cerebellar degeneration [44], and peripheral sensory loss [41].

3. Assessment of Deficient Finger Force Control in ALS

In a variety of disorders, impairments of anticipatory grip force adjustments have been reported. In particular, deficits of efficient grip force scaling and reduced temporal precision of the grip and load force coupling were observed in disorders of the basal ganglia [11,35], cerebellum [2,10,44], in children with cerebral palsy [8], during development [47], in the phase of aging [5] and when finger sensibility was impaired due to digital anesthesia [23,43] or due to polyneuropathy [38,40,41]. Consequently, the precision grip paradigm provides a useful tool in the understanding of normal sensorimotor processing and its dysfunction.

ALS is a progressive degenerative disorder of motor neurons in the spinal cord, brainstem, and motor cortex [28,56]. The disease manifests clinically with progressive muscular weakness, atrophy, and corticospinal tract signs in various combinations. In its most typical form, awkwardness in tasks requiring fine finger movements (e.g., difficulties with using a tool or buttoning a shirt), stiffness of the fingers, and weakness or wasting of the hand muscles are first indications of the disease. Abductors, adductors, and extensors of fingers and thumb tend to weaken before the long flexors, on which the hand grip depends. In its later stages, the disease presents the characteristic triad of atrophic weakness of the hands and forearms, spasticity of the arms and legs, and generalized hyperreflexia, all in the absence of sensory deficits. Thus, problems to use the hand during manipulative tasks in ALS should primarily result from less effective and uncoordinated force execution than from impaired processing of sensory feedback signals.

We analyzed the coordination between grip and load force profiles in patients with ALS performing vertical point-to-point arm movements with a hand-held instrumented object [34,42]. We used the holding – moving task to study grip force control in ALS, because the need for a complex temporal coupling of motor activity in the proximal arm and shoulder muscles responsible for transporting the object and in the fingers used to grasp it. In healthy subjects, this precise temporal coupling is reflected in the close coupling of grip and load force profiles (see Figure 1). Participants grasped a cylindrical and autonomous instrumented object between the tips of the thumb and other fingers on either side. Technical data about the object and a detailed description of the experimental procedure and data analysis have been provided elsewhere [35,37,38,40,41,43,44,45]. The object and the configuration of the hand and fingers used to grasp it are illustrated in Figure 2. The object incorporated a force sensor for grip force registration and linear acceleration sensors for registration of kinematic acceleration signals in three dimensions. The force sensor registered grip forces at two different sensitivities between 0-10 N (0.0025 N/bit) and 0-50 N (0.0125 N/bit). The linear acceleration sensors measured linear accelerations within a range of ±50 m/s^2. Subjects were instructed to move the object on a straight vertical line and to keep its orientation constant during movement. Subjects were instructed to move the object fast, but were not paced to move it at a certain speed. The amplitude of movement was 30 cm. Short breaks (approximately 1 second) were introduced in between single up and down (point-to-point) movements. The vertical movements were achieved largely by rotations of the upper arm about the shoulder joint and small movements of the forearm and wrist assured the motion of the object along a straight vertical line. Movements in the wrist contained medial and lateral deviations, but not flexion and extension; thus, the length of the long wrist and finger flexors was mainly kept constant during the movement.

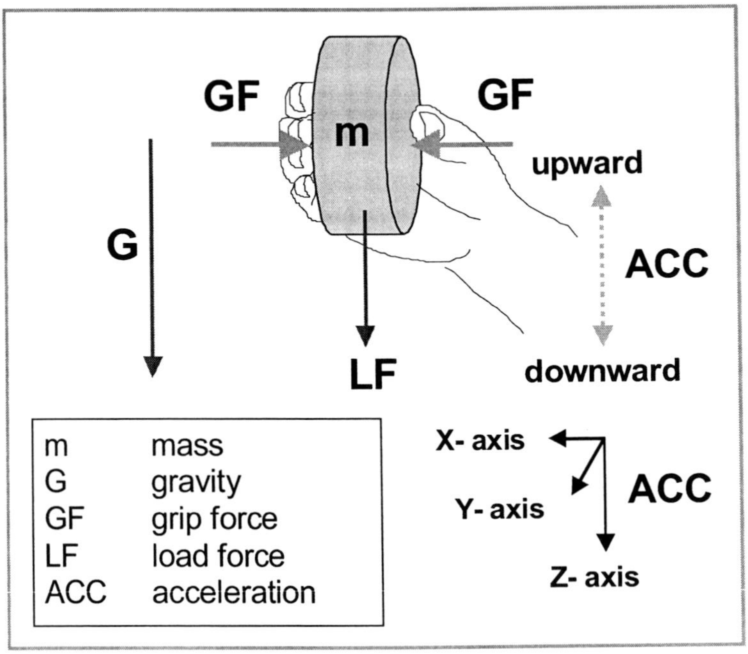

Figure 2. The instrumented object and the configuration of the hand and fingers used to grasp it. The forces produced during vertical point-to-point arm movements are illustrated. The object surface is covered with a medium grain sandpaper (no. 240). The object incorporated a force sensor to register grip force and three linear acceleration sensors to measure accelerations in three dimensions. m = mass (0.35 kg); G = gravity; ACC = kinematic acceleration in the direction of movement; GF = Grip Force; LF = Load Force ($m \times \sqrt{ACC_y^2 + (ACC_z + G)^2}$). The load force (FL) is calculated from the object mass and the vectorial summation of accelerations parallel to the grip surface, including gravity (along the object's Y- and Z-axis). Thus, the load force includes additional inertial loads, which arise from eventual movement components in the transversal (Y-) direction. Loading components acting in the direction of the applied grip forces (X-axis) are not included in the calculation of the object's load. These loads, acting orthogonal to gravity and kinematic acceleration were small and do not need to be compensated for by grip force to prevent the object from slipping.

Illustrative waveform data from consecutive upward and downward movements are shown in Figure 1 for a healthy subject. Acceleration, load force and grip force data are shown. Positive kinematic acceleration of the object (along the object's Z-axis, see Figure 1) is directed upward during the discrete vertical movements. The acceleration and load force data indicate that the subject complies with the instructions and performed single upward and downward movements with the hand-held object with 1 s breaks in between each movement during which the object is held stationary. The grip force profile parallels the load force profile exhibiting a maximum that coincides with a maximum in load force. In addition, the grip force level is similar or even smaller that the load force level, suggesting a precise scaling of the force magnitude according to the frictional condition at the skin-object interface. The object surfaces are covered with sandpaper and thus, the friction at the skin-object interface is high. Consequently, the grip force may drop below the load force level without danger of object slippage. Right hand to the grip force panel grip force is plotted against load force. The high correlation coefficients of the least square regression lines suggest a close temporo-spatial coupling between grip and load force profiles, regardless of movement direction.

In Figure 3, waveforms of grip and load force data are illustrated for three superimposed upward and downward movements performed by a patient with ALS and an age- and sex-matched control subject. The traces are fitted to coincide in the time point of maximum acceleration. In general, the patient produces smaller load forces, but greater grip forces when compared to the healthy control subject. During upward movements the patient and the control subject increase grip force right from the onset of movement (see the dashed vertical line in Figure 3). A maximum of grip force occurs closely in time with maximum load force for upward movements of both the patient and the control. Additional load oscillations are accompanied by additional grip force peaks occurring closely in time. The control subject exhibits a second grip force peak coinciding with a second load force peak occurring at the time of maximum deceleration of the upward movements. During downward movements, the grip force of the control subject starts to rise later during the movement course at the time of movement deceleration (see the arrowhead in the grip force panel for downward movements of the control subject in Figure 3). For the control subject, the grip force maximum coincides closely in time with maximum load force near the end of the movement. Similar patterns of grip force modulation with the movement-induced inertial load fluctuation have been described in detail for healthy subjects [13]. In contrast, the patient begins to rise grip force close to the onset of downward movements (see the arrowhead in the grip force panel for downward movements of the patient in Figure 2) and reaches its maximum close to or slightly before the maximum in load force during the deceleratory phase of the movement. This differences from a healthy grip force behavior were found in three of five ALS patients investigated [34,42]. In summary, the grip force control of ALS patients exhibits two major pathologies: (a) they apply inefficiently high grip forces against a hand-held object and (b) there is a desynchronisation of the temporo-spatial coupling between grip and load force profiles. These two major impairments will be discussed in detail.

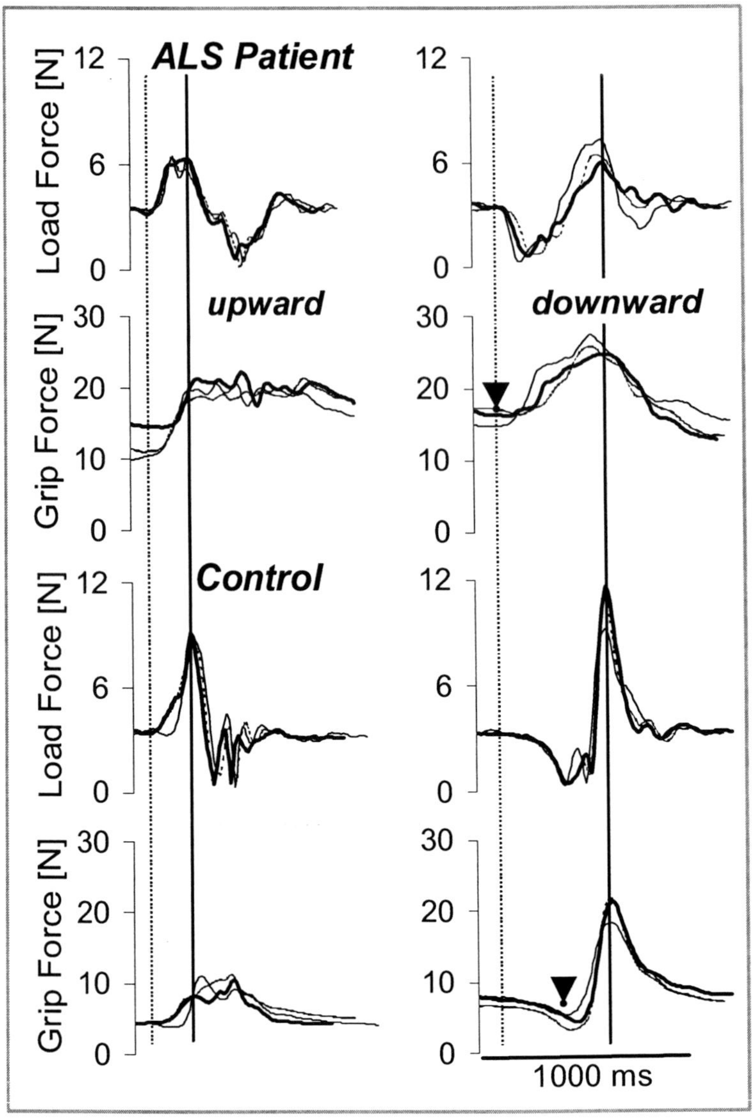

Figure 3. Illustrative data of load force and grip force during three consecutive upward (left) and downward movements (right) obtained from a patient with ALS (top) and a healthy age- and sex-matched control subject (bottom). The dashed vertical lines indicate the onset of vertical movements. The solid vertical lines indicate the maximum in load force coinciding with maximum acceleration. During upward movements both subjects' grip force increased right from the movement start. In contrast, during downward movements the patient's grip force started to rise earlier in the movement course (see the arrowheads in the grip force panels of the patient and control subject).

4. Inefficient Grip Force Scaling in ALS

When a grasped object is held unsupported in space, the grip force is precisely adjusted according to the load due to gravity [12,22]. In this situation, grip force is only slightly higher than the minimum required to prevent the object slipping. It is known that visual identification and sensory feedback from the grasping fingers can be used efficiently to select appropriate force levels. This selection is based on sensorymotor memories about previous object manipulations [12,24]. ALS patients produce greater grip forces than necessary to prevent the object slipping from the grasp during stationary holding the object and during the performance of vertical arm movements with the hand-held object (compare Figure 3). This observation suggests that the descending motor commands are processed with impaired force economy. As the registration and integration of sensory feedback signals from the moving arm and hand is suggested to be unaffected by motor neuron disease, one may argue that the selection of appropriate force levels is impaired in ALS.

The scaling of the grip force level appears to involve the sensory cortex [48,53] and the cerebellum [9], which project to the primary and several other motor cortices (supplementary motor area, premotor cortex and cingulate motor cortex) [21,27,32,49,50]. These former structures are unaffected in ALS and one might suggest that the efficiency of the grip force scaling was directly disturbed by deficient motor cortex and corticospinal tract function. Indeed, similar deficits of the elaborate motor function of the hand result from interruption of the spinal dorsal columns or disconnection between the first somatosensory and motor cortices compared to pyramidal tract lesions. An inefficient increase in grip force was also observed when the grasping digits were anesthetized [23,43], in the aging phase [5], and in disorders of the basal ganglia [11,35], peripheral sensory nerves [38,40,41] and cerebellum [2,10,44]. In all these studies either directly impaired sensibility or deficient registration and integration of sensory feedback signals into central force control programs had to be suggested. There are no deficits of proprioception and tactile sensibility in ALS and consequently the increase in grip force level cannot be assumed a strategy to compensate deficient afferent input. Rather, dysfunction of efficient grip force planning or a force overflow due to uncoordinated force output, e.g. due to symptoms of spasticity, have to be suspected. Interestingly, recent neurophysiological studies documented a hyperexcitability of the human motor cortex in ALS [57,58], which may at least in part result from decreased inhibition of cortical motor processing [57]. The grip force overflow observed in our ALS patients may be a first behavioral demonstration of motor cortex hyperexcitability as shown by transcranial magnetic stimulation [57,58]. Functional imaging studies demonstrated a functional reorganization of motor cortical structures in ALS [26], which may also result in a provisional and inefficient planning of the grip force magnitude during manipulative tasks.

Our patients uniformly reported problems of fine motor performance during everyday manual activities, such as rigidity and clumsiness of the fingers, resulting in dyscoordination of fine finger movements probably related to symptoms of spasticity. Thus, from the behavioral point of view it seems trivial that patients who experience insecurity of fine manipulative tasks and frequent object dropping due to clumsiness of the fingers may compensate their deficits by an increase in grip force. In ALS there is also an abnormal drive of the descending motor commands to the gamma motor neurons in the spinal cord [58], necessary for the precise tuning and coordination of muscle activity. The abnormal gamma motor neuron drive may hamper agonist-antagonist muscle activation or indirectly interfere with the sensory system, in particular proprioceptive feedback from muscle and joint receptors, resulting in disturbances of the subtle interplay between feedforward and feedback mechanisms in grip force control.

5. Dyscoordination of Grip and Load Force Profiles in ALS

In healthy subjects, grip force is modulated in parallel with the movement-induced inertial load fluctuations when performing arm movements with a hand-held object [13,14]. In particular, grip force rises early in upward and late in downward movements (see Figures 1 and 3). A maximum in grip force occurs at the time of maximum load force, which occurs at the onset of upward and near the end of downward movements. The precise matching of the grip force profile to the differential loading requirements of movement direction implicates that we can predict the consequence of our motor commands, namely the movement-induced load fluctuations, and regulate grip force in anticipation. To predict the consequences of a motor command requires a system that can simulate the dynamic behavior of the body and environment. [14,31,54,55]. Such a system is termed internal model as it models the behavior of the body and captures the causal relationship between actions and their consequences. Theoretical considerations and lesion data suggest that such an internal model may be located within the cerebellum [2,10,31,44].

The majority of our ALS subjects did not distinguish between upward and downward movements when regulating the grip force output. In particular, grip force increased right from the movement onset regardless of movement direction, indicating that the grip force profile was similar for upward and downward movements (see Figure 3). The problem to adjust the grip force profile to the differential loading requirements of movement direction implies that the grip force output was not programmed to match the temporal aspects of the load profile arising from the forthcoming movement. Similar deficits in the timing of the grip force profile according to the movement-induced load fluctuations have been described in patients with cerebellar lesions [2,10,44] and in children with developmental coordination disorder [19], which may affect the maturation of the cerebellum as well. Patients with cerebellar lesions show difficulties to select appropriate grip force levels and disturbances of the precise grip force coupling with the loads when performing arm movements with a hand-held object [2,10,44].

Indeed, the timing of voluntary movement has been considered to be a cerebellar function [49] and direct cerebellar involvement in the coordination between grip and load forces is supported by studies in the monkey, which have demonstrated changes in the activity of Purkinje cells during object manipulation [9]. The anatomical integrity of the cerebellum is not affected in motor neuron disease and the problem to time the grip force profile may result either from impaired integration of the movement plan into the movement execution system by deficient projections between cerebellum and motor cortices, or directly by impaired execution of the descending motor commands. The later may result in an undifferentiated grip force generation when hand-held objects are accelerated irrespectively of the actual loading condition, possibly overriding the precise motor output from a preserved internal model, implemented within the cerebellum. Indeed, the investigation of children with perinatal motor cortical lesions also demonstrated disruption of the temporal coupling between grip and load forces similar to that observed in patients with cerebellar disorders [8,15]. The functional anatomical connections between the cerebellum and the motor cortices give one possible explanation for the similar impairments of the temporal grip force regulation observed in patients with cerebella and motor cortical lesions. The cerebellum provides efferent projections to the motor cortices [21] and basal ganglia [32] from which it in turn receives afferent connections.

Alternatively, the uncoordinated grip force output observed in our ALS patients may result from reorganization processes within a well-documented network of multiple hand representations. Several cerebral motor cortices (primary motor, supplementary motor, premotor, and cingulate motor cortices) and the cerebellum cooperate when controlling human hand and finger movements. Studies on humans performing manipulative tasks using positron emission tomography and functional magnetic resonance imaging demonstrated that several motor cortices are organized in distributed and parallel patterns through basal ganglia-thalamo-cortical and cerebello-thalamo-cortical projections [21,25,27,32]. In simple motor tasks involving movements of the hand, all other motor cortices are active in concert with the primary motor cortex [27,25,50]. More complex sequential finger movements activate the supplementary motor area and also these cortical motor areas, which are active in simple motor tasks of the fingers [49]. Within this widely distributed motor network a provisional, but uncoordinated preparation, coordination and execution of the motor plan provided by an intact internal model, probably implemented in the cerebellum, could result in the deficient grip force regulation observed in ALS.

6. Therapeutic Considerations

In clinical examinations manual performance is usually tested using crude tasks, such as maximum force production and coordination of the hand and arm when grasping for objects [3,6]. Such gross measures of performance fail to establish which components are preserved providing a possible target for individual rehabilitation [30]. The precise adjustment of grip force according to the physical requirements of the manipulated object is a fundamental aspect of skilled motor performance of the hand [13,23]. The described method of recording and analyzing finger forces when moving a hand-held load is highly sensitive to demonstrate both physiological and pathological aspects of finger force control. When manipulating objects in daily life, such as using a fork when eating or a pen when writing, the ability to produce very high grip forces is not of crucial importance. On the contrary, the generation of inefficiently high grip forces hampers fine finger movements, facilitates early fatigue of hand muscles and may therefore contribute to a greater level of disability in activities of daily life [45].

Indeed, the generation of unnecessarily high finger forces when manipulating grasped objects is a common observation in patients with deficient hand function due to a variety of neurological disorders, such as stroke [16,18,30,45], basal ganglia disease [11,35], cereballar lesions [2,10,44], focal hand dystonia [46,51] and impaired sensory feedback [38,40,41]. Nevertheless, current rehabilitation concepts commonly focus on the measurement of maximum grip force to objectively evaluate the progress in rehabilitation. Based on our theory that an overflow in grip force contributes significantly to the disability in patients with mild to moderate sensory-motor dysfunction of the hand, it seems fruitful to define the reduction of unnecessarily high finger forces as the preferential goal in hand motor rehabilitation. A potential treatment scheme these patients should include the measurement of grip force during natural unencumbered arm movements with a hand-held load. The finding of uneconomically high grip force should motivate an individual training program to decrease the amount of force overshoot, facilitating fine finger movements and prevent early fatigue of affected hand muscles. Training programs targeting the reduction of grip force should be chosen according to the individual pathology. These training programs may include biofeedback methods, sensory discrimination training, behavioral approaches and the use of medication, such as BOTOX therapy. The question of what therapeutic approach is superior to another for a specific pathology should be addressed in future work.

References

[1] Asanuma, H., & Arissian, K. (1984). Experiments on functional role of peripheral input to motor cortex during voluntary movements in the monkey. *Journal of Neurophysiology, 52*, 212-227.

[2] Babin-Ratté, S., Sirigu, A., Gilles, M., & Wing, A.M. (1999). Impaired anticipatory finger grip-force adjustments in a case of cerebellar degeneration. *Experimental Brain Research, 128,* 81-85.

[3] Boissy, P., Bourbonnais, D., Carlotti, M.M., Gravel, D. & Arsenault, B.A. (1999) Maximal grip force in chronic stroke subjects and its relationship to global upper extremity function. *Clinical Rehabilitation, 13,* 354–362.

[4] Buys, E.J., Lemon, R.N., Mantel, G.W.H., & Muir, R.B. (1986). Selective facilitation of different hand muscles by single corticospinal neurones in the conscious monkey. *Journal of Physiology (London), 381*, 529-549.

[5] Cole, K.J., Rotella, D.L., & Harper, J.G. (1999). Mechanisms for age-related changes of fingertip forces during precision gripping and lifting in adults. *Journal of Neuroscience, 19*, 3238-3247.

[6] Colebatch, J.G., Gandevia, S.C. & Spira, P.J. (1989) Voluntary muscle strength in hemiparesis: distribution of weakness at the elbow. *Journal of Neurology, Neurosurgery and Psychiatry*, *49*, 1019–1024.

[7] Duque, J., Thonnard, J.L., Vandermeeren, Y., Sebire, J., Cosnard, G., & O. (2003) Correlation between impaired dexterity and corticospinal tract dysgenesis in congenital hemiplegia. *Brain*, *126*, 732-747

[8] Eliasson, A.C., Gordon, A.M., & Forssberg, H. (1995). Tactile control of fingertip forces during grasping in children with cerebral palsy. *Developmental Medicine and Child Neurology, 37*, 72-84.

[9] Espinoza, E., & Smith, A.M. (1990). Purkinje cell simple spike activity during grasping and lifting objects of different textures and weights. *Journal of Neurophysiology, 64*, 698-714.

[10] Fellows, S.J., Ernst, J., Schwarz, J.M., Töpper, R., & Noth J. (2001). Precision grip deficits in cerebellar disorders in man. *Clinical Neurophysiology, 112*, 1793-1802.

[11] Fellows, S.J., Noth, J., & Schwarz, J.M. (1998). Precision grip and Parkinson's disease. *Brain, 121*, 1771-1784.

[12] Flanagan, J.R. & Johansson, R.S. (2002) Hand movements. In: V.S. Ramshandran (Ed), Encyclopedia of the human brain, Vol 2. San Diego: Academic Press, pp. 399-414.

[13] Flanagan, J.R., & Wing, A.M. (1993). Modulation of grip force with load force during point-to-point movements. *Experimental Brain Research, 95*, 131-143.

[14] Flanagan, J.R., & Wing, A.M. (1997). The role of internal models in motion planning and control: Evidence from grip force adjustments during movements of hand-held loads. *Journal of Neuroscience, 17*, 1519-1528.

[15] Forssberg, H., Eliasson, A.C., Redon-Zouitenn, C., Mercuri, E., & Dubowitz, L. (1999). Impaired grip-lift synergy in children with unilateral brain lesions. *Brain, 122*, 1157-1168.

[16] Grichting B., Hediger, P., Kaluzny, P. & Wiesendanger, M. (2000) Impaired proactive and reactive grip force control in chronic hemiparetic patients. *Clinical Neurophysiology, 111*, 1661-1671

[17] Hepp-Reymond, M.C., & Wiesendanger, M. (1972). Unilateral pyramidotomy in monkeys: Effect on force and speed of a conditional precision grip. *Brain Research, 36,* 117-131.

[18] Hermsdörfer, J., Hagl, E., Nowak, D.A. & Marquardt, C. (2003). Grip force control during object manipulation in cerebral stroke. *Clinical Neurophysiology, 114*, 915-929.

[19] Hill, E.L. & Wing, A.M. (1999). Coordination of grip force and load force in developmental coordination disorder: A case study. *Neurocase, 5*, 537-544.

[20] Hillel, A.D., Miller, R.M., Yorkston, K., McDonald, E., Norris, F.H. & Konikow, N. (1989). Amyotrophic lateral sclerosis severity scale. *Neuroepidemiology, 8*, 142-150.

[21] Hoover, J., & Strick, P. (1999). The organization of cerebellar and basal ganglia outputs to primary motor cortex as revealed by retrograde transport of herpes simplex virus type 1. *Journal of Neuroscience, 19*, 1446-1463.

[22] Johansson, R.S. (1996). Sensory control of dexterous manipulation in humans. In: A.M. Wing, P. Haggard, & J.R. Flanagan (Eds.), *Hand and brain* (pp. 381-414). San Diego, CA: Academic Press.

[23] Johansson, R.S., & Westling, G. (1984). Roles of glabrous skin receptors and sensorimotor memory in automatic control of precision grip when lifting rougher and more slippery objects. *Experimental Brain Research, 56*, 550-564.

[24] Johansson, R.S., & Westling, G. (1988). Coordination of isometric muscle commands adequately and erroneously programmed for the weight during lifting tasks with precision grip. *Experimental Brain Research, 71*, 59-71.

[25] Kinoshita, H., Oku, N., Hashikawa, K., & Nishimura, T. (2000). Functional brain areas for the lifting of objects using a precision grip: A PET study. *Brain Research, 857*, 119-130.

[26] Konrad, C., Henningsen. H., Bremer. J., Mock, B., Deppe, M. Buchinger, C. Turski, P., Knecht, S., Brooks, B. (2002). Pattern of cortical reorganization in amyotrophic lateral sclerosis: a functional magnetic resonance imaging study. *Experimental Brain Research, 143*, 51-56.

[27] Kuhtz-Buschbeck, J.P., Ehrsson, H.H., & Forssberg, H. (2001). Human brain activity in the control of fine static precision grip forces: An fMRI study. *European Journal of Neuroscience, 14*, 82-390.

[28] Lawyer, T. Jr., & Netsky, M.G. (1953). Amyotrophic lateral sclerosis: Clinico-anatomic study of 53 cases. *Archives of Neurology and Psychiatry, 69*, 171-192.

[29] Lemon, R.N., Mantel, G.H.W., & Muir, R.B. (1986). Corticospinal facilitation of hand muscles during voluntary movement in the conscious monkey. *Journal of Physiology (London), 381*, 497-527.

[30] Mai, N. (1989) Residual control of isometric finger forces in hemiparetic patients. Evidence for dissociation of performance deficits. *Neuroscience Letters, 101*, 347–351.

[31] Miall, R.C., Weir, D.J., & Wolpert, D.M. (1993). Is the cerebellum a Smith predictor? *Journal of Motor Behavior, 25*, 203-216.

[32] Middleton, F., & Strick, P. (2000). Basal ganglia and cerebellar loops: Motor and cognitive circuits. *Brain Research Reviews, 31*, 236-250.

[33] Napier, J.R. (1956) The prehensile movements of the human hand. *Journal of Bone and Joint Surgery, 38B*, 902-913.

[34] Nowak, D.A. & Hermsdörfer, J. (2002) Impaired coordination between grip force and load force in amyotrophic lateral sclerosis: a case control study. *Amyotrophic Lateral Sclerosis and other motor neuron disorders, 3*, 199-207.

[35] Nowak, D.A. & Hermsdörfer, J. (2002). Coordination of grip and load force during vertical point-to-point movements with a grasped object in Parkinson's disease. *Behavioral Neuroscience, 116*, 837-850.

[36] Nowak, D.A. & Hermsdörfer, J. (2003) Predictability influences grip force control when catching a free-falling object. *Experimental Brain Research*, in Press

[37] Nowak, D.A. & Hermsdörfer, J. (2003). Digital cooling influences grasp efficiency during manipulative tasks. *European Journal of Applied Physiology, 89*, 127-133.

[38] Nowak, D.A. & Hermsdörfer, J. (2003). Selective deficits of grip force control during object manipulation in patients with reduced sensory feedback from the grasping digits. *Neuroscience Research, 47*, 65-72.

[39] Nowak, D.A. (2003) Different modes of grip force control: Voluntary and externally guided arm movements with a hand-held object. *Clinical Neurophysiology*, in Press

[40] Nowak, D.A., Glasauer, S. & Hermsdörfer, J. (2003). Grip force efficiency in long-term deprivation of somatosensory feedback: Observations in a deafferented woman. *NeuroReport, 14*: 1803-1807.

[41] Nowak, D.A., Glasauer, S. & Hermsdörfer, J. (2003). How predictive is grip force control in the complete absence of somatosensory feedback ? *Brain,* in Press.

[42] Nowak, D.A., Hermsdörfer, J. & Topka, H. (2003). When motor execution is selectively impaired: Control of manipulative finger forces in Amyotrophic Lateral Sclerosis. *Motor Control, 7*, 304-320.

[43] Nowak, D.A., Hermsdörfer, J., Glasauer, S., Philipp, J., Meyer, L., & Mai, N. (2001). The effects of digital anaesthesia on predictive grip force adjustments during vertical movements of a grasped object. *European Journal of Neuroscience, 14*, 756-762.

[44] Nowak, D.A., Hermsdörfer, J., Marquardt, C., & Fuchs, H.H. (2002). Grip and load force coupling during discrete vertical arm movements with a grasped object in cerebellar atrophy. *Experimental Brain Research, 145*, 28-39.

[45] Nowak, D.A., Hermsdörfer, J., Topka, H. (2003). Deficits of predictive grip force control during object manipulation in acute stroke. *Journal of Neurology, 250*, 850-860.

[46] Odergren, T., Iwasaki, N., Borg, J. & Forssberg, H. (1996) Impaired sensory-motor integration during grasping in writer's cramp. *Brain,119*,569-583.

[47] Paré, M., & Dugas, C. (1999). Developmental changes in prehension during childhood. *Experimental Brain Research, 125*, 239-247.

[48] Picard, N., & Smith, A.M. (1992). Primary motor cortical activity related to the weight and texture of grasped objects in the monkey. *Journal of Neurophysiology, 68*, 1867-1881.

[49] Rao, S., Harrington, D., Haaland, K., Bobholz, J., Cox, R., & Binder, J. (1997). Distributed neural systems underlying the timing of movements. *Journal of Neuroscience, 17,* 5528-5535.

[50] Roland, P.E., Larsen, B., Lassen, N.A., & Skinhoij, E. (1980). Supplementary motor area and other cortical areas in organization of voluntary movements in man. *Journal of Neurophysiology, 43,* 118-136.

[51] Serrien, D.J., Burgunder, J.M. & Wiesendanger, M. (2000) Disturbed sensorimotor processing during control of precision grip in patients with writer's cramp. *Movement Disorders,15*,965-972.

[52] Slavin, M.D., Jette, D.U., Andres, P.L., Munsat, T.L. (1998) Lower extremity muscle force measures and functional ambulation in patients with amyotrophic lateral sclerosis. *Archives of Physical Medicine and Rehabilitation*, *79*, 950-954.

[53] Strick, P.L., & Preston, J.B. (1982). Two representations of the hand area 4 of primate. II. Somatosensory input organization. *Journal of Neurophysiology, 48*, 150-159.

[54] Wing, A.M. (1996). Anticipatory control of grip force in rapid arm movement. In: A.M. Wing, P. Haggard, and J.R. Flanagan (Eds.), *Hand and brain: Neurophysiology and psychology of hand movements* (pp. 301-324). San Diego, CA: Academic Press.

[55] Wolpert, D.M., & Flanagan, J.R. (2001). Motor prediction. *Current Biology, 11*, 729-723.

[56] World federation of Neurology. (1994). El Escorial criteria for the diagnosis of amyotrophic lateral sclerosis. *Journal of Neurological Sciences, 124*, 96-107.

[57] Zanette, G., Tamburin, S., Manganotti, P., Refatti, N., Forgione, A., Rizzuto, N. (2002) Changes in motor cortex inhibition over time in patients with amyotrophic lateral sclerosis. *Journal of Neurology, 249,* 1723-1728.

[58] Zanette, G., Tamburin, S., Manganotti, P., Refatti, N., Forgione, A., Rizzuto, N. (2002). Different mechanisms contribute to motor cortex hyperexcitability in amyotrophic lateral sclerosis. *Clinical Neurophysiology, 113*, 1688-1697.

In: Amyotrophic Lateral Sclerosis: New Research
Editor: Christine A. Murray, pp. 279-301
ISBN 1-59454-179-5

Chapter XII

Satellite Potentials in Amyotrophic Lateral Sclerosis (ALS) – A Simulation Study

Ewa Zalewska[1*], Katarzyna Rowińska-Marcińska[2,3] and Irena Hausmanowa-Petrusewicz[2]

[1]Institute of Biocybernetics and Biomedical Engineering, Polish Academy of Sciences, Warsaw, Poland

[2]Neuromuscular Unit, Medical Research Center, Polish Academy of Sciences, Warsaw, Poland

[3]Department of Neurology, Medical University of Warsaw, Poland.

Abstract

The satellites of a motor unit potentials (MUP), i.e. late components distinct from the main component but time - locked to it, is a phenomenon found in electromyography. Satellite potentials are observed in EMG investigations in almost all neuromuscular disorders and occasionally in healthy muscles. In amyotrophic lateral sclerosis (ALS) satellite potentials are observed less frequently and have different features than in the case of other neurogenic processes.

The aim of this study was to analyse the parameters of satellite potentials and to model a possible pathomechanism underlying generation of satellites in ALS.

Motor unit potentials with satellites were characterized by the mean number of satellites per one motor unit potential, mean amplitude and duration of the main MUP component, mean amplitude and duration of the satellites. These parameters were compared between satellites recorded in the controls, ALS and spinal muscle atrophy (SMA, typ III).

* Correspondence concerning this article should be addressed to Dr. Ewa Zalewska Institute of Biocybernetics and Biomedical Engineering 02-109 Warsaw, Trojdena 4 str. Tel. +48 22 659-91-43; Fax. +48 22 659 70-30; E-mail: e.zalewska@astercity.net.

The prevalence index of satellites in SMA was significantly higher than that in ALS. In both, ALS and SMA, the prevalence index was significantly higher than that in the controls. The mean amplitudes and the mean duration of MUPs with satellites were significantly higher in SMA than in ALS, whereas there was no significant difference in the duration of the main components.
The mean number of satellites per one MUP, and the duration of satellites have larger values in SMA than those in ALS. A simulation study indicates that in ALS a satellite is more often a potential of a single fiber whereas in SMA - groups of muscle fibers of small diameters are the sources of satellites. The range of delay of satellites caused by slower neuromuscular transmission and conductivity in terminal axon sprouts have been estimated. The reduced number of satellites and muscle fibers contributing to a single satellite in ALS probably depend on a failure of the compensation process.

Keywords: Amyotrophic Lateral Sclerosis, Spinal Muscle Atrophy, satellite potentials, simulation study

Introduction

Amyotrophic lateral sclerosis (ALS) is a quickly progressing fatal, neurodegenerative disorder involving upper and lower motor neurons. The ongoing denervation-reinnervation-denervation that is characteristic of this process causes neurogenic changes in muscle structure, neuromuscular end-plates and presence of collateral twigs. These processes manifest themselves in characteristic features of electromyographic signals and therefore EMG studies are very important in the diagnosis as well as in the evaluation of the progress of disease. One of the electromyographic phenomenons observed in ALS are satellite potentials, also called late components [3,6,17,22].

The satellite potentials of a motor unit, defined as a delayed component time locked to the main component [17], are recorded in most neuromuscular diseases as well as in healthy muscles [2,3,6,8,9], being specific neither for neurogenic nor for myogenic disorders. Buchthal and Rosenfalck [3] found them in 3% of normal MUPs whereas Lang and Partanen [11] report this rate to be 10%. Only a few studies have been dedicated to satellite MUPs because, even though they are not so rare in EMG recordings, satellites are difficult to automatic analysis. The presence of satellites significantly perturbs the duration of MUP measured automatically [8,11,22]. The problem involved in automatic measurements of satellites is the reason why in most of EMG equipment such potentials are not evaluated and are excluded from the total number of MUPs. However, the presence of satellites as well as their characteristics might provide additional information about undergoing processes [1,6,8,9,11,19].

The prevalence of satellites in EMG records was analysed and described as a valuable method [2,6,8,18,19]. Finsterer [8] showed that the evaluation of MUPs with satellites increases the detection rate of neuromuscular disorders by up to13% when compared with traditional MUP analysis. Podnar and Fowler [18] have studied the sensitivity of MUP parameters in the diagnosis of multiple system atrophy (MSA). The authors concluded that satellites are a hallmark of the degenerative pathological process of MSA [18]. Rowinska et.

al [19] have found different characteristics of satellite potentials in various neuromuscular disorders and in the controls. The authors indicated differences in the satellites' occurrence as well as in satellites' characteristics between potentials in the controls, the Duchenne muscle dystrophy as well as between two neurogenic processes, eg. a quickly progressing process of amyotrophic lateral sclerosis (ALS) and a chronic neurogenic process, spinal muscle atrophy (SMA) type III. These results implicated the study of the origin of these differences. In our work we have limited analysis to two neurogenic processes, viz. ALS and SMA type III.

The ALS can be considered as a model of severe motor unit disintegration as a sequence of denervation-reinnervation-denervation. Mild chronic spinal muscle atrophy type III (Kugelberg – Welander disease) is another model of motor neuron disorder, much more stabilized and less progressive. In SMA some stages of disintegration and very effective reinnervation can be observed. The clinical characteristics of both these diseases have an opposite pathomechanism . ALS is a fatal, progressing disease with pronounced atrophy and weakness. SMA type III is a slowly developing mild, long lasting process with signs of compensation.

The introduction of new techniques into the electromyography, including recently developed simulation of muscle action potentials [13,14,25,26], provides some possibility of studing MUPs properties which have not been measured yet – that is adding new data important for research and diagnosis [15,20,26].

The aim of this study was to analyse differences in characteristics of satellite MUPs in ALS and SMA and to simulate the possible mechanisms of generating satellite potentials.

The paper has been divided into two parts. Part I presents electromyographic studies on satellites in the controls, ALS and SMA. Part II is dedicated to simulation studies of satellite potentials, in which we have tried to explain the differences between pathogenesis of satellite potentials in ALS and SMA.

Part I: Clinical Electrophysiological Studies

Characteristic Features of Motor Unit Potentials in ALS and SMA

Before discussing the electrophysiological pattern of ALS we should point out that the common denominator of all "motor neuron disorders" with various clinical features is an ideal term in electromyography without any nosological meaning. Interestingly, clinical electrophysiologists managed to distinguish between the specific EMG characteristics of ALS and other motor neuron disorders.

Based on long experience in the reorganization of motor units in ALS, remodelling of motor unit passes through three stages: (1) temporary denervation with decreased size of the motor unit, (2) compensatory reinnervation with enlargement of the surviving motor units with increased fiber density and (3) insufficient, ineffective compensatory innervation due to exhaustion of surviving motor neurons [7,10].

We must also assume that in ALS the real onset of the disease: before the weakness and wasting appear the process is subclinical till the loss of 30-50% of motor units. The study of the earliest denervation and reinnervation is possible in subclinically involved muscles In the

EMG recordings of the week muscles usually the later stages of the denervation – reinnervation process were seen.

The shape of MUP reflects the structural changes of motor unit. The characteristics of MUPs recorded in ALS and SMA have been widely described [5,6,7,21,23,24,28]. The high amplitude long duration MUPs registered in SMA reflect hypertrophy of muscle fibers and groups of small atrophic muscle fibers seen in muscle biopsy speciment. In SMA the new nerve-muscle junctions are stable, so jitter between MUPs components is not frequently seen. In ALS complex MUP with evident jitter and blocking within component were seen. In muscle speciment atrophy of muscle fibers without of hypertrophy is observed.

MUP, being a sum of single fiber potentials (SFPs), has a larger amplitude and longer duration with an increasing number of fibers.The increasing number of fibers due to reinnervation in both processes causes increase in MUP's size whereas delays in newly formed collaterals cause the irregular shape of the motor unit potential. The increased size of MUP is an important diagnostic criterion, whereas the shape of MUP has not yet been introduced into the quantitative analysis of MUPs in routine diagnostic examinations. The irregularity of MUP's shape is evaluated either using a number of turns and phases or an irregularity coefficient [22, 27]. Our previous studies on MUP irregularity in various neuromuscular disorders have shown that potentials in ALS are less irregular than MUPs in the neurogenic slowly progressing process - SMA [28]. This is probably due to the fact that in ALS, contrary to SMA, there is no significant fiber diameter dispersion [6,24]. The fiber diameter dispersion is considered to be the main factor of the MUP irregularity [29].

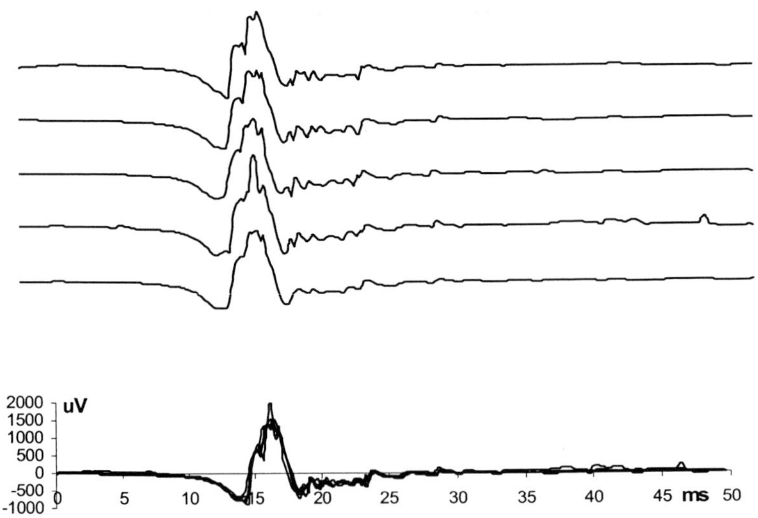

Figure 1. Consecutive MUPs recorded in ALS showing shape variability, "jiggle". Below the same potentials are superposed.

Another MUPs feature is the variability of consecutive MUPs' shapes often observed, especially in ALS recordings (Fig.1). Stålberg and Sonoo [21] called this shape variability as "jiggle" and proposed a method for its evaluation. Using a simulation study, assuming a jitter of individual muscle fiber of up to 300 μs, they found that jiggle increased in linear proportion to the increase in the jitter of individual single fiber action potentials [21].

Besides the shape variability of motor unit potentials observed in ALS, another electromyographic phenomenon is observed in this process, viz. satellite potentials of motor unit. As mentioned above, satellites are rarely analysed and evaluated in diagnostic examinations.

In what follows we present our clinical electrophysiological studies on MUPs with satellite potentials in control, rapid progressive (ALS) and chronic (SMA) neurogenic processes.

Material and Methods

The patient group comprised 25 (11 females and 14 males, aged 24-70 years, mean 54.2) cases of amyotrophic lateral sclerosis (ALS) and 29 (13 females, 16 males, aged 4-29 years, mean 13.2) cases with benign forms of spinal muscular atrophy (SMA). Altogether, EMG studies were performed on 131 muscles (54 patients). The control group comprised of 20 healthy subjects, aged-matched to the ALS group. The EMG in controls was recorded from 42 muscles (26 proximal and 16 distal) and 17 proximal normal muscles in aged - matched (to SMA group) children observed from other than neuromuscular reasons. Informed consent was obtained from each subject or the subject's parents.

A concentric needle EMG was performed in two proximal muscles (biceps brachii and rectus femoris) and in ALS distal muscles (interosseous I dorsalis and/or tibialis anterior). EMGs were recorded using a concentric needle electrode with the active surface of 0.07 mm^2 and electromyography Counterpoint (Dantec). Filter settings were 3 Hz and 10 kHz.

MUPs with satellites were characterized by the following parameters: number of satellites, duration of the whole potential, duration and amplitude of each separated spike components and duration of the isoelectric intervals between spikes.

The prevalence of the MUPs with satellites was evaluated by a prevalence index defined as the ratio of the number of needle insertions in which satellites were recorded to the total number of MUPs registration points.

The statistical analysis was performed using the Wilcoxin, chi-square and Pearson tests. Statistical significance was defined at the $p<0.05$ level.

Results

Characteristics of Satellites in ALS and SMA

The prevalence indexes characterizing the number of satellites recorded in ALS and SMA cases are given in Table 1 together with data for controls. The MUPs with satellites were recorded more frequently in SMA than in ALS. The prevalence index in SMA was 0.37, whereas that in ALS was 0.12. In both, ALS and SMA, the prevalence index was significantly ($p<0.05$) higher than that in controls (0,02).

The parameters of MUPs with satellite potentials were different in the SMA and ALS groups (Table 3). The amplitude of MUPs in SMA was significantly higher 2239 μV than that in ALS 1495 μV ($p<0.01$). The mean duration of MUPs with satellites was longer 28.7 in SMA than in ALS 21.2 ms. There was no significant difference between the mean duration of a single satellite component, however, the maximum duration was 13 ms in SMA and 8 ms in ALS. The mean value of the amplitude of satellites in ALS was shown to be higher, but the difference was not significant.

Table 1. Prevalence index of MUPs with satellites

Group	Number of investigated muscles	Number of muscles with satellites	Total number of MUPs with satellites	Prevalence index
ALS	77	43 (56%)	99	0.12 proximal 0.16 distal 0.07
SMA	54	45 (83%)	199	0.37
Control	42	15 (35%)	15	0,02

Table 2. Number and duration of satellite components

Group	Number of MUPs with satellites	Number of satellite components	Number of satellites per one MUP	Number of satellites 1-4 ms	Number of satellites > 5 ms
ALS	99	126	1.3 (1-3)	88 (70%)	38 (30%)
SMA	199	416	2.0 (1-6)	285 (68%)	131 (32%)
Control	15	15	1 (1)	14 (93%)	1 (7%)

Table 3. Parameters of MUPs in control, ALS and SMA

Parameter	ALS	SMA	Control
Duration of main spike in MUP	10.6 ms (4-25)	11.2 ms (3-32)	7.3 ms (5-11)
Amplitude of main spike in MUP	1495 μV (150-5000)	2239 μV (200-1500)	352 μV (180-700)
Mean duration of satellite in one MUP	3.6 ms (1-8)	4.0 ms (1-13)	3.8 ms (1-5)
Mean amplitude of satellite in one MUP with satellites	276 μV	227 μV	88 μV
Satellites jitter and blocking	+++	+	-

The mean number of satellite components per one MUP was 2 in SMA in comparison to 1.3 in ALS and 1.0 in controls ($p<0.01$). The maximum number of satellites in SMA was 6, whereas that in ALS was no more than 3. In controls not more than one satellite was recorded (Table 2).

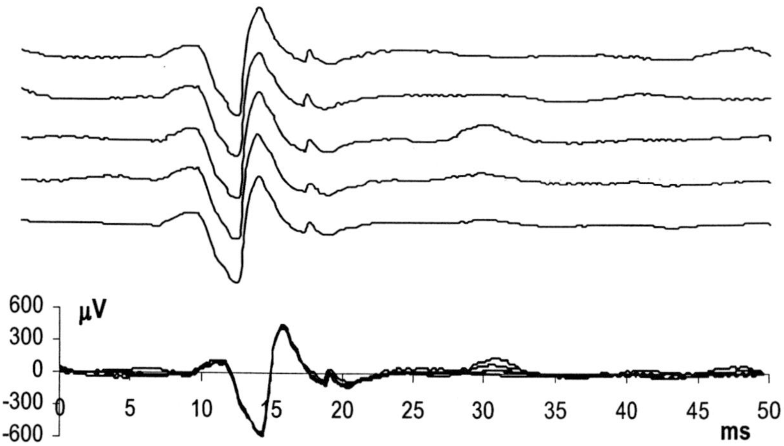

Figure 2. MUP with satellite in ALS. Satellite component seems to be a part of the main component. Below the same potentials are superposed.

In both, ALS and SMA, several satellites were jittering. The jitter of the satellite was more frequently observed in ALS than in SMA (Table 3).

In ALS, the results were not uniform. In the distal muscles (especially in severely involved interosseous I) the prevalence index was significantly lower (0.07) than in proximal muscles (0.16). The duration of MUPs with satellites was usually longer in proximal than in distal muscles in ALS.

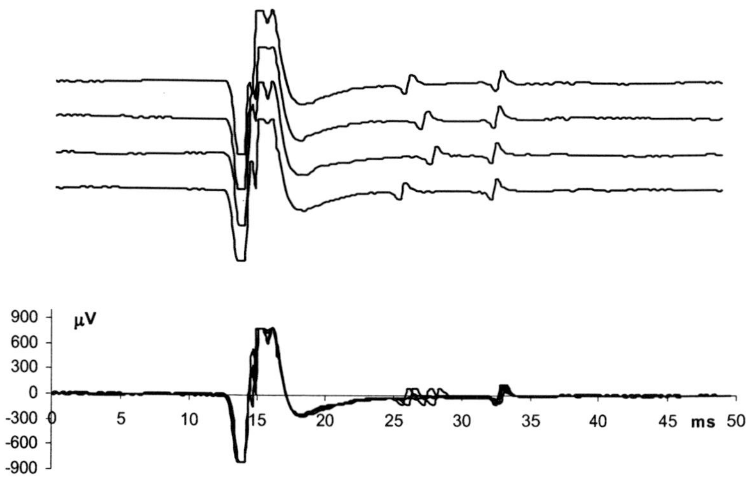

Figure 3. MUP in ALS with two satellite components. One of them shows a large jitter whereas the other one does not. Below the same potentials are superposed.

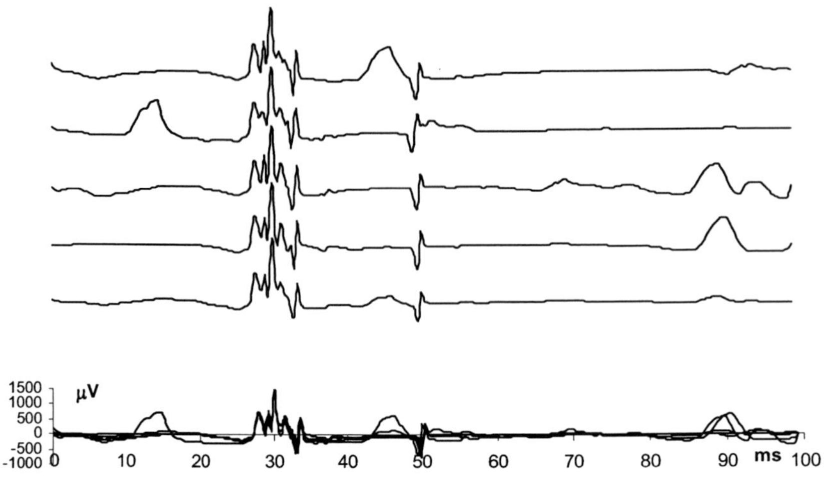

Figure 4. MUP in SMA with an irregular main component and a simple satellite potential. Below the same potentials are superposed.

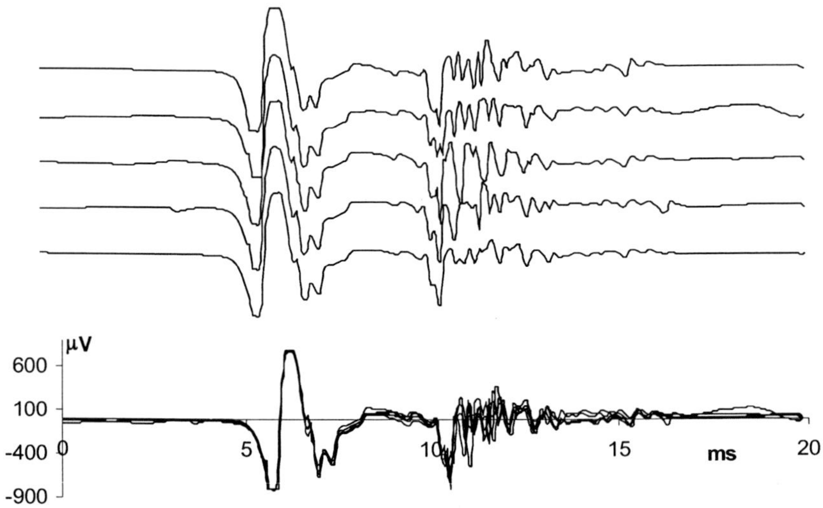

Figure 5. MUP in SMA with a smooth main component and an irregular longitudinal satellite component. Below the same potentials are superposed.

The following examples of MUPs with satellites illustrate the characteristics of MUPs with satellites revealed in ALS and SMA. Fig. 2 shows a MUP recorded in ALS case. The size of the main component indicates a reinnervation process. The small satellite seems to be a part of the main component. The satellite is slightly jittering.

Fig.3 presents a MUP recorded in ALS with two satellite components. One of them shows a large jitter whereas the other one does not.

MUPs recorded in SMA were more often irregular. Fig.4 shows a MUP with an irregular main component and one simple satellite. Fig.5, however, shows a MUP with a high, smooth component and an irregular, longitudinal satellite.

Our clinical EMG studies revealed significant differences between the characteristics of satellites in ALS and SMA. The most evident feature is the prevalence of MUPs with satellites much lower in ALS than in SMA but higher than in controls. The characteristics of satellites indicate a higher number of satellites per one MUP, their longer duration and delay in SMA. Part II presents a possible interpretation of these differences based on simulation studies.

Part II: Modeling Studies on Satellite Potentials

A simulation study has been carried out to explain the results of clinical studies presented in Part I, i.e. the evident differences in prevalence as well as in the characteristics of satellite potentials recorded in ALS and SMA.

We have analysed the generation of satellite potentials in motor units by simulating possible changes in neurogenic processes. The following factors influencing the propagation time of action potential in muscle fiber [2,4,6,24] have been considered:

- A decreased impulse propagation velocity along nerve terminals after primary nerve damage,
- Increased dispersion of end-plates along the muscle fibers due to long axonal sprouts,
- Delay in neuro-muscular transmission in newly formed collaterals,
- Slower conduction velocities in muscle fibers of smaller diameter.

We have also analysed the probable contribution of each factor in the delay of the satellite.

Method of Simulations

The model of motor unit structure adopted by Nandedkar and Stålberg [13,14,15,16,25,26,] was applied in the simulation study. In this model the random distribution of muscle fibers within the motor unit territory was assumed. Each muscle fiber, a source of a single fiber potential (SFP), has a given diameter and is located at a certain distance to the end-plate zone and to the electrode. The SFPs are triggered at the end plate zone and propagated along the fibers with the propagation velocity linearly proportional to the diameter of the fiber [13].

The motor unit action potential (MUP) recorded by a needle electrode is a sum of individual potentials. Each fiber contributes to the MUP dependent on three factors: fiber diameter, electrode to end-plate distance and muscle fiber to electrode distance. The equations describing these relationships were presented by the authors of the model [14,15].

In our studies, we have controlled the following parameters: density of muscle fibers, range of muscle fiber diameters, recording distance as well as muscle fibers distribution within the motor unit territory. In addition to the possibilities offered by the original model we have also considered a possible delay in axonal conduction or neuromuscular transmission.

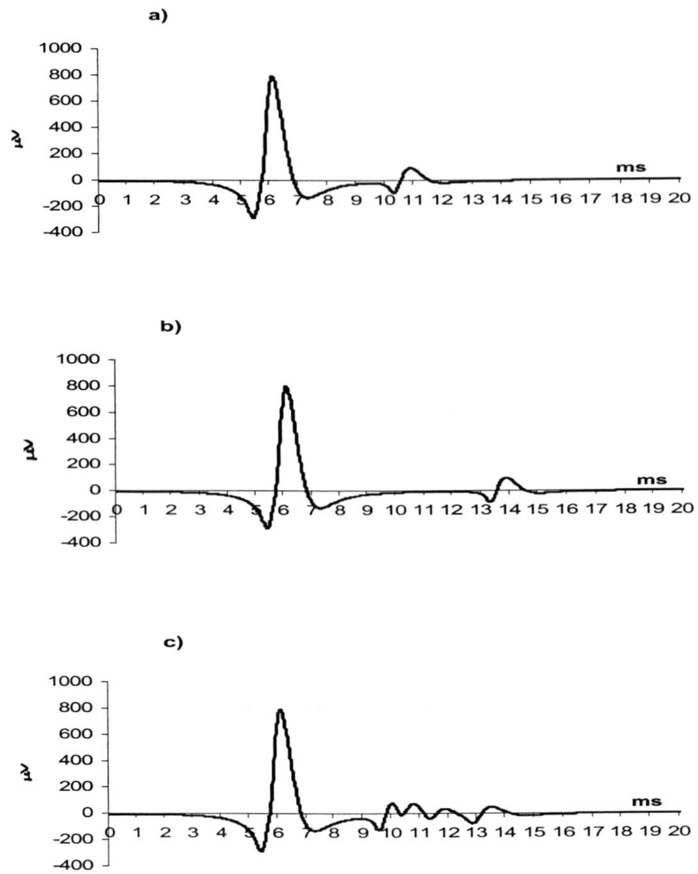

Figure 6. Simulated MUP with satellite. (a) SFPs from fibers of diameters in the range of 45-55 μm contribute to the main component. The satellite is a potential of one fiber of the diameter of 20 μm. The delay of the satellite calculated as an interval between the peaks is about 5 ms. (b) A simulated potential from Fig.6a modified by adding a delay caused by slower conduction in axon sprouts and immatured ectopic end plates assumed to be 3 ms. This modification results in a total delay of satellite about 8 ms and (c) The irregular potential is a result of the overlapping of SFPs from fibers of diameters in the range from 15 to 30 μm.

Simulation studies allowed us to simulate the potential that could be generated from a motor unit of the modeled structure. By modifying the structural characteristics listed above we have modelled a series of MUPs with satellites and we have analysed the relationships between these characteristics of the motor unit structure and MUPs parameters. Among other things the relationships between the amplitude or delay of satellites and the muscle fiber diameter the electrode to fiber distance and the recording distance have been analysed.

We have also applied an inverse procedure to that used in the simulation of MUP in a modelled structure of motor units. This inverse procedure has been developed to decompose the MUP into contributions from individual fibers. For a given real MUP we have approximated the number of fibers, their diameters and distances to the electrode and end -

plate zone so that the summation of simulated SFPs matched best the considered real MUP [30].

In our inverse procedure, we have used a standard multidimensional minimization method where the sum of differences between MUP and its model was minimized. In this algorithm, the initial guess assumes a certain number of fibers (typically 40 – 80) and a random distribution of their parameters. This distribution is then modified through consecutive minimization steps. Typically, about 100 iteration steps are necessary to obtain a satisfactory fit of a simulated MUP to a real MUP [30].

The result of this inverse analysis is a histogram indicating a probable number and diameters of muscle fibers and the approximated localization of muscle fibers contributing to the real potential under consideration.

Simulation of MUP with Satellites

In simulation studies we have assumed normal characteristics of motor unit structure, i.e. muscle fiber density of 5 fibers/mm^2 and a range of muscle fiber diameters from 45 to 55 μm. In this model, the normal end-plate dispersion of around 10 mm is also assumed. The pool of these fibers generates the main component of MUP (Fig.6). The satellite is a SFP and is generated by one additional fiber of the diameter of 20 μm located in the motor unit. As seen in Fig. 6a the difference in fiber diameters of about 20 μm results in the delay of about 5 ms between the main component and the satellite.

Other factors such as delays in axon sprouts, immature ectopic end - plates added to this model, will result in the increase in the delay of the satellite and/or the jiggle of the main component. Assuming this delay to be 3 ms the latency of the satellite will be about 8 ms (Fig. 6b).

When we assume that the satellite potential is formed by a group of fibers with a diameter within the range of 15-30 μm rather than by a single fiber, then the satellite potential could become irregular – as shown in Fig.6c. Such a satellite has a longer duration than that generated by one fiber.

Using the simulated potential presented in Fig.6 we have quantitatively analyzed the possible contribution of particular factors in the delay and also in the parameters of the satellite potential.

Factors Determining the Time Dispersion and Parameters of SFPs

The time dispersion of single fiber potentials reaching the electrode depends on the factors listed above. These factors may lead to the irregularity of recorded MUP and/or to the presence of satellite potentials. Some of these factors also determine the parameters of SFPs while others cause only a delay. Therefore, SFP parameters will also be considered in the following analysis of the possible contribution of factors influencing time dispersion of SFPs.

1. Changes in Parameters of a Single Fiber Potential

The amplitude and duration of a single fiber potential recorded by a concentric needle electrode depend on the fiber diameter as well as on the measurement conditions such as the fiber to electrode distance and the distance between the end-plate zone and the electrode (see Fig.7). The effect of these factors on parameters of a single fiber potential is summarized in Table 4.

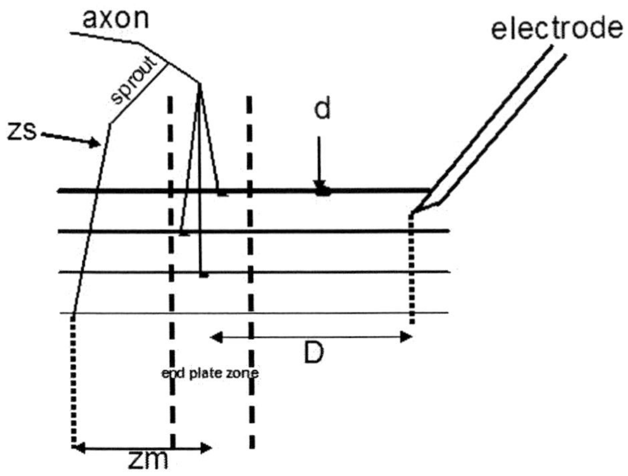

Figure 7 The propagation of action potentials along muscle fibers. The factors determining the propagation time from the end-plate zone to the electrode are marked as: Zs- is length of preterminal axonal sprout. Zm- is the distance between end-plate of new axonal sprout to the end-plate zone of this axon. D- is the distance between electrode and end-plate zone. d- is the fiber diameter.

Table 4. Factors determining the amplitude and duration of a single fiber potential

	Amplitude of SFP	Duration of SFP
Fiber diameter ↑	↑	↓
Fiber to electrode distance ↑	↓	↑

The factors from Table 4 determine the parameters of SFP as well as the propagation time. The relationships listed in Table 4 are impotrant for the interpretation of MUPs because they determine the degree of the overlapping of SFP that is crucial for the occurrence of separated components in MUP [29]. The remaining factors such as the changes in conduction velocity in axons as well as the neuromuscular transmission only affect the propagation time of the action potential rather than its parameters. All the above factors cause time dispersion of single fiber potentials reaching the electrode.

In what follows is presented the possible contribution of each factor to the delay of potentials.

2. Factors Determining Time Distribution of Muscle Fiber Potentials Reaching the Electrode

Fig. 7 schematically illustrates the recording of motor unit potential using a needle electrode. Factors determining propagation time are marked, and symbols used in the analysis are explained in this figure.

The muscle fiber diameter is the only a factor determining the propagation velocity in muscle fiber [13]. The larger the diameter the faster the velocity and the shorter the propagation time of the potential from the end-plate zone to the electrode. Other factors determining the propagation time are related to neuromuscular transmission and cause a delay at the start point of the action potential. The contribution weight of each factor will be determined in the sections below.

2.1. Slower conduction in smaller muscle fibers

The velocity of propagation of action potential along the muscle fiber is a linear function of the fiber diameter [13]. Assuming simultaneous generation the potentials in all muscle fibers will reach the electrode in the time determined by their diameters. The smaller the fiber diameter, the smaller the amplitude of the potential, longer duration and propagation time [29]. Therefore the potentials from the fibers of the diameter, for example of 50 μm and 20 μm will be recorded by the electrode as separated potentials with the time interval of approximately 3 ms. For a longer recording distance this interval will be also longer. Assuming that the velocity of the propagation of the action potential along muscle fiber is between 2 and 6 m/sec then the time dispersion between SFP reaching the electrode at a recording distance of D= 20 mm is approximately 6 ms.

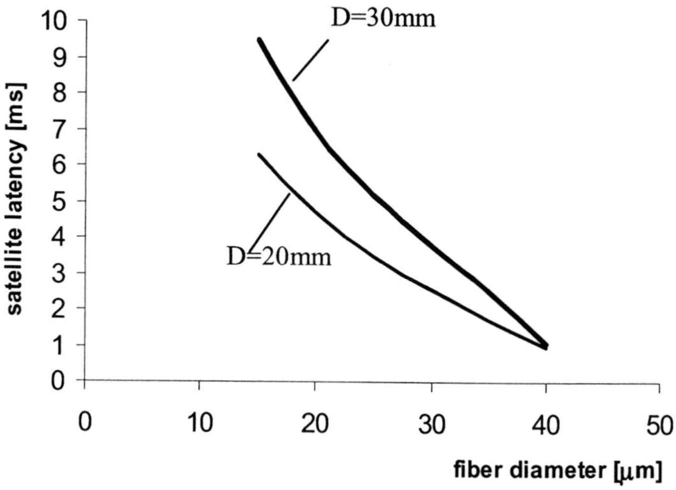

Figure 8. The interval between the peaks of the main and satellite components of MUP versus the diameter of the muscle fiber (origin of satellite component).

The time dispersion of single fiber potentials from muscle fibers of various diameters cause irregularity of MUP or presence of a satellite component delayed to the main component.

The relationship between the satellite latency and the fiber diameter was analysed quantitatively and the results are presented in Fig. 8. The latency of the satellite as a function of its fiber diameter was calculated for simulated MUP with a satellite shown in Fig. 6a. The satellite originated from one fiber and the latency was calculated as an interval between the peaks of the main component and the satellite. The plot of the satellite latency as a function of the fiber diameter is shown in Fig. 8.

The amplitude of the satellite also depends on fiber diameter. Fig.9 presents the relationship between satellite amplitude and the diameter of the muscle fiber. It is assumed that the satellite is the SFP.

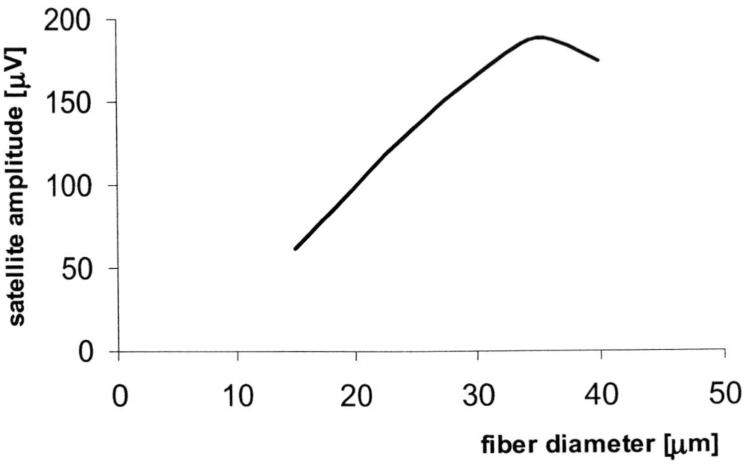

Figure 9. The relationship between diameters of the muscle fiber and the amplitude of its potential (for simulated potential shown in Fig 6a). Potentials from larger fibers have higher amplitude.

The plots in Fig. 8 are presented for various recording distances. The latency of satellite clearly depend on the recording distance. Amplitude of SFP does not depend on recording distance but the amplitude of satellite that is a sum of few SFPs will depend. In the next section this relationship will be analysed.

2.2 The recording distance

Another factor influencing the delay and amplitude of the satellite potential is the recording distance between the end-plate zone and the electrode. The longer the recording distance the larger the time dispersion of potentials propagating with various velocities (depending on their diameters).

The latency of satellite potentials increases with the recording distance. This latency may change in the range of 5 ms to 14 ms for the recording distance from 20 to 60mm (for MUP shown in Fig.6a).

2.3 Muscle fiber to electrode distance

Fig. 10 presents the dependence of the amplitude and latency of the satellite on the muscle fiber to the electrode distance. This distance has a bigger effect on the amplitude than on the latency of the recorded satellite.

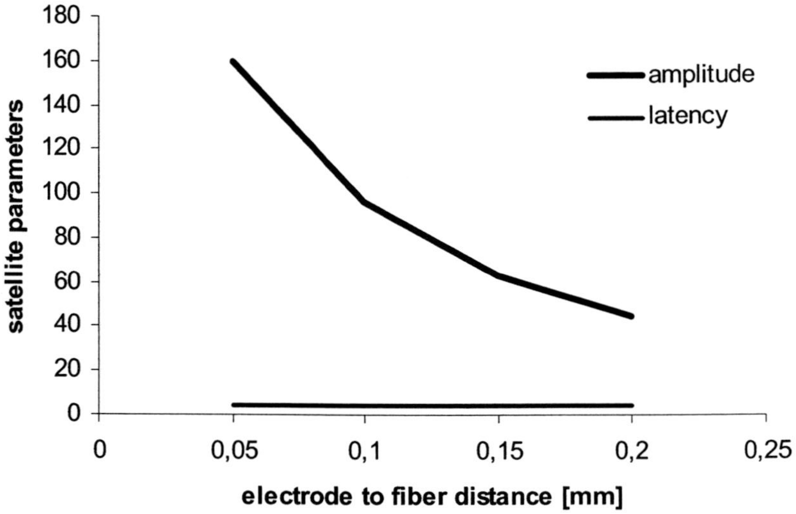

Figure 10. The amplitude and latency of the satellite potential recorded at various distances from the electrode (for MUP shown in Fig. 6a).

In summary, the muscle fiber diameter affects the parameters of a single fiber potential and determines the velocity of propagation of the potential along the muscle fiber. Therefore it determines the time of propagation from the end-plate zone to the electrode.

The propagation time of single fiber potentials is influenced, besides the fiber diameter and measurement conditions, by other factors related to changes in nerve conduction in affected terminal axons and to increased dispersion of end-plates. However, they do not affect SFP parameters. The possible contribution of these factors is presented and evaluated below.

2.4. Increased dispersion of end-plates

Axonal sprouts reinnervate denervated muscle fibers of other motor units and constitute new end-plates that may be located at a distance zm from the end-plate zone of the original motor unit (see Fig 7). Assuming a typical conduction velocity v in nerve terminals to be 3 m/s the axon sprout of the length zs that reinnervates a fiber of another motor unit at a distance zm from its end-plates will cause a delay of the potential of approximately (Fig.7):

$$td = zs/v + zs/vm,$$

where vm is the velocity of propagation in the muscle fiber assumed to be 3.5 m/s.

For example, for zs=20mm, zm=15mm the delay td it will be:

$$td=20[mm]/3[m/s] + 15[mm]/3.5[m/s] = 6.7\ ms+4.3\ ms = 11\ ms$$

In the model we have assumed a normal conduction velocity in an axon. However, this velocity may also be decreased due to nerve damage and there may be some additional delay in neuro-muscular transmission in newly formed collaterals.

Other factors that may contribute to the delay in individual SFP are: decreased velocity in the primary nerve, damage and delay in neuromuscular transmission in formed collaterals. It is difficult to estimate the effect of these factors separately. We may only consider their summarized effect.

All the factors described above have to be taken into account in the analysis of conditions of the possible generation of satellite potentials.

In summary, the factors presented above may contribute to the delay of satellite potential. Different contribution weight is the cause of various characteristics of a satellite recorded in neuromuscular disorders. In what follows we will try to establish the possible origin of the satellite in a given MUP. The aim of this analysis is to determine the role of undergoing processes that manifest themselves in satellite characteristic.

Analysis of a MUP With a Satellite in ALS

Let us consider an example of MUP with a satellite recorded in an ALS process that has some characteristic features. As follows from our clinical electrophysiological studies presented above, satellites often have small amplitude and short duration being located at a distance of a few ms from the main component.

Fig.11 is an example of a high amplitude MUP with one satellite. The overlapping of consecutive potentials does not show jiggle, which suggests that there is no significant time dispersion in neuromuscular transmission. The approximation of the number and diameters of muscle fibers indicate that the majority of fiber diameters range from 45 to 75 μm (Fig.11). The increased number of fibers contributing to the potential suggests that there exist a reinnervation process. There is a fiber 25 μm in diameter that may be a source of a satellite. The size of the potential required modification of the usually adopted values of the conductance parameters in the model.

The hypothesis that a satellite is a single fiber potential may be supported by the analysis of parameters of the satellite potential. We have performed a reconstruction of the satellite potential itself, which has also shown that a single fiber is a source of this component. The duration of 2 ms indicates the potential of one fiber.

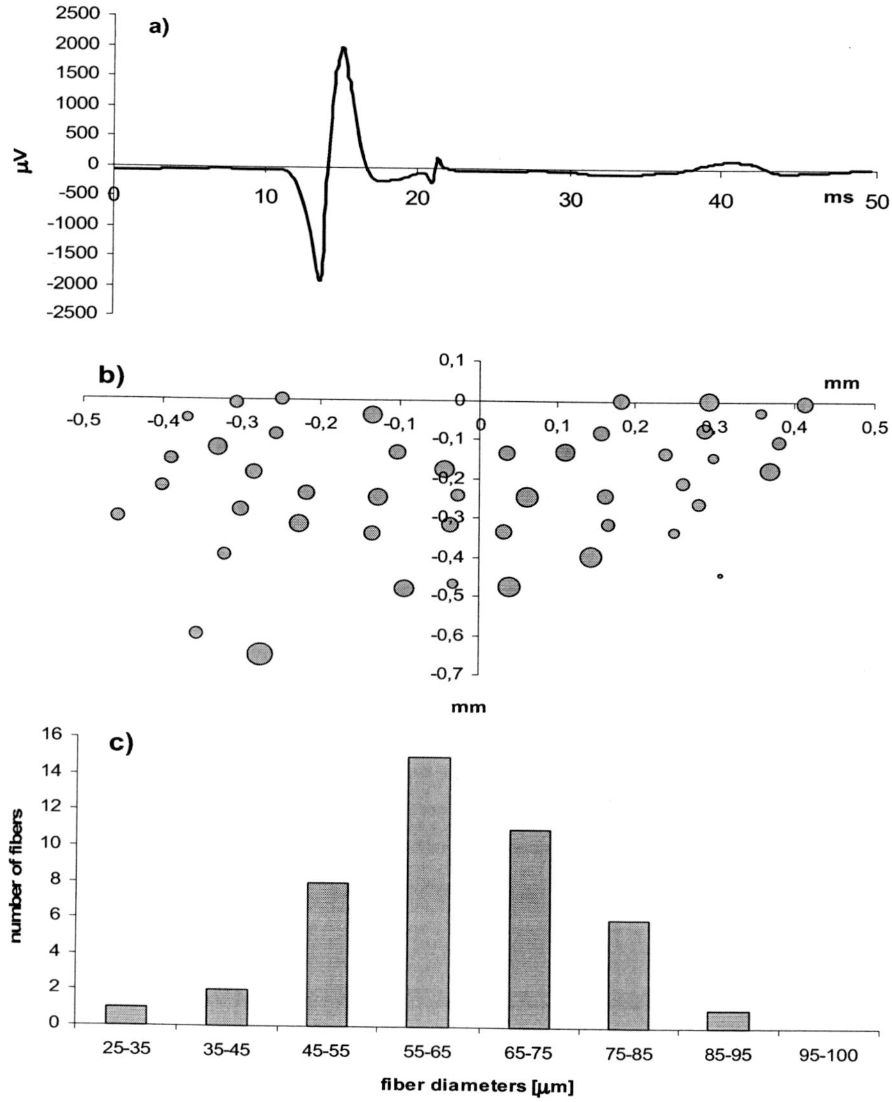

Figure 11 (a) MUP with satellite in ALS (b) approximated distribution of muscle fibers contributing into this MUP (c) histogram of muscle fiber diameters.

Analysis of a MUP with a Satellite in SMA

A MUP with an irregular component and four satellites has been analysed. The irregularity of the main component of MUP reflects the differentiation of muscle fiber diameters. The reconstruction method shows that the range of fiber diameters contributing to the main component is 55-95 µm. This indicates that there is a significant differentiation of fiber diameters that causes the irregularity. Satellites seem to be originated by a group of smaller diameter fibers (Fig.12).

The analysis of satellite potential itself indicates that it is generated by several fibers. This hypothesis is also supported by the duration and amplitude of these satellite potentials – they are larger and longer than those for a SFP.

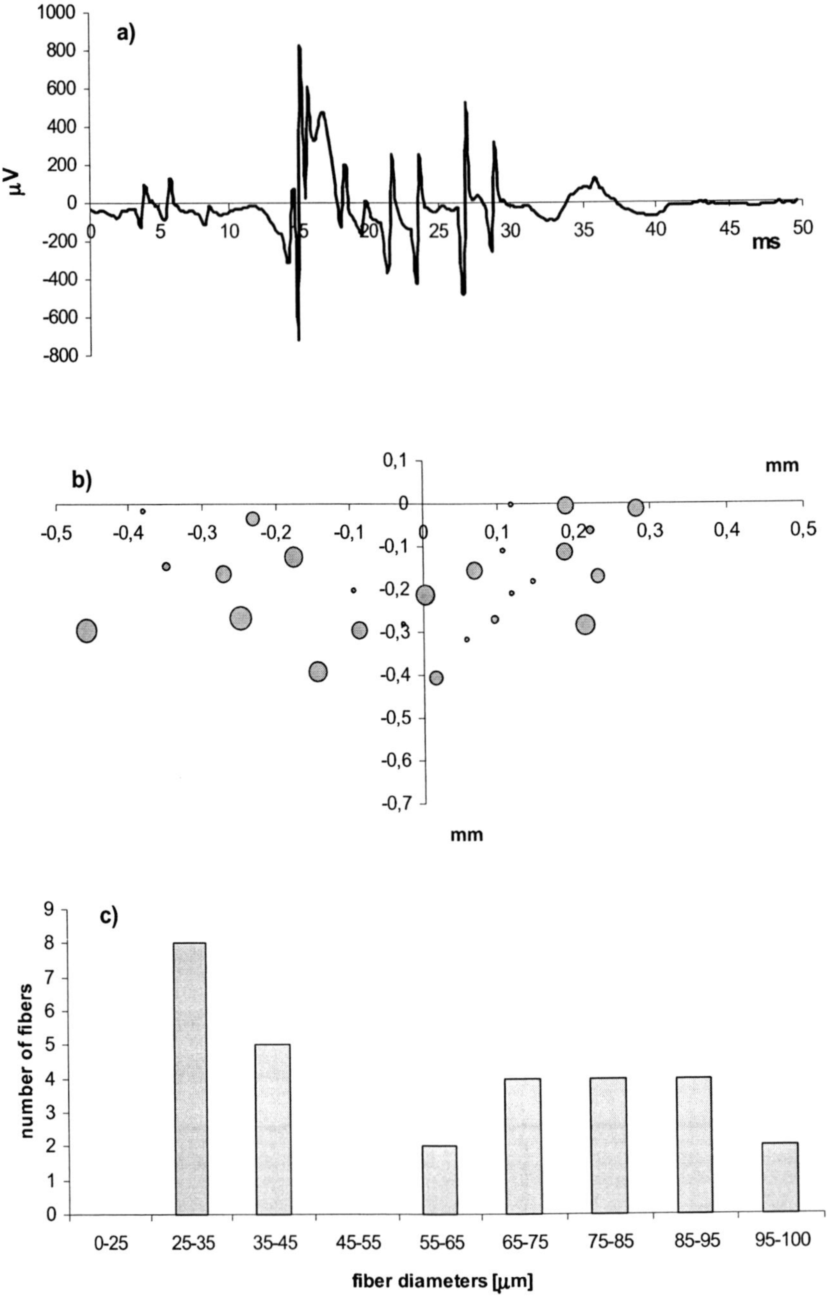

Figure 12 (a) MUP with satellite in SMA (b) approximated distribution of muscle fibers contributing into this MUP (c) histogram of muscle fiber diameters.

In summary, the analysis of examples of MUPs in ALS and SMA suggests that satellite potential may originate from a muscle fiber which is much smaller than other fibers (probably a denervated or reinnervated muscle fiber).

In the example of ALS potential analysed the duration and amplitude of the satellite suggest that it is a SFP. Of course, the possible delay caused by slower nerve conduction or neuromuscular transmission cannot be excluded. However, the absence of "jiggle" suggests that there are no significant transmission disturbances.

The analysis of an example of a SMA potential indicates significant differentiation of fiber diameters that manifests by irregularity of the main MUP component. This is also a reason why potentials from fibers of sufficiently smaller diameters (longer propagation time) are recorded as separated satellite components. The analysis of satellite components itself indicates that each component is an overlapping complex of a few SFP rather than one SFP.

In both examples, for ALS and SMA, the contribution of neuromuscular transmission delay is possible. However, the participation of this factor in the delay of a satellite could not be explicitly estimated using the present version of our model.

Discussion

Our results indicate that there are evident differences in the number and characteristics of satellite potentials in both neurogenic processes: ALS and SMA. We have found a much higher rate of MUPs with satellites in SMA than in ALS. The mean number of satellites per one MUP was higher in SMA. The mean duration of satellite components was longer in SMA.

In previous studies of satellite potentials [1,2,6,8,9,11] several hypothesis of their origin have been presented. It is suppoused that in neurogenic processes desynchronization of single fiber potentials is caused by slow impulse conduction in immature collateral nerve branches, immature neuromuscular junction and slower conduction in regenerating muscle fibers. Satellites are explained as potentials of single muscle fibers innervated by newly formed poorly myelinated nerve fibers, ectopic end plates or of regenerating muscle fibers. The above possible sources of satellites may be present in all neurogenic processes. Moreover, besides that there are several neurogenic changes in the motor unit that lead to the increase in MUP irregularity and the occurrence of satellites, some others changes have an opposite effect. The increase in muscle fiber density due to reinnervation and hypertrophy of muscle fibers result in the smoothing of MUP. In ALS, a relatively rapid progressive denervation-reinnervation process density of muscle fibers show an increase of the order of 2 to 4 and jitter increase of 30 to 100%. In SMA, the density of muscle fibers show an increases by a factor of 4 to 9 [24]. Reinnervation increases fiber density and therefore the number of SFPs summarized into the MUP. The more SFPs are overlapped the smoother will be the MUP. Hypertrophy of muscle fibers leads to a decrease in the time dispersion of SFPs because conduction velocity increases proportionally to fiber diameter. When a recording distance is assumed to be D=20 mm, the interval between SFPs from fibers of d1=40 μm and d2=50μm will be 1 ms whereas the interval between SFPs from fibers of larger diameters of 60 μm and

70 μm will be shortened to about 0.5 ms. This shows that potentials of larger muscle fibers will tend to overlap and therefore smooth the MUP.

The differences in satellite characteristics found in our studies suggest that there are different contributions of various factors determining SFPs time dispersion in the processes under consideration. The different severity of pathological processes in acute and chronic diseases seems to be responsible for these differences, in spite of similar changes affecting nerve and muscle fibers.

Considering the possible contribution of each of the above factors, there is a question of the range of possible latency caused by slower nerve conduction and neuro-muscular transmission. According to our calculations this latency may be estimated about 10 ms. The same value of 10 ms has been estimated by Desmedt [6]. Finsterer and Mamoli [9] have pointed out that the neurogenic pathomechanism is unlikely to explain the satellite latency of 40 ms. It would imply the end-plate scatter of 120-160 mm and nerve terminals of 60-80 mm length on the assumption of normal nerve conduction velocity of 1.5-2 m/s. This may suggest the contribution of another factor.

Our simulations indicate that the fiber diameter is an additional factor that may cause a delay of a satellite. As shown in our studies, a satellite may be a potential of one fiber with a smaller diameter that seems to be observed more often in an ALS potential while it might be generated by a group of smaller fibers that shown example of SMA potential. This hypothesis might be supported by the fact that in a chronic SMA process there is a large variability of fiber diameters whereas this is not the case in an ALS process [6,24].

This hypothesis can be strongly supported by the results of biopsies. Terminal branches from a single axon innervate several neuromuscular junctions producing fibers type grouping. Denervation in ALS causes to appear a large number of small groups of atrophic muscle fibers. In SMA there are hypertrophied muscle fibers, small fibers clustered in larger atrophic groups. Small fibers in one group vary moderately in size. In chronic denervation with reinnervation the muscle fibers of same type are grouped.

These biopsy data may provide some explanation of the phenomenon that in ALS satellites there are usually SFP, whereas in SMA the satellite is a sum of potentials of several fibers. In SMA, it may originate from a group of reinnervated atrophic fibers. In the case of several satellites observed in SMA, consecutive satellites may originate from different groups of fibers. As follows from biopsy denervated-reinnervated muscle fibers in one group have similar diameters. They vary, however, from one group to another. Each satellite component may originate from a different pool of reinnervated muscle fibers [6,24].

It should also be emphasized that neurogenic factors such as slower nerve conduction and neuromuscular transmission should be of much less importance in a chronic SMA process than in the early stage of denervation-reinnervation in an ALS process. The jitter that provides information on the stability of the reinnervation process was small in our EMG recordings in SMA, which indicates the maturity of reinnervated neuromuscular junctions. Therefore, these neurogenic factors are not sufficient for the generation of several satellites with relatively long latency. Groups of fibers of smaller diameters seem to be the source of these components.

Another question concerning satellites is whether MUP irregularity and satellites result from the same processes. Finsterer and Mamoli [8] concluded that satellite potentials were more often found in combination with normo- than with polyphasic MUP, which may suggest that satellite potentials and polyphasic MUPs derive from different pathophysiological mechanisms. However, our results seem to point to an opposite answer. Simulation studies indicate similar factors create polyphasic as well as satellite components. Both phenomena reflect the desynchronization of the potentials generated by muscle fibers belonging to one motor unit and are the result of motor unit reorganization. An increase in the number of phases or turns reflects decreased synchrony in the generation of SFPs (axonal and neuromuscular transmission delays) as well as delays in propagation of action potential along muscle fibers (decreased fiber diameter). The relationships between factors influencing the MUP irregularity have been quantitatively analysed by a simulation study [29]. These relationships could also be applied to approximate structural conditions of a motor unit that makes it possible to generate separate satellite components,

Lateva et.al [12] have performed a simulation study on the origin of satellites in normal muscles. The authors put forward a hypothesis that satellite potentials are generated by pairs of muscle fibers connected at one of the muscle/tendon junctions. One of the fibers receives neural innervation while the other does not. However, this simulation study was performed with to use of a model with a monopolar needle electrode.

The differences between two neurogenic processes, ALS and SMA, in respect to structural and functional changes during the progression of a process are well known [5,6,24]. The results presented in this paper show different characteristics of satellites in ALS and SMA. Except for explanations of the generation of satellites in neurogenic processes reported in previous studies [2,6,9,24] we have shown a significant role of atrophic denervated-reinnervated muscle fibers. Modelling studies made it possible to analyse contributions of various factors determining delay and parameters of satellite potentials and therefore extend our knowledge on this electromyographic phenomenon, which may help to increase diagnostic yield of the analysis of satellites.

References

[1] Antonini G, et. al. Satellite potentials on EMG: Neurophysiologic evidence of axonal transaction in MS? *Neurology*, 2001;57:1126-1128.

[2] Borenstein S, Desmedt JE. Late components of the motor unit potential in muscle disease, in Kunze K, Desmedt JE (eds): Studies in Neuromuscular Diseases. Basel, Karger, 1975.

[3] Buchthal F, Rosenfalck A. On the structure of motor units. In: Desmedt JE ed. New development in electromyography and clinical neurophysiology vol. 1, Basel Karger 1973, 71-85.

[4] Cohen HM et. al. A computer model of denervation-reinnervation in skeletal muscle. *Muscle Nerve*, 1987;10: 826-836.

[5] Daube JR. Electrodiagnostic studies on amyotrophic lateral sclerosis and other motor neuron disorders. *Muscle Nerve*, 2000; 23;10:1488-1502.

[6] Desmedt JE. Plasticity of motor unit organization studied by coherent electromyography in patients with nerve lesions or with myopathic or neuropathic

deseases. *Prog Clin Neurophysiol, vol.9*, Ed. J.E.Desmedt, Karger, Basel 1981, 250-304.

[7] Emeryk-Szajewska B, Kopec J, Karwanska A. The reorganization of motor units in different motor neuron disorders. *Electromyogr Clin Neurophysiol*, 2003;43, 23-31.

[8] Finsterer J, Mamoli B. Satellite potentials: definition, normal values and validity in the detection of mild myogenic lesions. *Electroencephalogr Electromyogr*, 1992;23:20-28.

[9] Finsterer J, Mamoli B. Satellite potentials as a measure of neuromuscular disorders. *Muscle Nerve*, 1997;5:585-592.

[10] Hecht BM, Kasatkina LE. Electromyograpic analysis of different stages of denervation and reinnervation. *Wiss. Z. Ernst Moritz-Arndt Univ.* 1983;32, 27-31.

[11] Lang AH, Partanen USJ. "Satellite potentials" and the duration of motor unit potentials in normal, neuropathic and myopathic muscles. *J Neurol Sci*, 1976;27:513-524.

[12] Lateva ZC, Mc Gill KC. Satellite potentials of motor unit action potentials in normal muscles: a new hypothesis for their origin. *Clin Neurophysiol*, 1999; 110:1625-1633.

[13] Nandedkar SD, Stålberg E. Simulation of single fiber action potentials. *Med Biol Eng Comput,* 1983; 21:158-165.

[14] Nandedkar SD, Sanders DB, Stålberg EV, Andreassen S. Simulation of concentric needle EMG motor unit action potentials. *Muscle Nerve*, 1988; 2:151-159.

[15] Nandedkar SD, Sanders DB, Stålberg EV. EMG of reinnervated motor units: a simulation study. *Electroencephalogr Clin Neurophysiol*, 1988; 70:177-184.

[16] Nandedkar SD. Models and simulations in electromyography. *Muscle Nerve* 2002:Suppl 11, S46-S54.

[17] Nomenclature Committee AAEE: Glossary and terms in clinical electromyography. *Muscle Nerve*, 1987;9:G1-G53.

[18] Podnar S, Fowler CJ. Sphincter electromyography in diagnosis of multiple system atrophy:technical data. *Muscle Nerve*, 2004;29;151-156.

[19] Rowinska-Marcinska K, Ryniewicz B, Hausmanowa-Petrusewicz I, Karwanska A. Diagnostic value of satellite potentials in clinical EMG, *Electromyogr Clin Neurohysiol*, 1997;37:483-489.

[20] Sandberg A, Hansson B, Stålberg E. Comparison between concentric needle EMG and macro EMG in patients with a history of polio. *Clin Neurophysiol*, 1999:110, 1900-1908.

[21] Stålberg E, Sonoo M. Assesment of variability in the shape of the motor unit action potential, the "jiggle", at consecutive discharges, *Muscle Nerve*, 1994;17:1135-1144.

[22] Stålberg E, Andreassen, S, Falck, B, Lang, H, Rosenfalck, A, Trojaborg, W. Quantitative analysis of individual motor unit potentials: a proposition for standardized terminology and criteria for measurement. *J Clin Neurophysiol*, 1986; 3(4): 313-348.

[23] Stålberg E, Dioszeghy P. Scanning EMG in normal muscle and in neuromuscular disorders. *Electroencephalogr Clin Neurophysiol*, 1991;81;6: 403-416.

[24] Stålberg E, Fawcett PRW: Electrophysiological methods for the study of the motor unit in Spinal Muscle Atrophy. Progressive Spinal Muscle Atrophies, ed. Gamstorp I and Sarnat HB, Raven Press, New York, 1984, 111-134.

[25] Stålberg E, Karlsson L. Simulation of the normal concentric needle electromyogram by using a muscle model. *Clin Neurophysiol*, 2000; 112:464-471.

[26] Stålberg E, Karlsson L. Simulation of EMG in pathological situations. *Clin Neurophysiol*, 2001; 112:2118-2132.

[27] Zalewska E, Hausmanowa-Petrusewicz I. Evaluation of MUAP shape irregularity - a new concept of quantification. *IEEE Trans Biomed Eng*, 1995;42: 616-620.

[28] Zalewska E, Rowińska-Marcińska K, Hausmanowa-Petrusewicz I. Shape irregularity of motor unit potentials in neuromuscular diseases. *Muscle Nerve*, 1998; 21: 1181-1187.

[29] Zalewska E, Hausmanowa-Petrusewicz I, Stålberg E: Modeling studies on irregular motor unit potentials. *Clin Neurophysiol*, 2004;11;3:1543-1556.

[30] Zalewska E, Hausmanowa-Petrusewicz I. Approximation of motor unit structure from the analysis of motor unit potential (in preparation).

In: Amyotrophic Lateral Sclerosis: New Research
Editor: Christine A. Murray, pp. 303-322

ISBN 1-59454-179-5

Chapter XIII

Magnetic Resonance Spectroscopic Investigation in Amyotrophic Lateral Sclerosis (ALS)

Kazuo Abe*
Department of Neurology, Osaka University, Osaka 565-0871, Japan

Abstract

It has long been known that central nervous lesions of amyotrophic lateral sclerosis (ALS) may extend beyond the spinal cord and the brain stem to involve the cerebral hemisphere. However, roles of degenerative changes of cerebral hemisphere have been controversial. Although it is a case that ALS has both upper and lower motor neuron signs and upper motor neuron signs may be resulted from degeneration in the motor related cerebral, whether degenerative changes in cerebral hemisphere develop higher cognitive dysfunction is not clear. Recent advent of neuroimaging techniques enables us to investigate these cerebral involvements in vivo and to study correlation between results of neuroimage and cognitive dysfunction. Among them magnetic resonance spectroscopy (MRS) present us a useful information about on-going changes of metabolites in the brain of ALS. We have investigated metabolites in the brain of patients with ALS by using MRS. In our reports, we described that the NA (*N*-acetylaspartate and *N*-acetylaspartylglutamate)/ Cr (creatine and phosphocreatine), ratio was reduced in the motor area and the frontal lobe in patients with ALS. And the NA/Cr ratio in the brain had significant correlations with clinical signs including cognitive functions. Addition to our studies, several attempts have been conducting this field of investigation. From reviewing our studies and literally evidences, we believe that the reduced NA/Cr ratio was a marker of cortical neuronal loss and dysfunction in ALS. Here, we introduce MRS investigations to detect abnormalities in the CNS of ALS, mainly according with

* Correspondence concerning this article should be addressed to Dr. Kazuo Abe, Department of Neurology, Osaka University Graduate School of Medicine, D-4, 2-2 Yamadaoka, Suita, Osaka 565-0871, Japan. Tel; 81-6-6879-3571; Fax; 81-6-6879-3579; E-Mail; abe@neurol.med.osaka-u.ac.jp.

ourselves, and discuss usefulness of MRS to detect and to evaluate pathologic process in the brain of ALS.

Keywords: amyotrophic lateral sclerosis (ALS), magnetic resonance spectroscopy (MRS), proton MRS (lH-MRS), NA (N-acetylaspartate and N-acetylaspartylglutamate), Cr (creatine and phosphocreatine), Cho (glycerophosphorylcholine, phosphorylcholine), Glx (glutamate + glutamine), mI (Myo-Inositol).

Introduction

Amyotrophic lateral sclerosis (ALS) is the most common and well-recognized form of motor neuron disease. It affects adults and has a progressive course leading to death. Its occurrence is mostly sporadic, a familial form being recognized in only 5-10% of patients [1-3]. At some time during the illness, the patients show a combination of upper (UMN) and lower (LMN) motor neuron signs [1-3]. The pathological basis of these signs is destruction of motor neurons in the spinal cord and brain stem, with associated peripheral and cranial nerve axonal degeneration, and in the cortex, associated with corticospinal and corticobulbar tract degeneration [4-6]. The etiology and pathogenesis of ALS remain unknown [3, 7-14].

According to the current diagnostic criteria, the EI Escorial Criteria of the World Federation of Neurology (WFN), there must be an absence of radiological abnormalities in the skull and spine, no significant abnormalities of the brain or spinal cord on MRI and no compressive lesions of the spinal cord or roots [15]. However, since ALS has been known to have neuropathological abnormalities in the central nervous system (CNS), imaging devises may be able to detect such abnormalities. Some abnormalities have been reported to be detected on T2-weighted images, such as high signal in the corticospinal and corticobulbar tracts and low signal in the motor cortex, particularly the precentral gyrus [16, 17]. Other neuroimaging techniques including SPECT, PET can also be reported to detect abnormalities in the central nervous system (CNS) [18,19]. Magnetic resonance spectroscopy (MRS) is a possible neuroimaging technique and has an advantage to present useful information about on-going changes of metabolites in the CNS of ALS. [20-25]. Literally, the usefulness of proton MRS (^{1}H-MRS) has been recognized in the study of the natural history [20-24], efficacy of treatment [26] and clinical outcome [25] of ALS.

In this review, we introduce MRS investigations to detect metabolites abnormalities in the CNS of ALS, mainly according with our previous report [25], and discuss usefulness of MRS to detect and to evaluate pathologic process in the CNS of ALS.

Neuroimages in ALS

The diagnosis of sporadic amyotrophic lateral sclerosis (ALS) is based on a combination of clinical and electrophysiological findings, and exclusion of other conditions that might produce the clinical picture. There is no definitive diagnostic test for the disease, and there is no established technique for demonstrating CNS involvement except for the clinical neurological examination. For these reasons, there has been an interest in the use of neuroimaging devices including MR imaging, MRS, single photon emission computed tomography (SPECT) or positron emission tomography (PET) to diagnose ALS and to monitor its clinical course.

MRI has been detected some characteristic features of CNS involvement in ALS, such as hyperintensity in the corticospinal tracts on proton density-weighted images and hypointensity in the motor cortex on T2-weighted images [17,26]. These features, however, are present in less than half of patients with clinically diagnosed ALS, and motor cortex hypointensity can be observed in normal volunteers and in subjects with other neurodegenerative diseases.

Functional neuroimaging techniques including SPECT and PET have also been conducted and found reduced cerebral blood flow in the frontal lobes including motor cortices [18, 27]. However, its high cost and ionizing radiation complications of these techniques may be a problem.

Proton MRS (^{1}H-MRS)

MRS uses similar technology as the more familiar MRI, but differs by allowing the measurement of the concentrations and synthesis rates of individual metabolites within precisely defined regions (ROI; region of interest) in the human brain. The basis of its chemical specificity is that the resonance frequency of an MRS active nucleus depends not only on the local magnetic field strength, but also on its chemical environment, a phenomenon referred to as chemical shift. MRS studies can be performed using several nuclei that have a property known as magnetic moment. Although the nuclei most commonly used in MRS studies are the proton (^{1}H), phosphorus (^{31}P), and carbon (^{13}C) nuclei, because of its inherent physical properties and high natural abundance, the ^{1}H nucleus provides the greatest sensitivity for in vivo MRS studies. MRS has disadvantage in its low spatial resolution method, with a resolution of approximately 1 to 4mm^3 in animal and 7 to 40 mm^3 in human. Also, MRS disadvantage in its low sensitivity in comparison with methods using radioactive tracers and therefore detects only compounds with a concentration of greater than 100□μM. Therefore, in present, neurotransmitters such as dopamine, serotonin, and acetylcholine cannot be measured using MRS methods. However, the lack of the need to use radioactive tracers and its safety allows MRS to be used in cross-sectional and longitudinal. [28-32] More importantly, MRS studies of normal developmental processes can be performed.

MRS can identify metabolites in the brain such as NA, Cr, Cho, Glx and mI (Figure 1). The main components of NA are *N*-acetylaspartate and *N*-acetylaspartyl glutamate, both of which are exclusively located in neuron in the central nervous system [33] and NA is recognized as a neuronal marker. Previously reported MRS studies demonstrated that the decrease of NA is reversal in some disease, such as carbon monoxide poisoning [34]. However, in most of diseases, decrease of NA is an indication of irreversible neuronal loss and functional impairment of neurons. The components of Cr, creatine and phosphocreatine are involved in energy metabolism via the creatine kinase reaction generating ATP.

Generally, the sum of these metabolites is constant, and therefore Cr has been used as a reference metabolite [35]. The Cho signal arises from glycerophosphorylcholine, phosphorylcholine, etc. These metabolites are involved in phospholipid synthesis and degradation, and are thought to reflect membrane synthesis and degradation. Although glutamate + glutamine (Glx) is abundantly present in the central nervous system and work as primary excitatory neurotransmitter, there have been few studies changes of Glx in the brain. This may be due to methodological problem, such as lower sensitivity, poor spectral resolution, and shorter T_2 relaxation time. Myo-Inositol (mI) is primarily located in glial cells and a possible glial marker [34] or plays a role in osmoregulation [37]

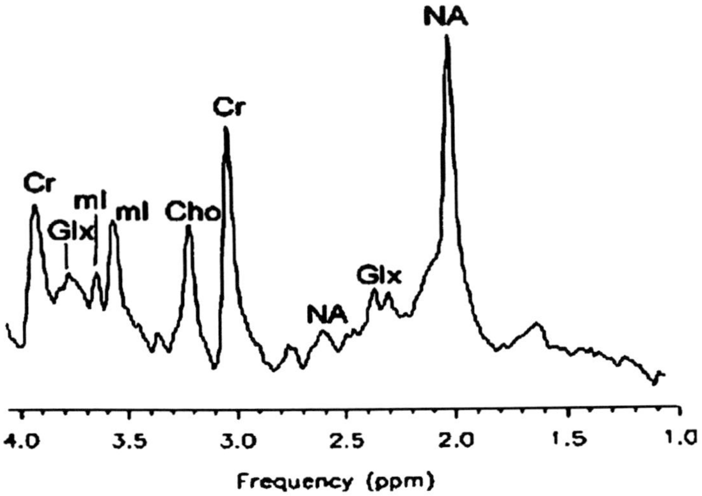

Figure 1. A representative data of ^{1}H-MRS by a three-Tesla system. Measurements were carried out in a whole body three-Tesla system with a maximum gradient strength of 40mT/m at a slew rate of 150T/m/s (Signa VH/*i*, GE Medical Systems, Milwaukee, WI, US). MRS data were acquired using PRESS with water presaturation by using chemical shift selective (CHESS) pulses, and with following parameters: TR = 6 sec, TE= 25 ms, a spectral width of 2500 Hz, 2048 data points, and 64 excitations. Before acquiring each spectrum, the magnetic field was adjusted by manual shimming and the receiver gain and the transmit gain were adjusted manually. A single 8-ml (2 x 2 x 2 cm) ROI was positioned in the frontal white matter. NA: N-acetyl group, Glx: glutamate + glutamine, Cr: creatine + phosphocreatine, Cho: choline-containing compounds, mI: *myo*-inositol

According to selection of ROIs, there are two major methods for MRS acquisition; single voxel MRS and MRS imaging (MRSI) (Figure 2). For MRS investigation, determination of ROIs is an essential (Table), and single voxel MRS essentially has a problem in choice of ROIs. In case of small ROIs, we cannot get clear signals. While in case of relatively large ROIs, the heterogeneity of the tissue composition within ROI is not negligible. The volume of a ROI varies from 1ml to 10ml or more in *in vivo* proton MRS, which are not small enough to locate a ROI within solely one tissue (for example, gray matter or white matter), and

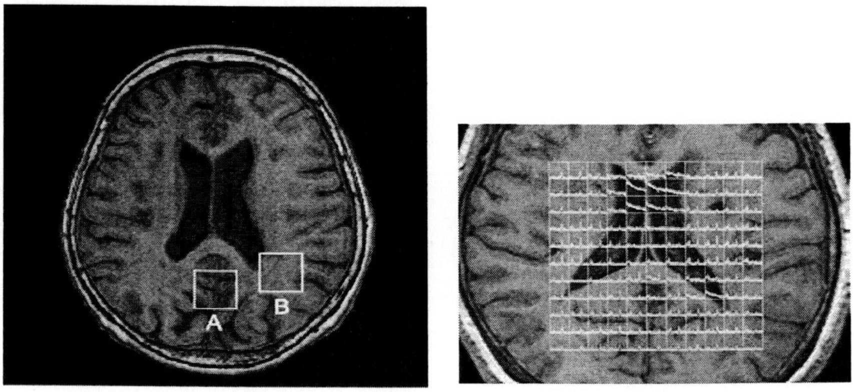

Single voxel MRS

MRS Imaging

Figure 2. Selection of ROIs in a single voxel MRS (left) and a MRS imaging (MRSI, right).

Table. Comparison of Single voxel MRS and MRS imaging.

	SINGLE VOXEL	SPECTROSCOPIC IMAING
Echo Time	Short or Long	Usually long
Detectable Compounds	NAA, Cho, Cr, Lac, inositols, Glx, Glc, lipids, Macromolecules	NAA, Cho, Cr, Lac
Typical Voxel Sizes (cm3)	4-20	1-4
Typical Scan Times (minutes)	5-10	6-30
Shimming	Localized	Global
Water/Lipid suppression	Better	Worse
Commercially Available	Most Vendors	Some Vendors
Quantitation	Yes	Maybe
Multiple Voxels	3 or 4 at most	Many voxels

inevitably contains other tissues not be aimed. As the metabolite concentrations have been reported to be different between the gray matter and the white matter this undesirable tissue contamination can cause the inaccuracy of the measurement. However, small ROIs such as in MRSI (Figure 2 right), we may not get clear metabolite peaks. In previous MRS studies, investigators prefer to use single voxel MRS for getting clear metabolite peaks. The other hand, an advantage of MRSI is that spectra are acquired from an array of voxels, each of which is several times smaller than the typical (8-mL) acquisition volume in single voxel MRS. Thus, 2-dimensional (and 3-dimensional) MRSI offers the opportunity to obtain spectral data from a relatively small area of interest, such as the primary motor strip. A disadvantage of MRSI has been lower spectral resolution and signal-to-noise ratio in each spectrum of the array compared with typical single voxel MRS, making quantitation of data more difficult in MRSI studies. Reminding these advantage and disadvantage of each method is needed in clinical investigation.

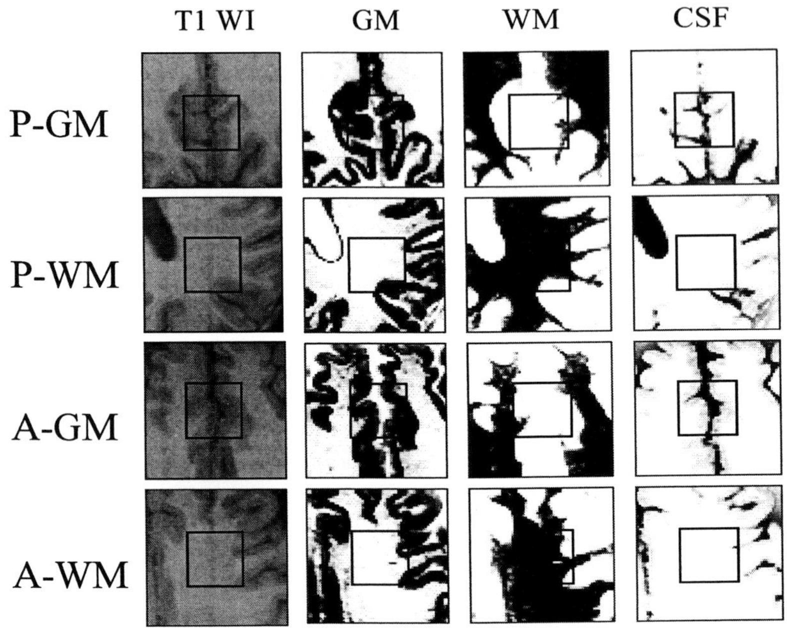

Figure 3. Segmentation of each ROI into gray matter, white matter and CSF by using SPM99 . We segmented ROIs into gray matter, white matter and CSF in the posterior white matter (P-WM), the anterior white matter (A-WM), the posterior grey matter (P-GM) and the anterior grey matter (A-GM) . MRI: T1-weighted Image: axial 3D Fast inversion recovery SPGR, TR 10.8ms, TE 3.7/Fr ms, FA 15 degree, BW 15.6kHz, FOV 20x20cm, 1.3mmthk/0.0sp, Matrix 256x192, 1NEX T2/PD-weighted Image: axial 2D Fast spin echo, TR 5000ms, TE 17.0/102.0ms, ETL 12, FOV 20x20cm, 5.0mmthk/0.0sp, Matrix 256x256, 1NEX. MRS: single voxel PRESS, TR=6sec, TE=25ms, spectral width = 2500Hz, data points = 2048, NEX=64, voxel size= 8 cm^3 (2 x 2 x 2 cm).

To conquer inhomogeneity within selected ROIs, we had started a trial to evaluate MRS signals separately from the gray matter, the white matter, and the cerebrospinal fluid (CSF). Using T2 weighted images, we segmented images by SPM99 (Statistical Parametric Mapping, The Welcome Department of Cognitive Neurology, London) to gray matter, white matter, CSF and other tissues. Sequently, we choose ROIs and calculated respectively percentages of gray matter, white matter, CSF and other tissues (Figure 3). We set a variable, gray matter fraction (GMF) as the fraction of the volume of the gray matter to the volume of total brain tissue (the sum of the gray matter and the white matter) in a ROI. The presumed multiple regression model as below for each metabolite within ROIs.

$$[\mathbf{C}]_i = b_0 + b_1 \times [\mathbf{AGE}]_i + b_2 \times [\mathbf{GMF}]_i + e_i \text{ for } i = 1, 2, \ldots, n$$

In the equation, [C] is the concentration of metabolite C (mMol), $\boldsymbol{b_0}$ is a coefficient constant, $\boldsymbol{b_1}$, and $\boldsymbol{b_2}$ are regression coefficients of predictors, $\boldsymbol{n}$ is the total number of spectra, and $\boldsymbol{e}$ is a random error. The regression equations of each metabolite of all ROIs were statistically evaluated. This approach enables us to evaluate an individual single voxel MR spectrum more precisely by considering both age and the tissue composition [38].

Proton MRS (^{1}H-MRS) Investigation in ALS

In this section, we first introduce our previous ^{1}H-MRS investigation in ALS [25] and discuss our results and others.

We studied fourteen clinically definite ALS patients (8 men and 6 women, mean age 65.8±9.9 SD, range 48-72 years old) satisfying EL Escorial criteria for ALS [15] and fourteen age- and sex- matched normal controls without neurological deficits (8 men and 6 women, mean age 59.3±12.8 SD, range 44-72 years old).

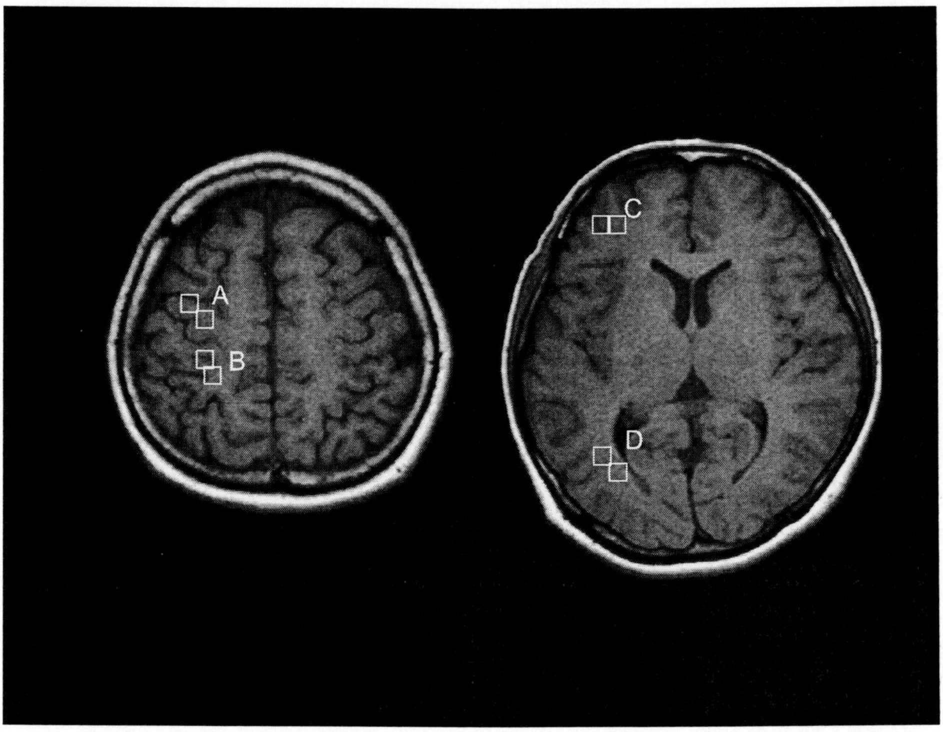

Figure 4. Location of Volume of Interests (VOIs). Eight 2-ml VOIs were positioned in the motor area (A), in the parietal Lobe (B), in the frontal lobe (C), and in the occipital lobe (D).

All patients were neurologically examined and severity of disease was evaluated using manual muscle strength test (full score is 110), Norris limb scale (full scale is 63), and Norris bulbar scale (full score is 39) [40, 41]. Cognitive function was screened by using Mini Mental State Examination (MMSE) [42]. To assess the frontal lobe function, we use Wisconsin Card Sorting Test (WCST) [43]. In order to exclude the possibility that abnormalities of neuropsychological functions in patients with ALS has been caused by associated depression or anxiety, patients and controls were rated with Zung's self rating depression scale (SRS) [44].

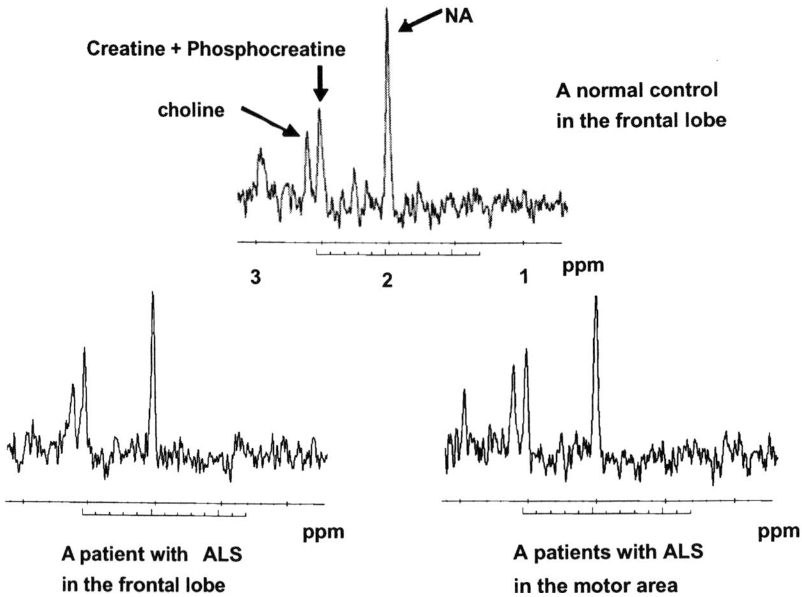

Figure 5. Representative results of ^{1}H-MRS in patients with ALS. In patients with ALS, peak of NA was reduced in the motor area lobe and in the frontal lobe in comparison to normal controls.

MR imaging and ^{1}H MRS studies were performed with a 1.5-T MR-Imaging system (Signa Advantage, General Electric Medical Systems, Milwaukee, WI) using a standard quadrature head coil. We obtained a set of T1-weighted axial images parallel to the orbito-meatal line and placed the volume of interest (VOI) in motor area, frontal lobe, parietal lobe and occipital lobe with attention to avoid the partial volume effect from parenchymal atrophy (Figure 4). Each VOI was a cubic shape whose size was 2ml. After localized shimming of the VOI, ^{1}H-MRS was performed using a stimulated echo acquisition mode sequence for volume selection with a chemical shift selective pre-sequence for water suppression. Acquisition parameters were a repetition time (TR) of 1500 msec and an echo time (TE) of 140 msec, with the number of acquired point of 1024, and acquisition of 256. After acquisition, the MRS data were transferred to a SUN computer (SPARC Station 330, Model 547, SUN Microsystems, Mountain View, California) and were processed by using a SA/GE processing software (General Electric Medical Systems, Milwaukee, WI). The process included zero filling to 2048 data points, 3 Hz line broadening and fast Fourier transformation (FFT). After zero-order phase correction and cubic baseline correction, Lorenzian fit for the peak area determination by the Marquardt-Levenberg method was used to measure the areas of spectra from each VOI [25]. For our calculations we used the NAA peak at 2.01 ppm, the Cr peak at 3.02 ppm and the Cho peak at 3.22 ppm (Figure 5). Although other investigations also identified the Glx signals in the region between 2.0 and 2.50 ppm, we could not clearly identify Glx peak. Since the absolute concentration of the metabolites could not be determined, the metabolic signal intensity ratio (NA/Cr or Cho/Cr) for each VOI was calculated. Nonparametric statistics, the Kruskal-Wallis and Man-Whitney tests were used to assess the differences in the NA/Cr ratios between patients and normal controls. The Spearman's rank correlation was used to test a possible linear relationship between the clinical rating scores and ^{1}H-MRS findings. All statistical analyses were carried out by a statistic software (STAT View 4.5-J, Hulinks Inc., Tokyo) using a microcomputer (Power Mac G4, Apple computer Inc., Cupertino, CA). Statistical significance was defined as $p<0.05$.

In patients with ALS, the brain NA/Cr ratio was reduced in the motor area (1.69±0.14 vs. 2.23±0.26, $p<0.01$) and in the frontal lobe (1.74±0.232 vs. 2.27±0.15, $p<0.01$) in comparison to normal controls (Figure 6). On the other hand, the NA/Cr ratio was unchanged in the parietal and occipital lobes of patients with ALS as compared with controls.

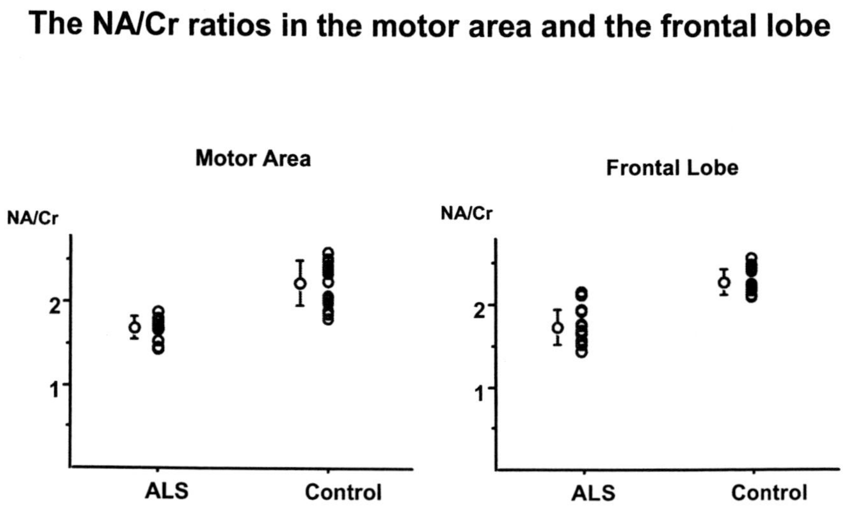

Figure 6. The NA/Cr ratios in the motor area and the frontal lobe. In patients with ALS, brain NA/Cr was reduced in the motor area lobe (1.69±0.14 Vs 2.23±0.26, $p<0.01$) and in the frontal lobe (1.74±0.232 Vs 2.27±0.15, $p<0.01$) in comparison to normal controls.

Patients with ALS had lower scores on MMT (75.7±6.6 Vs 110±0.0, $p<0.001$), Norris limb scale (51.0±4.5 vs. 63±0.0, $p<0.001$), and Norris bulbar scale (28.6±3.4 vs. 39±0.0, $p<0.001$) in comparison to normal controls. There was a significant correlation between the NA/Cr ratio in the motor area and Norris Limb Scale ($r=0.50;p<0.01$). These findings are consistent with the neuronal loss in the motor area in patients with ALS. There was no significant difference between patients with ALS and controls concerning the total score of MMSE (28.8±1.2 Vs 29.4±0.91). Patients with ALS had lower achievement in the number of WCST (2.64±1.7 vs. 5.86±0.73, $p<0.001$) in comparison to normal controls. There was a significant correlation between the frontal lobe NA/Cr ratio in the frontal lobe and the achieved number of WCST ($r=0.71;p<0.05$).

Degeneration of upper motor neurons in the cerebral cortex is a fundamental pathological change in patients with ALS [4-6, 44]. However, there have been controversies about reduction of NA, a neuronal marker, in the motor area and the frontal lobe in patients with ALS. In spinal cords obtained at autopsy, the levels of NA measured by high-performance liquid chromatography were decreased by 40% in ALS compared with controls [5], but there were no changes in the levels of NA in the frontal or the motor area. [45,46] In contrast to these findings in postmortem brain tissue, in vivo [1] H-MRS studies [28] have suggested a decrease in NA within the motor area of ALS patients. The explanation for the NA discrepancy between postmortem measurements and in vivo[1] H-MRS in the motor area of ALS patients remains unclear. However, cortical changes may be different patients to patients and there may be wide variations. Literally, low NA/ Cr in vivo has been observed in various types of neurological disorders and appeared to result from either a decrease in the intracellular volume of neurons per unit volume of brain or a decrease in the concentration of NA within neurons due to metabolic dysfunction [45-48]. Since the concentration of NA within neurons relates number of exciting neurons, discrepancy may be due to difference of number of exciting neurons between postmortem and in vivo measurements. This study suggests that a decrease in the NA concentration in the motor area and frontal lobe from patients with clinically definite ALS compatible with the degenerative changes following the loss of neurons in this region and that significant correlation between decrease in the NA concentration and clinical features. Other investigations using single voxel ^{1}H-MRS have also detected neuronal damage or loss in the motor cortex in ALS [20-25, 32, 49-53]. As noted in previous studies, NA/Cr ratios were decreased in the motor cortex in ALS. Cho/Cr ratios might also elevate in ALS [21]. There was considerable overlap between ALS and control values, although Chan et al. [22] found that 79% of ALS patients had NA/Cr ratios below a value of 2.5.

Degenerative changes in motor cortices and motor related cerebral structures may have been widely accepted, but concerning other cerebral structures relating especially with cognition there have been controversies. Abe et al. [18, 54] demonstrated reduction of isotope uptakes in the frontal lobes in ALS patients with cognitive dysfunction and suggested there might be wide range of cortical degeneration in ALS patients. Other investigations also support existence of cognitive dysfunction in ALS patients, which had been one of "negative" signs in ALS patients [3], and involvements of cerebral structures relating with cognition also demonstrated by investigations using ^{1}H-MRS [25]. The other hand, Ellis et al. [55] used automated image analysis to quantify volumes of cerebral gray and white matter in 16 ALS patients who demonstrated a reduction in NA/Cr ratios measured by ^{1}H-MRS in the subcortical white matter in the motor cortex region in the patients with bulbar-onset ALS. They found that ALS patients revealed localized deficits in gray matter volume centered on Brodmann areas 8, 9, and 10 bilaterally, and axonal degeneration in the subcortical white matter in the motor region in patients with bulbar-onset ALS. They considered it consistent with a "dying back" process affecting cortical motoneurons in bulbar-onset ALS. However, other investigations supported that neurons in cerebral cortices in ALS patients primarily degenerated, although there may be wide range of degeneration among them. [54, 56, 57] Thus, we consider that degeneration in cerebral cortices in ALS patients may be primal degenerative change and may relate with disease process.

Addition to cerebral cortices, ^{1}H-MRS has been applied to the brainstem [23, 58]. Pioro et al. tried to detect in vivo differences in signal intensities of specific metabolites in the medulla of ALS patients. They found that elevated Glx in the medulla of ALS patients and hypothesized that Glx excitotoxicity in ALS pathogenesis because the higher Glx signal in the medulla correlated with more dysarthria and dysphagia of patients. However, difficulty of localizing adequate ROIs in the medulla or other brainstem regions may weak their hypothesis. The main challenges of single voxel ^{1}H-MRS of the CNS structures contained in the posterior cranial fossa are the proximity of bone, causing inhomogeneity of the main magnetic field and difficult shimming, and the small size of the VOIs required to avoid partial volume effects with adjacent CNS structures and CSF spaces, implying low signal-to-noise ratio. Other possible sources of poor quality spectra include motion of the brain, vessels, and CSF [59]. Recent challenge by Mascalchi M et al. tried to evaluate the feasibility of single voxel ^{1}H-MRS of the CNS structures contained in the posterior cranial fossa and to determine the distribution of the normal metabolite ratios, concentrations, and T2 relaxation times in the midbrain, pons, medulla, dentate nucleus and cerebellar vermis. They concluded that single voxel ^{1}H-MRS enables an in vivo biochemical analysis of the CNS structures contained in the posterior cranial fossa but with the exception of the medulla. To evaluate metabolites in the he medulla may require further development of ^{1}H-MRS method, although the medulla contains hypoglossal nuclei that is a major involved region of ALS pathological process [60].

Quantitation of Metabolites Measured by ^{1}H-MRS

In the previous ^{1}H-MRS studies, since the absolute concentration of the metabolites could hardly be determined, the metabolic signal intensity ratio (for example NA/Cr or Cho/Cr) for each VOI has been calculated. There is no indication that potential correlations between NA, Cho, and Cr concentrations were investigated. Without measurement of absolute concentrations, the comparisons assessing lateralization, disease duration, disease severity, and progression of disease severity have not been able to be conducted. To compensate this weakness, some investigations of semi-quatitation of metabolites measured by ^{1}H-MRS have been conducted.

An easy and comprehensive quatitation method is to determine metabolite concentrations using the water signal as an internal standard. However, water is not necessarily an ideal internal standard and this method may not be standard method for quatitation of metabolites. Provencher SW [61] introduced the LCModel method for analyzing an in vivo spectrum as a Linear Combination of Model spectra of metabolite solutions in vitro. The LCModel analyzes the spectra as a linear combination of the *in vitro* model spectra of metabolite solutions acquired with the same MR system and the same parameters as human spectra except for TR, which was changed to 10sec for the prolonged T_1 relaxation time of metabolites in the solution. In measurement, before or after the acquisition of human data, spectra from 8-ml (2 x 2 x 2 cm) ROI located in an approximately 500ml spherical container of 50mMol *N*-acetylaspartate solution were acquired with the same parameters as *in vivo* acquisition except for TR of 10sec, and these spectra were used as external standards for the quantitative analysis. The differences of the receiver gain and the transmitter gain of each spectrum were corrected in the LCModel. Thomas NA et al expanded LC model into two-dimensional (2D) MRS techniques that improved spectral dispersion enabling the detection of several brain metabolites at low concentrations that have not been resolved using the conventional one-dimensional (1D) MRS techniques. [62]

Assessment of Efficacy of Treatment by ¹H-MRS

¹H-MRS has also been used for assessment of drug treatment in many kind of neurological diseases including Parkinson's disease [29]. In such a investigation, we could evaluate metabolic changes in brain region where drugs affected (Figure 7, 8). The other hand, since there has been lack of specific drug therapy for ALS, assessment of efficacy of treatment by ¹H-MRS has been few. However, when riluzole was approved as an effective drug for ALS treatment, some trials to assess efficacy of treatment using ¹H-MRS were reported [63-67].

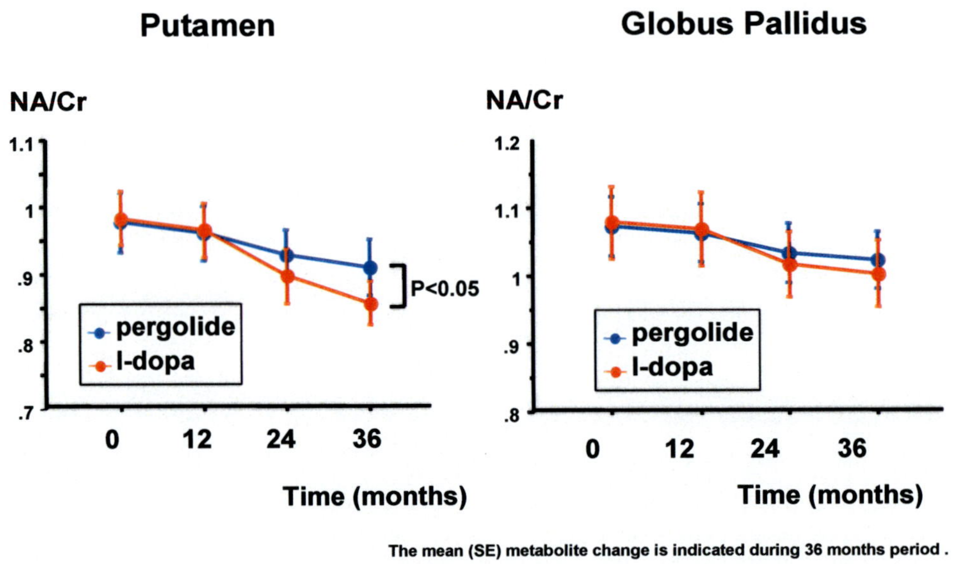

Figure 7. Serial change of the NA/Cr in the putamen and globus pallidus. In the putamen, the NAA/Cr ratio in the pergolide-treated Parkinson's disease (PD) patients showed significant differences in the rate of decrement compared with levodopa-treated PD patients ($P<0.05$). The Cho/Cr ratio in the pergolide-treated PD patients showed significant differences in the rate of increment compared with levodopa-treated PD patients ($P<0.05$).

Since there have been concepts of energy dysregulation and oxidative stress and their complicated interdependence have rapidly evolved to assume primary importance in understanding the pathophysiology of numerous neurological disorders, neuroprotective strategies addressing specific bioenergetic defects hold particular promise in the treatment of these conditions including Huntington's disease, Parkinson's disease, mitochondrial cytopathies and other neuromuscular diseases. All of which, to some extent, share 'the final common pathway' leading to cell death through either necrosis or apoptosis [68]. In a series of observation, there has been a hypothesis that mitochondrial pathology is an early observation in motor neurons and skeletal muscle of ALS patients. Based on this hypothesis, Vielhaber et al. [64, 65] observed the effects of a 1-month oral administration of creatine on 15 patients with sporadic ALS, most of whom had mitochondrial pathology in skeletal muscle and measured metabolites changes by using ¹H-MRS. Upon creatine supplementation they observed in the controls a decline in the NA/Cr, NA/Cho, Glx/Cr, and Glx/Cho metabolite ratios. In contrast, in the ALS patient group the NA/Cr, NA/Cho metabolite ratios remained unchanged, while the Glx/Cr, and Glx/Cho metabolite ratios decreased. Consequently they considered that creatine supplementation causes an increase in the diminished NA levels in ALS motor cortex as well as an increase of choline levels in both ALS and control motor cortices. They also considered that a deficiency of enzymes of mitochondrial respiratory chain in the ALS motor cortex which might affect motor neuron survival. Using an animal model of familial ALS, Snow et al. [66] investigated the effects of riluzole (Ril), Cr and a combination of these treatments on the onset and progression of clinical signs and neuropathology. Based on the results, they considered that treatment with Ril and Cr were both effective in delaying disease onset and clinical disability. Kalra S et al. [69] tried to evaluate effect of gabapentin therapy for ALS using ^{1}H-MRS. They found that the NA/Cr ratio was decreased in the precentral and postcentral gyri of ALS patients compared with healthy controls. However, the change in the NA/Cr ratio was not different between treated patients and untreated patients in any of the regions studied. They concluded that no improvement in neuronal integrity was detected in motor and nonmotor cerebral regions after GBP treatment. Kalra S et al. also evaluated intrathecal BDNF in ALS. However, they could not find effective changes in NA [70].

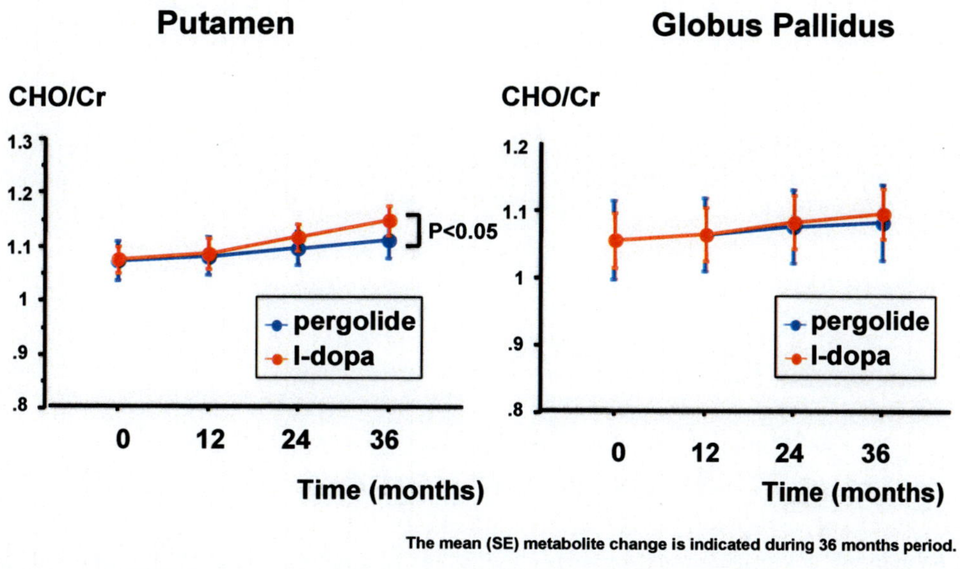

Figure 8. Serial change of the CHO/Cr in the putamen and globus pallidus. In the globus pallidus, the NAA/Cr ratio in the pergolide-treated PD patients and levodopa-treated PD patients did not show significant differences in the rate of decrement for two treatment (P=0.4). The Cho/Cr ratio in the pergolide-treated PD patients and levodopa-treated PD patients did not show significant differences in the rate of increment for two treatment (P=0.18).

All of these assessments by ^{1}H-MRS supported the superiority of ^{1}H-MRS in reproducibility and accuracy of measurement. These types of assessment by ^{1}H-MRS will increase and may be useful for clinical assessment of ALS treatment [71, 72].

Longitudinal Assessment of Clinical Course by ^{1}H-MRS [20-24, 32, 73]

Longitudinal assessments of clinical course by using ^{1}H-MRS have also been conducted (Figure 5, [29]). Functional neuroimaging techniques including SPECT and PET have also been adapted in longitudinal assessment of clinical course of ALS patients [54, 73]. However, high cost and ionizing radiation complications of these techniques may prevent us from repetitively using them to follow longitudinal changes in ALS patients. On the other hand, ^{1}H-MRS may be safe and cost effective in follow up studies [29, 54, 74]. Pioro and colleagues [75] performed 2 examinations, 8 months apart, on 1 patient who demonstrated marked clinical deterioration during the same time interval. They found a 23% decrease in NA/Cr in the motor region and lesser decreases in adjacent cerebral regions. Pohl et al. [76] obtained serial spectral results on 16 patients with ALS and found that NA/Cho, but not NA/Cr, showed a significant decrease (9%) during a mean interval of 12 months, and a significant correlation with progression of disease severity. A significant decrease (10%) in NA in 3 patients with ALS during a mean interval of 11 weeks has also been reported.1 interestingly, the NA/Cho and NA decreases were detected in patients with ALS undergoing treatment with riluzole during the interval between spectroscopic examinations. Suhy et al. [32] tried to determine (1) the reproducibility of metabolite measurements by ^{1}H-MRS in the motor cortex; (2) the extent to which ^{1}H-MRS imaging (MRSI) detects abnormal concentrations of NA, Cho, Cr in early stages of ALS; and (3) the metabolite changes over time in ALS. The interclass correlation coefficient of NA was 0.53 in the motor cortex tissue and 0.83 in nonmotor cortex tissue. When cross-sectional data for ALS patients were compared with those for controls, the NA/Cr ratio in the motor cortex region was significantly reduced.

As was the case for disease severity analyses, comparisons between the results of different investigators are complicated by the lack of uniformity in technique and method of ^{1}H-MRS.

Higher Magnetic Field MR Apparatus Has Merits in Measurement of ^{1}H-MRS?

Advent of MR technology provides us higher magnetic field MR apparatus than ever. Several years before, 3.0 Tesla units may be highest apparatus in clinical usage. However, since there may be higher magnetic field apparatuses, some say 3.0 Tesla may be middle magnetic field. In this situation, a question that higher magnetic field MR apparatus has benefits in measurement of ^{1}H-MRS may be raised. In our personal experience, we use 1.5 Tesla units and a 3.0 Tesla unit and felt some benefit in ^{1}H-MRS at 3.0 Tesla to detect some metabolites including Glx. Theoretically, ^{1}H-MRS at a higher field strength has the advantages of higher signal-to-noise ratio and improved spectral resolution. In deed we can easily detect Glx and mI that have hardly detect clearly ^{1}H-MRS using 1.5 Tesla apparatuses [74]. The other hand, Kantarci K, et al. [77] compared the ability of single-voxel ^{1}H-MRS at

1.5 and 3 T to diagnostically discriminate among cognitively normal elderly subjects, patients with mild cognitive impairment (MCI), and patients with Alzheimer disease (AD). Average line widths and interexamination variability of metabolite ratios were higher at 3.0 Tesla than at 1.5 T. Although consistent quantification of Glx/Cr and glutamine (Gln) /Cr peak ratios occurred at 3.0 Tesla but not at 1.5 Tesla, they concluded that the diagnostic performance of ^{1}H-MRS was not better at 3.0 Tesla than at 1.5 Tesla. Accumulation of ^{1}H-MRS data may solve this question.

Conclusions

Degeneration of CNS is a fundamental pathological change in patients with ALS [4-6]. However, there has been controversial about origin of degeneration. Eisen A, et al suggested cortical degeneration in ALS may be resulted from dying back process of degeneration in spinal neurons [76]. However, a lot of investigation support cortical degeneration in ALS is primary one [17, 79] and cognitive dysfunction including forgetful, attention deficits, and character changes may be contributed cortical degeneration in the frontal lobe of ALS patients [56,78,80]. Neuropathological examination may elucidate correlation between degeneration in the CNS of ALS patients and clinical signs [81]. However, correlation between on going degeneration in the CNS of ALS patients and clinical signs may need another currently available technology. Measurement of changes of metabolites including NA, Cr, Cho, Glx, and mI in the CNS in patients with ALS is a reliable marker of neuronal degeneration and ^{1}H-MRS may be a promising neuroimaging technique to detect changes of metabolites in CNS and elucidate pathogenesis of ALS. In addition, its superiority in reproducibility and accuracy and the lack of the need to use radioactive tracers and its safety, ^{1}H-MRS may be useful in objective and quantitative measurement of neuronal degeneration in clinical trial of drugs for ALS.

Acknowledgement

I appreciate Drs. Terakawa Haruhiko, Hikita Tachio, Mihara Masahito, Watanabe Yoshiyuki, and Fujita Norihiko for their cooperation in our MRS studies.

References

[1] Friedman AP, Friedman D. Amyotrophic lateral sclerosis. *J Nerv Ment Dis* 1950; 111: 1-18.

[2] Lawyer Jr T. Netsky MG. Amyotrophic lateral sclerosis. A clinicoanatomic study of fifty-three cases. *Arch Neurol Psychiatry* 1953; 69: 171-192.].

[3] Rowland LP, Shneider NA. Medical Progress: Amyotrophic Lateral Sclerosis. *N Engl J Med* 2001; 344:1688-1700.

[4] Lassek AM. The human pyramidal tract II. A numerical investigation of the Betz cells of the motor area. *Arch Neurol Psychiatry* 1940; 44: 718-729.

[5] Smith MC. Nerve fiber degeneration in the brain in amyotrophic lateral sclerosis. *J Neurol Neurosurg Psychiatry* 1960; 23: 269-282.

[6] Brownwell B, Oppenheimer DR, and Hughes JT. The central nervous system in motor neuron disease. *J Neurol Neurosurg Psychiatry* 1970; 33: 338-357

[7] Rosen DR, Siddique T, Patterson D, et al. Mutations in Cu/Zn superoxide dismutase gene are associated with familial amyotrophic lateral sclerosis. *Nature* 1993;362:59-62.

[8] Majoor-Krakauer D, Ottman R, Johnson WG, Rowland LP. Familial aggregation of amyotrophic lateral sclerosis, dementia, and Parkinson's disease: evidence of shared genetic susceptibility. *Neurology* 1994;44:1872-1877.

[9] Cruz DC, Nelson LM, McGuire V, Longstreth WT. Physical trauma and family history of neurodegenerative diseases in amyotrophic lateral sclerosis: a population-based case-control study. *Neuroepidemiology* 1999;18:101-110.

[10] Brait K, Fahn S, Schwarz GA. Sporadic and familial parkinsonism and motor neuron disease. *Neurology* 1973;23:990-1002.

[11] Pullen AH, Humphreys P. Ultrastructural analysis of spinal motoneurones from mice treated with IgG from ALS patients, healthy individuals, or disease controls. *J Neurol Sci* 2000;180:35-45.

[12] Vincent A, Drachman DB. Amyotrophic lateral sclerosis and antibodies to voltage-gated calcium channels -- new doubts. *Ann Neurol* 1996;40:691-693.

[13] Verma A, Berger JR, Snodgrass S, Petito C. Motor neuron disease: a paraneoplastic process associated with anti-hu antibody and small-cell lung carcinoma. *Ann Neurol* 1996;40:112-116.

[14] Hays AP, Roxas A, Sadiq SA, et al. A monoclonal IgA in a patient with amyotrophic lateral sclerosis reacts with neurofilaments and surface antigen on neuroblastoma cells. *J Neuropathol Exp Neurol* 1990;49:383-398.

[15] Brooks BR. El Escorial World Federation of Neurology criteria for the diagnosis of amyotrophic lateral sclerosis: Subcommittee on Motor Neuron Diseases/Amyotrophic Lateral Sclerosis of the World Federation of Neurology Research Group on Neuromuscular Diseases and the El Escorial "Clinical Limits of Amyotrophic Lateral Sclerosis" workshop contributors. *J Neurol Sci* 1994;124(suppl):96-107.

[16] Imon Y; Yamaguchi S, Yamamura Y, Tsuji S, Kajima T, Ito K, Nakamura S. Low intensity areas observed onT2-weighted magnetic resonance imaging of the cerebral cortex in various neurological diseases. *J Neuol Sci* 1995;134: S27-S32.

[17] Abe K, Fujimura H, Kobayashi Y, Fujita N, Yanagihara T. Degeneration of the pyramidal tracts in patients with amyotrophic lateral sclerosis. A premortem and postmortem magnetic resonance imaging study. *J Neuroimaging* 1997;7:208-212.

[18] Abe K, Fujimura H, Toyooka K, T Hazama, Hirono N, Yorifuji S, Yanagihara T. Single photon emission tomographic investigation of patients with motor neuron disease. *Neurology* 1993;43: 1569-1573.

[19] Dalakas MC, Hatazawa J, Brooks RA, Di Cjiro G. Lowered cerebral glucose utilization in amyotrphic lateral sclerosis. *Ann Neurol* 1987; 22: 580 - 586.

[20] Comi G, Rovaris M, Leocani L. Review: neuroimaging in amyotrophic lateral sclerosis. *Eur J Neurol* 1999;6:629-637.

[21] Block W, Karitzky J, Traber F, Pohl C, Keller E, Mundegar RR, Lamerichs R, Rink H, Ries F, Schild HH, Jerusalem F. Proton magnetic resonance spectroscopy of the primary motor cortex in patients with motor neuron disease: subgroup analysis and follow-up measurements. *Arch Neurol* 1998; 55: 931-936.

[22] Chan S, Shungu DC, Douglas-Akinwande A, Lange DJ, Rowland LP. Motor neuron diseases: comparison of single-voxel proton MR spectroscopy of the motor cortex with MR imaging of the brain. *Radiology* 1999; 212: 763-769.

[23] Pioro EP, Majors AW, Mitsumoto H, Nelson DR, Ng TC. ^{1}H-MRS evidence of neurodegeneration and excess glutamate+glutamine in ALS medulla. *Neurology* 1999; 53: 71-79.

[24] Sarchielli P, Pelliccioli GP, Tarducci R, Chiarini P, Presciutti O, Gobbi G, Gallai V. Magnetic Resonance imaging and ^{1}H-magnetic resonance spectroscopy in amyotrophic lateral sclerosis. *Neuroradiology* 2001;43:189-197.

[25] Abe K, Takanashi M, Watanabe Y, Tanaka H, Fujita N, Hirabuki N, Yanagihara T. Decrease in N-acetylaspartate/creatine ratio in the motor area and the frontal lobe in amyotrophic lateral sclerosis. *Neuroradiology* 2001;43:537-541.

[26] Bowen BC, Pattany PM, Bradley WG, et al. MR imaging and localized proton spectroscopy of the precentral gyrus in amyotrophic lateral sclerosis. *Am J Neuroradiol.* 2000;21:647-658.

[27] Chan S, Kaufmann P, Shungu DC, Mitsumoto H. Amyotrophic lateral sclerosis and primary lateral sclerosis: evidence-based diagnostic evaluation of the upper motor neuron. *Neuroimaging Clin N Am* 2003;13:307-26.

[28] Kalra S, Cashman NR, Genge A, Arnold DL. Recovery of N-acetylaspartate in corticomotor neurons of patients with ALS after riluzole therapy. *NeuroReport* 1998;9: 1757-1761.

[29] Rothman DL, Behar KL, Hetherington HP, Shulman RG. Homonuclear ^{1}H double-resonance difference spectroscopy of the rat brain in vivo. *Proc Natl Acad Sci USA* 1984; 81: 6330-6334.

[30] Novotny EJ Jr, Fulbright RK, Pearl PL, Gibson KM, Rothman DL. Magnetic resonance spectroscopy of neurotransmitters in human brain. *Ann Neurol* 2003;54(Suppl 6): S25-S31.

[31] Terakawa H, Abe K, Kubota T. Longitudinal effect of dopamine agonist versus levodopa therapy on Parkinson's disease progression: Proton magnetic resonance spectroscopic study. *Ann Neurol* 2003;54(Suppl 7): S41.

[32] Suhy J, Miller RG, Rule R, Schuff N, Licht J, Dronsky V, Gelinas D, Maudsley AA, Weiner MW. Early detection and longitudinal changes in amyotrophic lateral sclerosis by H-1 MRSI. *Neurol* 2002;58: 773-779.

[33] Moffett JR, Namboodiri MA, Cangro CB, Neale JH. Immunohistochemical localization of *N*-acetylaspartate in rat brain. *Neuroreport* 1991;2:131-4.

[34] Kamada K, Houkin K, Aoki T, Koiwa M, Kashiwaba T, Iwasaki Y, Abe H. Cerebral metabolic changes in delayed carbon monoxide sequelae studied by proton MR spectroscopy. *Neuroradiology* 1994;36:104-6.

[35] Charles HC, Lazeyras F, Krishnan KR, Boyko OB, Patterson LJ, Doraiswamy PM, McDonald WM. Proton spectroscopy of human brain: effects of age and sex. *Prog Neuropsychopharmacol Biol Psychiatry* 1994;18:995-1004.

[36] Brand A, Richter-Landsberg C, Leibfritz D. Multinuclear NMR studies on the energy metabolism of glial and neuronal cells. *Dev Neurosci* 1993;15:289-98.

[37] Videen JS, Michaelis T, Pinto P, Ross BD. Human cerebral osmolytes during chronic hyponatremia. A proton magnetic resonance spectroscopy study. *J Clin Invest* 1995;95:788-93.

[38] Hattori N, Abe K. Umeda M, Fukunaga M, Inoue N, Someya Y, Matsui M, Sakoda S, Sawada S. Age-related changes of cerebral metabolite concentrations: a quantitative proton MR spectroscopic study. *Proceedings of 11th Annual Meeting of ISMRM.*

[39] Al-Chalabi A, Leigh PN. Recent advances in amyotrophic lateral sclerosis. *Curr Opin Neurol* 2000; 13:397-405

[40] Wade DT. Motor and sensory impairments. In Wade DT. Measurement in neurological rehabilitation. Oxford, New York, Tokyo: *University of Oxford Press*, 1992:50-58.

[41] Norris FH Jr, Calanchini PR, Fallat RJ, Panchari S, Jewett B. The administration of guanidine in amyotrophic lateral sclerosis. *Neurology* 1974; 24:721-728.

[42] Folstein MF, Folstein SE. " Mini - Mental State ": a practical method for grading the cognitive state of patients for the clinic. *J Psychiatr Res* 1975; 12: 189 - 193.

[43] Nelson HE. A modified card sorting test sensitive to frontal lobe defects. *Cortex* 1976; 12: 313 - 324.

[44] Zung WWK. A self rating depression scale. *Arch Gen Psychiatry* 1965; 12: 63 - 70.

[45] Tsai GC, Stauch-Slusher B, Sim L, Hedreen JC, Rothstein JD, Kuncl R, Coyle JT Reductions in acidic amino acids and N-acetylaspartylglutamate in amyotrophic lateral sclerosis CNS. *Brain Res* 1991;556:151-156.

[46] Plaitakis A, Constantakakis E. Altered metabolism of excitatory amino acids, N-acetyl-aspartate and N-acetyl-aspartyl-glutamate in amyotrophic lateral sclerosis. *Brain Res Bull* 1993;30:381-386.

[47] Hammer RP Jr, Tomiyasu U, Scheibel AB. Degeneration of the human Betz cell due to amyotrophic lateral sclerosis. *Exp Neurol* 1979;63:336-346.

[48] Arnold DL and Matthews PM. *Practical aspect of clinical applications of MRS in the brain.* In Young IR and Charles HC, eds. MR spectroscopy: Clinical Applications and Techniques. London: Martin Dunitz Publishers, 1995:139-159.

[49] Block W, Traber F, Flacke S, Jessen F, Pohl C, Schild H. In-vivo proton MR-spectroscopy of the human brain: Assessment of N-acetylaspartate (NAA) reduction as a marker for neurodegeneration. *Amino Acids* 2002;23:317-323.

[50] Pioro EP. MR spectroscopy in amyotrophic lateral sclerosis motor neuron disease. *J Neurol Sci* 1997;152(Suppl 1): S49-S53.

[51] Gredal O, Rosenbaum S, Topp S, Karlsborg M, Strange P, Werdelin L. Quantification of brain metabolites in amyotrophic lateral sclerosis by localized proton magnetic resonance spectroscopy. *Neurol* 1997;48: 878-881.

[52] Ellis CM, Simmons A, Glover A, Dawson JM, Williams SCR, Leigh PN. Quantitative proton magnetic resonance spectroscopy of the subcortical white matter in motor neuron disease. *Amyotroph Lateral Sc* 2000; 1: 123-129.

[53] Pohl C, Block W, Traber F, Schmidt S, Pels H, Grothe C, Schild HH, Klockgether T. Proton magnetic resonance spectroscopy and transcranial magnetic stimulation for the detection of upper motor neuron degeneration in ALS patients. *J Neurol Sci* 2001;190: 21-27.

[54] Abe K, Fujimura H, Toyooka K, Yorifuji S, Yanagihara T. Imaging in motor neuron disease. *Neurology* 1994;44: 1186-1187, 1994.

[55] EllisC M, SucklingJ, AmaroEJr, BullmoreE T, SimmonsA, WilliamsS C, LeighP N. Volumetric analysis reveals corticospinal tract degeneration and extramotor involvement in ALS. *Neurology* 2001;57: 1571-1578.

[56] Abe K. Cognitive function in amyotrophic lateral sclerosis. *Amyotroph Lateral Sc* 200;1: 343-347.

[57] Portet F, Cadilhac C, Touchon J, Camu W. Cognitive impairment in motor neuron disease with bulbar onset. *Amyotroph Lateral Sc* 2001;2 : 23-29.

[58] Cwik V A, Hanstock C C, Allen P S, Martin W R. Estimation of brainstem neuronal loss in amyotrophic lateral sclerosis with in vivo proton magnetic resonance spectroscopy *Neurology* 1998;50:72-77.

[59] Hattori N, Abe K. Umeda M, Fukunaga M, Inoue N, Someya Y, Matsui M, Sakoda S, Sawada S. Estimation of the cerebral metabolite concentrations in pure gray matter and white matter by in vivo proton MR spectroscopy. *Proceedings of 11th Annual Meeting of ISMRM.*

[60] Mascalchi M, Brugnoli R, Guerrini L, Belli G, Nistri M, Politi LS, Gavazzi C, Lolli F, Argenti G, Villari N. Single-voxel long TE 1H-MR spectroscopy of the normal brainstem and cerebellum. *J Magn Reson Imaging* 2002;16: 532-537.

[61] Provencher SW. Estimation of metabolite concentrations from localized in vivo proton NMR spectra. Magn Reson Med 1993; 30:672-9.

[62] Thomas MA, Hattori N, Umeda M, Sawada T, Naruse S. Evaluation of two-dimensional L-COSY and JPRESS using a 3 T MRI scanner: from phantoms to human brain in vivo. *NMR Biomed* 2003;16:245-251.

[63] Kalra S, Genge A, Arnold DL. Improved corticoneuronal integrity in amyotrophic lateral sclerosis after one day of riluzole treatment. *Neurology* 2001;56: A236

[64] Vielhaber S, Kaufmann J, Kanowski M, Sailer M, Feistner H, Tempelmann C, Elger CE, Heinze HJ, Kunz WS. Effect of creatine supplementation on metabolite levels in ALS motor cortices. *Exp Neurol* 2001; 172 : 377-382.

[65] Vielhaber S, Kaufmann J, Kunz WS. Creatine effects in ALS Motor cortices revealed by in vivo localized proton magnetic resonance spectroscopy. *J Neurol Sci* 2002;199: 6.

[66] Snow RJ, Turnbull J, Da Silva S, Jiang F, Tarnopolsky MA. Creatine supplementation and riluzole treatment provide similar beneficial effects in copper, zinc superoxide dismutase (G93A) transgenic mice. *Neuroscience* 2003;119: 661-667.

[67] Bensimon G, Lacomblez V, Meininger V. ALS/riluzole study group: a controlled trial of riluzole in amyotrophic lateral sclerosis. *N Engl J Med* 1994; 330: 585–591.

[68] Baker SK, Tarnopolsky MA. Targeting cellular energy production in neurological disorders. *Expert Opin Inv Drug* 2003;12: 1655-1679.

[69] Kalra S, Cashman NR, Caramanos Z, Genge A, Arnold DL Gabapentin therapy for amyotrophic lateral sclerosis: Lack of improvement in neuronal integrity shown by MR spectroscopy. *Am J Neuroraidol* 2003; 24: 476-480.

[70] Kalra S, Genge A, Arnold DL. A prospective, randomized, placebo-controlled evaluation of corticoneuronal response to intrathecal BDNF therapy in ALS using magnetic resonance spectroscopy: feasibility and results. *Amyotroph Lateral Sc* 2003;4: 22-26.

[71] Carter GT, Krivickas LS, Weydt P, Weiss MD, Miller RG. Drug therapy for amyotrophic lateral sclerosis: Where are we now? *I Drugs* 2003;6: 147-153.

[72] Dib M. Amyotrophic lateral sclerosis - Progress and prospects for treatment. *Drugs* 2003; 63: 289-310.

[73] Kalra S, Arnold DL. Imaging: MRS, MRI, PET/SPECT. *Amyotroph Lateral Sc* 2002;3 : S73-S74.

[74] Hattori N, Abe K, Sakoda S, Sawada T. Proton MR spectroscopic study at 3 Tesla or glutamate/glutamine in Alzheimer's disease. *Neuroreport* 2002; 13: 183-186.

[75] Pioro EP, Antel JP, Cashman NR, Arnold DL. Detection of cortical neuron loss in motor neuron disease by proton magnetic resonance spectroscopic imaging in vivo. *Neurology.* 1994;44:1933-1938.

[76] Pohl C, Block W, Karitzky J, et al. Proton magnetic resonance spectroscopy of the motor cortex in 70 patients with amyotrophic lateral sclerosis. *Arch Neurol* 2001; 58:729-735.

[77] Kantarci K, Reynolds G, Petersen RC, Boeve BF, Knopman DS, Edland SD, Smith GE, Ivnik RJ, Tangalos EG, Jack CR. Proton MR spectroscopy in mild cognitive impairment and Alzheimer disease: Comparison of 1.5 and 3 T. *Am J Neuroradiol* 2003;24: 843-849.

[78] Eisen A, Weber M. The motor cortex and lateral amyotrophic sclerosis. *Muscle Nerve* 2001;24: 564-573.

[79] Kiernan JA, Hudson AJ. Changes in sizes of cortical and lower motor neurons in anyoptrophic lateral sclerosis. *Brain* 1991;114(pt 2):843- 853

[80] Abe K. Structural and functional changes in patients with motor neuron disease. *J Neurol Neurosurg Psychiatry* 1996;61: 234-235, 1996

[81] Tsuchiya K, Ikeda K, Mimura M, Takahashi M, Miyazaki H, Anno M, Shiotsu H, Akabane H, Niizato K, Uchihara T, Tominaga I, Nakano I. Constant involvement of the Betz cells and pyramidal tract in amyotrophic lateral sclerosis with dementia: a clinicopathological study of eight autopsy cases. *Acta Neuropathol* 2002;104: 249-259.

In: Amyotrophic Lateral Sclerosis: New Research
Editor: Christine A. Murray, pp. 323-346
ISBN 1-59454-179-5

Chapter XIV

Molecular Genetic and Biochemical Studies of Russian Patients with Sporadic Motor Neuron Disease

V. I. Skvortsova[1,*], P. A. Slominsky[2], G. N. Levitsky[1], M. I. Shadrina[2] and S. A. Limborska[2]

[1]Department of Fundamental and Clinical Neurology,
Russian State Medical University, Moscow, Russia
[2]Institute of Molecular Genetics, Russian Academy of Sciences,
Moscow, Russia.

ABSTRACT

We conducted molecular genetic and biochemical study of 73 patients with sporadic motor neuron disease (MND) with definite diagnosis according to the Revised El Escorial Criteria (1998). According to the Norris classification (1993), 57 patients (78%) had amyotrophic lateral sclerosis (ALS) form of the disease, and among them 35 had cervical onset (47.9%), 5 had truncal onset (6.8%), 13 had lumbar onset (17.8%) and 4 had diffuse onset (5.5%) of the disease. The remaining 16 patients (22%) had progressive bulbar palsy (PBP). All patients were assessed by the Norris ALS Score (1974) each six months until death. Patients with slow, moderate and rapid progression lost <4.5, 5-10 and >10 degrees each 6 months respectively ($r = -0.96$, $p < 0.0001$) and comprised 40 (54.8%), 21 (28.7%) and 12 (16.5%), respectively.

The search for mutations in CuZn-superoxide dismutase gene showed that 3 individuals (4.1%) were the carriers of mutations. One female aged 67 was homozygous for the D90A mutation, whereas another female aged 55 was heterozygous for this mutation. The last female aged 71 was heterozygous for the G12R mutation. All patients had

* Correspondence concerning this article should be addressed to Dr. Veronika I. Skvortsova, Department of Fundamental and Clinical Neurology, Russian State Medical University, 127387, Lenskaya str., 15, block 3, Moscow, Russia., E-mail: vskvor@sl.ru.

lumbar onset of ALS. The D90A homozygous patient had very slow progression lasting 24 years, and the heterozygous one deteriorated rapidly. That corresponded to the original findings by P.M. Andersen, who first described D90A associated ALS cases. However, we found identical haplotypes within polymorphic markers on both 21st chromosomes of the D90A homozygous and well as of D90A heterozygous ALS patient (D21S263-1, D21S223(SOD-1)-3, D21S63-10, D21S262-4, D21S261-2). No cases of ALS in association with D90A heterozygosity and this so-called Scandinavian haplotype have been reported before. This was the first case when D90A heterozygosity was detected in an individual with ALS who has the "protective" Scandinavian haplotype shown to be typical only for the autosomal-recessive D90A carriers. The D90A heterozygous patient was thought to develop the disease due to ALS-causative factor other than D90A mutation with pathogenically strong action against the putative "protective" properties of the haplotype. The patient with G12R mutation had more rapid progression and elder age of onset than the Italian cohort of G12R ALS patients, although the same clinical phenotype.

The study of alanine-9-valine (A9V) manganese-superoxide dismutase gene signal sequence polymorphism showed that there were no differences between frequencies of A9V alleles in patients and 50 neurologically normal controls from Moscow.

The study of S/L-polymorphism of heavy neurofilament subunit gene (NEFH) showed that the homozygosity for short (S) allele had higher frequency in the MND group than in 45 neurologically normal controls (33.9% vs 6.7%, $\chi^2 = 10.37$, $p < 0.005$). Patients with different variants of S/L-polymorphism showed no difference in age or site of onset. A statistically significant correlation was established between the loss of total clinical score and the NEFH genotypes (Spearman correlation, $R = 0.335$, $p < 0.03$). The lowest values of loss of total clinical score were observed in patients with the LL genotype (mean ± SD, 18.8 ± 12.4), and the highest ones in patients with the SS genotype (mean ± SD, 31.1 ± 16.3). The dissimilarity in mean values of loss of total clinical score in the patients with LL and SS genotypes was statistically significant (Newman–Keuls test $q = 3.671$, $p < 0.05$).

The activities of CuZn-superoxide dismutase in erythrocytes measured by Beauchamp and Fridovich (1971) of MND patients did not differ from those in control group, but was higher in S allele carriers vs LL genotype carriers (^730 vs ^677 U/g Hb; px2 < 0.05). Also, the content of thiobarbituric acid substances (TBARS) in cerebrospinal fluid measured by Ohkawa and Heikkila (1979) was higher in the SS genotype carriers vs controls (^0.425 vs ^0.307 nmol/ml, $p < 0.05$).

These findings suggested that the SS genotype of the NEFH gene in the Russian population is a predisposition factor for both sporadic MND and oxidative stress possibly mediated by abnormal pro-oxidative interaction between short NEFH and CuZn-SOD.

Introduction

According to the modern concept of motor neuron disease (MND) etiology, it is a fatal progressive degeneration of upper and lower motoneurons developing due to interaction of hereditary and exogenous factors [1]. Sporadic cases represent as many as 90%, and 10% are hereditary or familial. The only proven causative gene is CuZn-superoxide dismutase (SOD-1). However, mutations in this gene can explain only 25% of familial and about 5–7% of sporadic cases. Identical clinical features of sporadic and familial MND suggest their common elements of pathogenesis, hence rare familial cases present interest for further etiological elucidation [2]. It was shown experimentally that MND associated with SOD-1 gene mutations develops due to novel and yet unknown cytotoxic property of the mutant protein rather than oxidative stress following enzymatic activity changes [1]. Besides, in some MND patients mutations were found in other functionally different genes (heavy neurofilaments, apurine-apyrimidine endonuclease, "survival motoneuron") and generalized skin abnormalities were found in all patients [1, 2]. All this leads to the concept that MND is a common syndrome that can be caused by variegated genetic defects leading to selective motoneuron loss, extraneural and spotty extramotor and abnormalities [2].

Over 100 SOD-1 mutations are known worldwide to date [3]. In the majority of cases there is no correlation between the mutation and disease phenotype (site and age of onset, duration of the disease) within and between families. Many SOD-1 mutations were shown to have low penetrance, so hereditary MND cases, which they cause, can be falsely taken for sporadic [1]. In Russia single familial cases were described by S. N. Davidenkov [4], who suggested low penetrance in several familial MND cases as early as in 1933. Autosomal recessive homozygous D90A mutation (aspartate to alanine substitution in codon 90) was shown to produce uniform phenotype of lumbar ALS with very slow progression with the highest prevalence in Scandinavia, and heterozygous relatives of these patients were never affected. However, autosomal dominant D90A cases were shown to produce variable phenotype and typical rapid progression [1]. Such a dissociation can be explained by the presence of so-called Scandinavian haplotype (D21S263, D21S223 (SOD-1), D21S63, D21S262, D21S261), inherited by homozygous D90A carriers 43 generations ago [5]. P.M. Andersen et al. [1] and A. Al-Chalabi et al. [5] supposed that this haplotype is linked with putative "protective" factor that suppressed the cytotoxic effects of mutant SOD-1 protein, which explains the uniform phenotype, very long duration of the recessively inherited disease in D90A homozygous carriers and absence of MND in their heterozygous relatives. The cases of autosomal dominant MND with typical rapid progression and variable phenotype associated with heterozygous D90A mutation was explained by absence of Scandinavian haplotype and elder age of the mutation [5]. Here we present two earlier reported ALS cases of homozygosity and heterozygosity for D90A from Moscow [6].

Findings about the role of oxidative stress in sporadic MND are contradictory. There is a paucity of studies where antioxidant status and oxidative markers in MND were assessed simultaneously [7, 8] and where oxidative markers in CSF were measured in vivo [7, 9]. The majority of authors found the presence of oxidative stress but preserved antioxidant status in MND, and they showed no correlation of oxidative and antioxidant biochemical markers with clinical features of MND [10]. However, many therapeutic trials of antioxidants in MND showed negative results [11]. The contradictory character of these findings makes it expedient to further specify how oxidative markers and antioxidant system are altered in sporadic MND, to determine if any alterations are specific and to judge whether it is important to compensate them by therapeutic intervention.

The paradoxical absence of oxidative stress signs in MND cases associated with SOD-1 mutations but not in sporadic cases leads to further research for defects in genes encoding other antioxidant enzymes in MND, such as manganese superoxide dismutase (SOD-2), located in mitochondria. This inducible enzyme is encoded by a gene on 6q25. Two groups of authors revealed alanine-9-valine polymorphism (A9V) in the second exon, which is responsible for transport of the enzyme from cytosol to mitochondria. One of the homozygous polymorphic variants (it is still unrecognized which one of two) was shown to destabilize alpha-helical conformation of the enzyme, the preservation of which determines its proper mitochondrial targeting [12]. Two independent studies of association between homozygous variants of this polymorphism and MND in American and Scandinavian populations came to contradictory conclusions [12, 13].

Autopsy studies performed on MND sufferers have revealed aggregation and abnormal assembly of neurofilaments (NF) in the perikarya and proximal axon of the motor neurons [14]. Neurofilaments are the most abundant structural proteins specific to neuronal cells. There are three NF subunits of light, medium and heavy molecular weight: NEFL, NEFM and NEFH. NEFM and NEFH have a tail domain that contains a repeated motif, X-lysine-serine-proline-Y-lysine, where X is a single amino acid and Y is one to three amino acids. In humans, there are two common variants of the NEFH tail, one with 45 motif repeats, called the long (L) allele, and another with 44 repeats, termed the short (S) allele [15]. Various deletions of the NEFH tail have been revealed in MND patients. All cases of deletions in the L allele were associated with the disease; however, no association between deletions in the S allele and MND has been reported. Another study of familial and sporadic MND revealed no deletions in the NEFH gene, but described point mutations in patients and control subjects [16]. Experimental studies on transgenic mice with CuZn-superoxide dismutase (SOD-1) mutation suggested a protective role of NEFH and a negative role of NEFL in MND pathogenesis, as the increased survival of mice was associated with increased expression of human NEFH and decreased expression of NEFL [17]. These findings suggest a possible role of the NEFH gene in MND pathogenesis.

Here we present complex molecular genetic and biochemical study of the markers discussed above in Russian sporadic MND patients.

Patients and Methods

With informed consent, blood samples were drawn from 73 patients with idiopathic motor neuron disease. All patients were Russians from Moscow, Tver and St. Petersburg populations. The study was adopted by the Ethics Committee of the Russian State Medical University. The control group for genetic markers comprised 50 randomly sampled healthy individuals from Moscow. The control group for biochemical markers comprised 39 healthy individuals from Moscow. The comparison group for biochemical markers comprised 25 patients with spondylotic myelopathy. All patients, control and comparison subjects had compatible basic demographic values (Table 1).

All MND patients were seen at the Department of Fundamental and Clinical Neurology of the Russian State Medical University. Patients with spondylotic myelopathy were also seen at the Department of Neurology and Neurosurgery of Moscow State Odontological Medical University. Baseline assessment included medical history, physical and neurological examination, electromyography and MRI scans of brain and whole spinal cord. Diagnosis was made according to the Revised El-Escorial Criteria [18] including MRI findings, concentric needle electromyography (EMG) and electroneurography (ENG) of muscles and nerves of the neck and upper and lower extremities.

According to a family history, all patients within age range 28–72 years had sporadic MND. According to the Norris classification [19] and related authors we subdivided our patients into 5 groups. Sixteen patients had progressive bulbar palsy (22%) and 57 (80%) had amyotrophic lateral sclerosis (ALS), among them were 35 patients with cervical onset (47.9%), 5 patients with truncal onset (6.8%) , 13 patients with lumbar onset (17.8%) and 4 patients with diffuse onset (5.5%). No patients had progressive muscular atrophy or primary lateral sclerosis.

Table 1. Demographic values of MND patients, control group and patients with spondylotic myelopathy

Group	All MND patients	Control group (biochemical values)		Comparison group (biochemical values)	
		Blood donors	CSF donors	Blood donors	CSF donors
Total	73 (100%)	22 (100%)	17 (100%)	17 (100%)	8 (100%)
Males	37 (49.3%)	10 (47.8%)	8 (47%)	10 (58,8%)	4 (50%)
Females	36 (50.7%)	12 (52.2%)	9 (53%)	7 (41.2%)	4 (50%)
Average age	55±10.9	56±10.9	54.4±8.7	53±14	53±12

p > 0.1 for all groups.

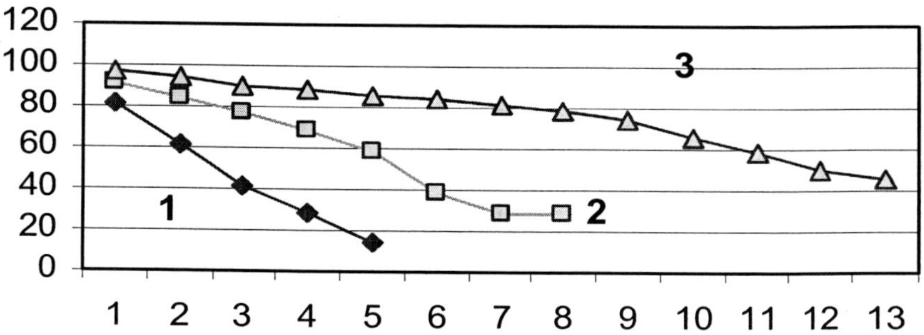

Figure 1. Progression rates according to Norris ALS Score in the united group of MND patients. X axis shows periods of assessment (6 months), Y axis shows degrees by Norris ALS Score. 1 — rapid; 2 — moderate; 3 — slow.

Progression rates were assessed by the Norris ALS Score [20] each 6 months up to the fatal end. We determined rapid, moderate and slow progression rates which significantly differed according to the comparison of two regression lines ($r = -0.96$; $p < 0.001$; $r = -0.97$; $p < 0.001$; $r = -0.98$; $p < 0.001$). There were 40 patients with rapid progression (54.8%), who lost over 10 degrees by Norris ALS Score each 6 months, 21 patients with moderate progression (28.7%), who lost from 5 to 10 degrees, and 12 patients with slow progression

(16.5%), who lost less than 5 degrees each 6 months respectively (Figure 1). Also, the loss of total clinical score was calculated for the first year since onset.

We studied all 5 exons of the SOD-1 gene as described previously [5]. For the study of haplotypes in patients with SOD-1 mutation we used 5 closely linked polymorphic markers (D21S263, D21S223, D21S63, D21S262, D21S261), which locate at 0.1, 0.2, 0.82, 0.82 and 0.47 cM distances from the SOD-1 gene respectively. DNA preparations with known haplotype, kindly given by Professor P.M. Andersen, were used for the haplotype analysis. We also performed the study of alanine-9-valine polymorphism (A9V) in exon 2 of the SOD-2 gene and the S/L-polymorphism of the heavy neurofilament subunit gene (NEFH).

Table 2. Primer sequences and annealing temperatures used for amplification of each polymorphic marker

D21S263	TTGGCTTTGGAACCAG CATCAGCAAGGGTCCTC	64°C 1 min
D21S223	GAAAGAAGCACAGAGGGGT CTCACTCACATTTAACTTGGG	67°C 1 min
D21S63	TCATGACGAGCACAGTAGAGT CAGGATTATTTAGGCTAGAAC	65°C 1 min
D21S262	TCTATGAGACAGGGCCAC ATATTCCGTGTTGATTGTTGTT	65°C 1 min
D21S261	AAAACACCTTACCTAAAACAGCA AGATGATGGTGAGTCCTGAG	69°C 1 min
SOD-2	AGCCCAGCCTGCGTAGAC TACTTCTCCTCGGTGACG	95°C 1 min 62°C 1 min 72°C 1 min
NEFH	GTGGTGGAGAAGTCTGAGAA CTTTGACTTTCACCTCCTGGG	95°C 1 min 61°C 1 min 72°C 1 min 30 s, 72°C 10 min.

DNA was extracted from peripheral leukocytes by standard methods, using proteinase K/phenol–chloroform extraction [21]. Primer sequences and annealing temperatures are cited in Table 2 (Human Genome Database, www.gdb.org, 22, 23]. PCR was performed in 20 μL reaction volumes containing 100–200 ng of the genomic DNA, 50 mM Tris-HCl (pH 8.8), 15 mM $(NH_4)_2SO_4$, 5 mM $MgCl_2$, 0.01% gelatin, 0.01% Tween-20, 0.2 mg/ml BSA, 5% glycerin, 5 pM of the appropriate primers and 200 μM of each dNTP. One of the primers was labeled with $[^{33}P]\gamma ATP$ before being used in the PCR reaction. Labeling reactions were performed in 20 μL buffer, containing 2 μL 10× kinase buffer, 50 pmol of appropriate primer, 50 μCi $[^{33}P]\gamma ATP$, and 2.5 U T4 polynucleotide kinase (Sileks, Russia). After initial denaturation (5 min, 94°C), 2.5 U Taq DNA polymerase (Sileks, Russia) was added, and the samples were PCR amplified (30 cycles of 1 min at 94°C, 1 min at 61°C and 1 min at 72°C). After the last cycle, the reaction mixture was incubated for 10 min at 72°C and chilled to 4°C for 10 hours. The PCR products were then electrophoresed on an 8% non-denaturing polyacrylamide gel containing 0.5× TBE buffer. After electrophoresis, the gel was autoradiographed overnight. In order to check whether the revealed conformities of allelic distribution were connected with the stratification of the compared cohorts or not, the analysis of M235T polymorphism of the angiotensinogen (ANG) gene and of Ins/Del polymorphism of the angiotensin converting enzyme (ACE) gene was performed as described [24, 25].

We also measured superoxide dismutase (SOD-1) activity in erythrocytes, total SOD activity in cerebrospinal fluid (CSF) and thiobarbituric acid reactive substances (TBARS) in blood serum and CSF of MND patients with SOD-1 mutations and 84 neurologically normal controls, matched by age and gender, from whom blood and CSF samples were drawn with informed consent.

Superoxide dismutase activity in erythrocytes was measured on a Perkin-Elmer 555 spectrophotometer (UK) using a model of auto-oxidation of 6-hydroxydopamine by Cohen and Heikkila [26]. Superoxide dismutase was extracted from erythrocytes as follows: 0.2 ml of packed erythrocytes underwent lysis in 0.8 ml cooled distilled water, then 163 μL of lysate was added to 1 ml of cooled distilled water (Methods in Enzymology, 1984). After that samples were immediately chilled at –20°C and stored for not more than a month before detection of enzymatic activity. Prior to detection, erythrocytes was exposed to 0.5 ml of chloroform–ethanol mixture (in 3:5 volume ratio) chilled beforehand at –20°C. After the denaturation procedure sedimentation of coagulated proteins was performed on a centrifuge. Superoxide dismutase activity of extracts was detected on a Perkin-Elmer 555 spectrophotometer (UK) using the model of auto-oxidation of 6-hydroxydopamine by Cohen and Heikkila (1974) as follows. In the control assay 0.1 ml 4 mM solution of 6-hydroxydopamine in 0.1 M HCl were added to 1.9 ml of the reaction mixture (100 mM KCl and 100 mM Hepes-Tris pH 7.3 in 25°C), immediately mixed and the kinetics of colored product accumulation was registered at 485 nm. Addition of extraction product did not influence the slope of the kinetics curve proportional to the velocity of superoxide anion radical generation. When 50 μL of erythrocyte extract was added the curve slope decreased in proportion to SOD-1 content, i.e. 1 unit of SOD-1 activity corresponded to 50% decrease in colored product generation velocity. Activity was expressed in units of activity per g of hemoglobin (U/g Hb).

Total SOD activity in CSF was measured following Beauchamp and Fridovich [27] using a model of kinetics of inhibition of nitrotetrazolium blue reduction by superoxide anion in a xanthine–xanthine oxidase system by spectrophotometry. CSF samples were immediately chilled at –20°C and stored for not more than a month before detection of enzymatic activity. Total SOD activity in CSF was measured following Beauchamp and Fridovich (1971): 2 ml of 0.05 M K-phosphate buffer, 20 μL of Triton X-100 solution, 20 μL of $2.5x10^{-3}$ M nitrotetrazolium blue solution, 20 μL 10^{-2} M xanthine solution and 20 μL of xanthine oxidase (Fluka, Germany) were put into the measuring cuvette. The same ingredients were put into the reference cuvette except for the xanthine oxidase solution. The inhibition kinetics of nitrotetrazolium blue reduction in the xanthine–xanthine oxidase system were measured in 560 nm on an M-400 spectrophotometer (Germany). The unit of SOD activity corresponded to the amount of enzyme required for 50% inhibition of nitrotetrazolium blue reduction under the conditions of detection. Activity was expressed in units of activity per g of hemoglobin (U/g Hb).

Registration of TBARS in blood serum and CSF was performed following Ohkawa et al. [28] in the reaction with 2-thiobarbituric acid on a Hitachi-850 spectrofluorimeter (Japan). TBARS content was expressed in nmol/ml.

Statistical analysis was made with Biostat software (Hungary, 1999). Frequencies of allelic variants were compared using the χ^2 test. The Mann–Whitney U-test was used to compare biochemical values in a pair of groups, and the results were described by medians and intervals between I and IV quartiles. Differences between progression rates were assessed by comparison of two regression lines. A $p < 0.05$ was considered significant.

Results

We found one homozygous missense mutation GAC → GGC in codon 90 of exon 4 of the SOD-1 gene, resulting in aspartic acid to alanine substitution (D90A) in one female patient; the same heterozygous mutation was found in her clinically unaffected daughter. We found heterozygous D90A mutation in another patient and her clinically unaffected father, and heterozygous missense mutation GGC → CGC in codon 12 of exon 1 of the SOD-1 gene, resulting in glycine to arginine substitution (G12R) in one more patient, and the same mutation was found in her clinically unaffected son. Clinical description of these patients is given below.

Homozygous D90A

Patient T., a 68-year-old female, fell ill at the age of 45 in 1978. Before the disease onset, T. had complained of lumbago for two years. Initial symptoms were fatigue, random fasciculations, muscle cramps, weakness and wasting of the left leg muscles and, two years later, right leg muscles, and gait disturbances. The first neurological examination conducted in our clinic in 1981 revealed lower paraparesis with low muscle tone, distal muscle atrophy, spontaneous and induced fasciculations along with brisk tendon reflexes and extensor plantar responses. Cognitive, bulbar, respiratory and cerebellar functions, eye movements, pelvic sphincter and sensory innervation were spared. Physical examination revealed no evidence for a non-neurological etiology to explain the symptoms. Hematological and CSF tests showed no inflammatory process. The stated pathological symptoms correlated with typical ALS findings found by EMG. There was no history of CNS infection, CNS intoxication or trauma.

The patient's parents and grandparents died in their seventies and eighties from old age or unrelated diseases. Three generations of T's relatives lived in the town of Dmitrov near Moscow and her father's relatives have also been Moscovites for three generations.

T's symptoms have been slowly progressing for 8 years and appeared refractory to various therapeutic approaches. In 1989, T became unable to walk and was admitted to our clinic again. Upper paraparesis with fasciculations, distal atrophies, low muscle tone and hyperreflexia added to lower flaccid paraplegia with areflexia and extensor plantar responses, thus presenting a worsening progression. In addition, mild dysphonia, dysphagia and rightward paresis of the soft palate, along with a brisk jaw jerk, were observed. CT scans made in 1995 with no myelographic technique revealed marked spinal cord atrophy, especially in the lumbar region. Since then the disease has been progressing slowly but irretrievably. Spinal automatism reflexes became prominent in the legs. Slight bilateral ataxia in hands began in 1997 and is also slowly progressing. This finding is suggestive for concomitant spinocerebellar tract and posterior column degeneration. The patient has not developed difficulties with micturition.

Needle EMG revealed chronic partial denervation, reduced pattern of recruitment and enlargement of motor unit potentials (MUPs) duration and amplitude up to +9.4% and 1945 μV in neck muscle and up to +14.8% and 3161 μV in left adductor pollicis brevis. No MUPs could be recruited from the lateral gastrocnemius muscles. Stimulation ENG revealed signs of generalized axonopathy of hypoglossal and median nerves. No M-responses could be elicited from nerves of the low extremities. Sensory potentials and conduction velocities were normal. Forced vital capacity was 105% from predicted.

Table 3. Activity of SODs and concentration of TBARS in MND patients with and without SOD-1 mutations and controls

Biochemical values	MND patients with SOD-1 mutations	MND patients, no SOD-1 mutations	The control group
SOD-1 activity in erythrocytes, U/g Hb	^710 (642.5; 746)[1]	^699 (688; 700)	^689 (651.5; 744.5)
Total SOD activity in CSF, U/g protein	^0.845 (0.6; 1. 54)[2]	^1.3 (1.11; 1.65)	^0.78 (0.51; 1.22)
TBARS concentration in serum, nmol/ml	^1.24 (0.8; 2.0)[1]	^ 0.96 (0.9; 1.11)	^0.77 (0.64; 1.13)
TBARS concentration in CSF, nmol/ml	^0.33 (0.28; 1.06)[1]	^0.42 (0.33; 0.71)	^0.307 (0.22; 0.36)

[1]$p > 0.1$ vs patients without mutations and controls; [2]$p = 0.06$ vs patients without mutations and controls; ^ median and the interval between quartiles I and IV.

The loss of Norris ALS Score was 1.02 degrees per six months for the period of 264 months of the disease, indicating slow progression rate. The diagnosis was made: "Motor neuron disease associated with homozygosity for D90A mutation. ALS, lumbar onset, very slow progression with concomitant involvement of spinocerebellar tracts and posterior columns". The patient died in June 2002 of pneumonia after hip fracture with consequent osteosynthesis. Total duration of the disease was 288 months.

Additional biochemical studies of SODs and TBARS are presented in Table 3.

Heterozygous D90A

Patient V., 55-year-old female, fell ill in November, 1997 when weakness and wasting appeared firstly in the right and several months after in the left leg and gait unsteadiness appeared. Once she fell down when skiing. After that random fasciculations throughout all muscles, and a year later wasting and weakness of the right arm appeared. In July, 1998 weakness and wasting began in the left arm, gradually atrophies of spinal and brachial muscles added and fasciculations reduced. In August, 1998 the patient underwent clinical and EMG examination and MND was diagnosed. Lumbar puncture and CT scan of brain were negative. Symptoms gradually progressed. In January, 1999 she was examined inpatient in the neurological department of the Russian State Medical University. Distal flaccid tetraparesis with low muscle tone in distal and spasticity in proximal muscles was revealed in the neurological status. It was up to 3 degrees in proximal and up to 2-3 degrees in distal sections of extremities predominantly leftwards. Marked atrophies, rare fasciculations and cramps were observed. Tendon reflexes were brisk except Achilles reflexes which were absent. There were no cognitive, bulbar, cerebellar, respiratory, sensory and autonomic disorders. Prominent akairia was seen.

The patient's mother was a refugee and V's birth took place in a train without doctor and equipment during a Nazi air raid and their carriage narrowly escaped bombing. In 1967 V had a mechanical injury with a consequent cellulitis of the right calf. Skin autotransplantation was performed. Since June 1998 extensive trophic ulcer developed there. She had varicose vein disease in legs for 10 years. Several months before the disease onset V had painted her country house with fire-safe ochre containing lead and had felt sick as if "being poisoned".

She had no history of chronic progressive movement disorders. Her mother died at the age of 45 of hemorrhagic stroke. Her 96-year-old father is alive; he has no MND, but suffers from spondylosis and neurosensory numbness. She has a healthy brother from her mother's first spouse, and the brother has two children. V's grandparents were able to maintain their daily activities until death and died in their seventies and eighties. Three generations of the patient father's and mother's relatives have lived in the town of Petropavlovsk (Kazakhstan) and in Byelorussia, respectively.

No non-neurological pathology was found to explain the symptoms. Blood, urine and CSF tests were normal. Biochemistry panel revealed twofold increase in creatine kinase (274 units, normal value is below 121 units) and hyperproteinemia up to 96 g/L (normal 60–80 g/L) due to mild hypergammaglobulinemia (10.7%).

Needle EMG revealed chronic partial denervation, reduced pattern of recruitment and enlargement of MUP duration and amplitude up to +19.1% and 1560 μV in neck muscle and up to +29.4% and 4345 μV in left adductor pollicis brevis. In the left lateral gastrocnemius muscle spontaneous activity of muscle fibers prevailed on fasciculations and only 17 MUPs were recruited with duration and amplitude enlargement up to +35% and 1765 μV respectively. Stimulation ENG revealed signs of generalized axonopathy of hypoglossal, median and to greater extent peroneal nerves. Sensory axonopathy with demyelination of sural nerves was revealed and ratios between H-reflexes to M-response amplitudes were mildly enlarged only leftwards.

Brain MRI revealed signs of Vallerian degeneration of corticospinal tracts from the posterior limbs of internal capsules and downwards on T2-weighted and fat and liquid attenuation inversion recovery images along with moderate external hydrocephalus. Cervical MRI revealed spondylosis of C_{4-7} without compression of CSF spaces and intramedullary changes. Spirometry performed in February, 1999 revealed normal FVC (93%). V. rejected the follow-up spirometry.

In March, 2000 in the neurological status V. had akairia and depression. Vision and eye movements were spared. The lower jaw was inclined rightwards and there was obvious paresis in chewing muscles leftwards. She was not able to blow cheeks. Palate and jaw jerks were brisk. Soft palate had normal excursion. V had severe nasophonia and moderate dysphagia. The tongue slightly deviated rightwards and its mobility was reduced, but no obvious fasciculation or atrophy was seen. Bilateral Marinesco signs were elicited. Flaccid paresis of neck extensors up to 2 degrees and flexors up to 3 degrees was observed. She had flaccid distal tetraplegia and spastic proximal tetraparesis up to 3 and 4 degrees, more pronounced leftwards. Marked atrophies of truncal and extremity muscles were seen along with rare induced fasciculations. Tendon reflexes were absent, except decreased knee reflexes. Abdominal and plantar responses were absent. Convincing sensory and cerebellar signs were not detected.

The follow-up assessment by the Norris ALS Score on the 24th, 30th and 36th months from the onset were 71, 54 and 26 degrees respectively. During these intervals V. lost 8.6–11.5 degrees, indicating moderate to rapid progression (5–10 or over 10 degrees per 6 months).

Additional biochemical studies of SODs and TBARS are presented in Table 3.

V. was treated with piriditol, L-carnitine, lecytine, B and E vitamins, Cerebrolysin, fluoxetine and acetylcysteine. She rejected gastrostomy. The diagnosis was made: "Motor neuron disease associated with heterozygosity for D90A mutation. ALS, lumbar onset, rapid progression". V. died in May, 2000.

Heterozygous G12R

Patient C., 71-year-old female, fell ill in March, 1997 at the age of 69, complaining of pain in iliofemoral joints and muscle cramps in calves followed by gait unsteadiness and stiffness and generalized fasciculations. A month later her right heel began to "shuffle", and three months later the same appeared in the left heel. Six months later wasting and clumsiness appeared in her right arm, and after a month in the left one. Symptoms gradually progressed. A year after onset, she started to use a cane while walking. Two years after onset, she stopped going outdoors and could only move around her room. Problems with grooming, writing, eating and hair brushing appeared gradually. In February, 1999 she complained of nasal voice tune, speech problems and choking with liquids. At that time she was admitted to the neurological clinic of the Russian State Medical University.

She had a history of urolithiasis, chronic pyelonephritis and moderate arterial hypertension. In 1993 she had commotion, when she fell down on ice, and in 1994 she was hit in a car accident and received a conservative treatment at the neurosurgical department for frontal bone fracture and cerebral contusion. She had obnubilation, hemispheric meningism, episodes of frustration and mild paresis of her left heel. These symptoms regressed after a fortnight. Since then she complained of diffuse headaches and received acetazolamide.

She had no history of contacts with heavy metals, polio or tick bite. She worked as a weaver.

She had no convincing family history of chronic progressive movement disorders. She had a healthy 39-year-old son and 18-year-old granddaughter. She was born in the town of Noginsk (Moscow district) and had no siblings. Her father died during World War II, and her mother died acutely of a "heart attack" at the age of 57. Her mother's relatives live in Siberia and she was aware neither about their, nor about her grandparents' health status.

She had arterial hypertension and stranguria on physical examination. Blood tests, biochemistry panel and CSF test were normal. There was mild leukocyturia in the urine test. Her cranial X-ray revealed the askew line of the former frontal fracture. Chest X-ray was normal, and lumbar spondylogram revealed spondylosis of L5-S1. Spirometry revealed forced vital capacity decrease to 88% of predicted. Needle EMG findings corresponded to chronic partial denervation due to motoneuron loss. The most prominent increase in duration and amplitude of motor unit potentials (MUPs) was detected in her right calf (up to +18.4% and 4600 μV, normal values are ±13% and 300–1000 μV, respectively). Stimulation ENG revealed generalized motor axonopathy of hypoglossal, median and peroneal nerves, being the most prominent in the latter with motor conduction velocity decreased to 25–30%. Sensory potentials and conduction velocities were normal. Increased ratio of H-reflex to M-response amplitude was found in her left gastrocnemius muscle indicating pyramid deficiency. Brain MRI with 0.15 T field strength revealed multiple vascular lesions hyperintensive on T2-weighted images and mildly hypointensive on T1 weighted images, leukoareosis of periventricular spaces and moderate external hydrocephalus prevailing in frontal and temporal regions. Cervical spine MRI revealed backward protrusions of C_{4-5}, C_{5-6} and C_{6-7} without dural compression, CSF space deformities and intramedullary changes.

There were no general cerebral and meningeal signs or cognitive, eye movement and sensory disorders. Masticatory and mimic muscles were spared. Jaw jerk and palate reflexes were brisk, soft palate movements were intact. There were fasciculations and decreased mobility of the tongue, mild spastic dysarthria, nasal voice and mild dysphagia for liquids. She had spastic tetraparesis up to 3-4 degrees by the Medical Research Council Scale in upper extremities and up to 2-3 degrees in lower extremities. Paresis of heels was flaccid and prevailed in the peroneal group and rightwards. There were moderate atrophies of muscles on extremities and signs of right shoulder joint arthrosis. Diameters of right extremities were lower than of left. There were generalized induced fasciculations and cramps. Tendon reflexes were symmetrically brisk except Achilles reflexes, which were absent. Babinsky sign was elicited leftwards, abdominal reflexes were absent.

Biochemical studies of SODs and TBARS are presented in Table 3.

The neurological diagnosis was as follows: "Motor neuron disease. Amyotrophic lateral sclerosis, lumbar onset with predominant UMN involvement. Chronic ischemic brain disease and post-traumatic encephalopathy. Respiratory deficiency, 1st stage. Diffuse spondylosis". Rilutek was inaccessible. She received L-carnitine, B vitamins, tizanidine, Cerebrolysin, fluoxetine, dipyridamole and treatment of shoulder joint arthrosis. Speech and dietary therapy was prescribed. She rejected gastrostomy.

After discharge she was observed as outpatient. Her Norris ALS Scores on the 23th, 29th and 34th months after onset were 63, 36 and 18 degrees respectively. During these intervals she lost 9.6–14.4 degrees, indicating rapid progression (over 10 degrees per 6 months). Half a year after discharge the patient stopped moving and eating independently. Marked spastic tetraparesis with hyperreflexia up to 1–2 degrees in legs and 2–3 degrees in hands was observed without prominent increase in amyotrophic syndrome. Severe dysarthria and dysphagia developed with rightward paresis of soft palate, sialorrhea and dyspnoea at rest. She died in March, 2000. Total duration of the disease was 35 months.

Table 4. Results of haplotyping of D90A mutation carriers

Marker	Haplotypes					
	D90A homozygous patient		D90A heterozygous patient		D90A heterozygous patient's father	
D21S263	**1**	**1**	**1**	2	**1**	5
D21S223	**3**	**3**	**3**	2	**3**	3
D21S63	**10**	**10**	**10**	10	**10**	13
D21S262	**4**	**4**	**4**	5	**4**	6
D21S261	**2**	**2**	**2**	2	**2**	2

Interestingly, we revealed, that both homo- and heterozygous D90A as well as V's father had identical Scandinavian haplotype (Table 4). Biochemical tests on SODs activity and TBARS level showed that there were no significant differences between these parameters in patients and control values (Table 3).

Analysis of alanine-9-valine (A9V) polymorphic variants of SOD-2 gene distribution performed in 62 patients revealed AA, AV and VV genotypes in 21%, 50% and 29% of patients respectively. In control group individuals with AA, AV and VV genotypes comprised 18%, 54% and 28% respectively. There were no significant differences between frequencies of these genotypes in MND patients and controls. The frequencies of A and V alleles in patients and controls also did not differ (Table 5).

There were no differences in frequencies of forms, sites and ages of onset, and progression rates of MND in patients with different A9V-polymorphic variants.

Results of the study of S/L-polymorphism of the heavy neurofilament subunit gene (NEFH) are presented in Table 6. We found L and S alleles both in the control group and in sporadic MND patients. It is necessary to note that we only identified L and S alleles, and did not reveal any deletions in the L and S alleles.

Table 5. Analysis of Ala9Val polymorphism of SOD-2 gene in MND patients and the control group from Moscow

	MND patients		Controls		χ^2	P
	N	Frequency, %	N	Frequency, %		
Ala	57	46	45	45	0.022	NS
Val	67	54	55	55		
Ala/Ala	13	21	9	18	0.16	NS
Ala/Val	31	50	27	54	0.18	NS
Val/Val	18	29	14	28	0.013	NS

Table 6. Distributions of NEFH genotypes and alleles variants in MND patients and the control group from Moscow

	MND patients		Controls		χ^2	P
	N	Frequency,%	N	Frequency,%		
L	61	49.2	63	63	**4.27**	**P<0.05**
S	63	50.8	37	37		
LL	20	32.2	16	31.1	0.015	NS
SL	21	33.9	31	62.2	8.91	**P<0.01**
SS	21	33.9	3	6.7	11.93	**P<0.001**

As shown in the first two lines of Table 6, the L alleles had a higher (63%) and S alleles had a lower (37%) frequency in the control group. In patients, the frequency of the L alleles was 49.2% and that of the S alleles was 50.8%. The comparative allele distributions carried out with the standard χ^2-test revealed statistically significant divergences between the patients and controls ($\chi^2 = 4.27$).

The last three lines of Table 6 demonstrate the genotype distribution for patients and controls. We identified 20 patients with the LL genotype, 21 with the LS genotype and 21 with the SS genotype. In the control group, there were 16 LL, 31 LS and 3 SS genotypes. The genotype distributions in both groups did not deviate from the Hardy–Weinberg equilibrium. The SS genotype frequency was significantly higher in patients (33.9%) compared with the control group (6.7%). Statistical estimation by the standard χ^2 test of the difference in the SS genotype frequency between these groups gave the most significant results ($\chi^2 = 11.93$ and $p < 0.001$).

On the other hand, the distribution of the alleles of the A9V polymorphism in SOD-2 gene (Table 5), of the M235T polymorphism in angiotensinogen gene and of I\D polymorphism of angiotensin converting enzyme gene did not differ from the control group.

Table 7. Antioxidant enzymes and oxidative markers in MND patients and controls and comparison groups

Studied groups		SOD-1 activity in erythrocytes (U/g HB)	Total SOD activity in CSF (U/g HB)	TBARS in CSF (nmol/ml)	TBARS in blood serum (nmol/ml)
Control group		^689 (651.5; 744.5)	^0.780 (0.510; 1.220)	^0.307 (0.217; 0.36)	^0.77 (0.64; 1.13)
Spondylotic myelopathy		^705 (642; 737)	^0.595[1] (0.512; 1.097)	^0.638[1] (0.425; 1.23)	^1.02[1] (0.76; 1.61)
MND group		^707[1] (666.5; 724)	^0.875[1] (0.557; 1.772)	^0.329[2](0.282; 1.064)	^1.2[2] (0.77; 1.99)
Site of onset	Cervical onset ALS	^ 703[1] (665.5; 733.5)	^0.845[1] (0.597;1.54)	^0.426[1,4] (0.342; 1.11)	^1.08[1] (0.71; 1.68)
	Lumbar onset ALS	^705[1] (691; 743.5)	2.0[2] (1.46; 2.33)	^ 0. 876[1] (0.557; 0.938)	^1.26[1] (1.04; 2.0)
	Truncal onset ALS	^ 691[1] (658,5; 717.5)	^0.375[1] (0.322; 0.427)	^0.549[1](0.35; 0.7)	^1.67[1] (1.14; 1.73)
	Diffuse onset ALS	^690[1] (660; 710)	^0.965[1] (0.932; 0.997)	^0.461[1] (0.348; 0.579)	^1.34[1] (1.3; 1.42)
	PBP	^707[1] (641; 727.5)	^0.785[1] (0.513; 1.5)	^0.275[1] (0.256; 0.302)	^0.96[1] (0.8; 1.45)
Progression rate	Rapid	^713[1] (666; 747.5)	^0.89[1] (0. 565; 1.78)	^0.326[1] (0.281; 0.506)	^1.24[2] (0.79; 1.59)
	Moderate	^701[1] (648.5; 722.5)	^0.78[1] (0.565; 1.06)	^0.315[1] (0.276; 1.06)	^1.16[2] (0.9; 1.96)
	Slow	^ 701[1] (689; 782)	^2.0[2,3] (2.0; 2.11)	^0.815[5] (0.526; 1.25)	^1.08[1] (0.9; 1.19)
Age of onset	<40 years	^711[1] (721; 682)	^0.38[1] (0.25; 0.9)	^0. 281[1](0.246; 0.6)	^1.06[1] (0.96; 1.11)
	40—60 years	^711[1] (746.5; 653.5)	^0.92[1] (0.58; 1.79)	^0.393[2] (0.315; 1.045)	^1.08[1] (0.71; 1.92)
	>60 years	^677.5[1] (626.5; 713.25)	^0.86[1] (0.635; 1.43)	0.315(0.275; 1.057)	^1.27[2] (0.96; 1.65)

p > 0.1 vs controls and the comparison groups; [2] p < 0.05 vs controls; [3] p < 0.05 vs rapid and moderate progression rates; [4]p < 0.01 vs controls and patients with PBP; [5] p < 0.1 vs controls; ^ - the median and the interval between quartiles I and IV.

Figure 2 illustrates how the loss of total clinical score was distributed between patients with LL, LS and SS genotypes. A statistically significant correlation was established between the loss of total clinical score and the NEFH genotypes (Spearmen correlation, $R = 0.335$, $p < 0.03$). The lowest values of loss of total clinical score were observed in patients with the LL genotype (mean ± SD, 18.8 ± 12.4), and the highest values of total clinical score were observed in patients with the SS genotype (mean ± SD, 31.1 ± 16.3). The dissimilarity in mean values of loss of total clinical score in the patients with LL and SS genotypes was statistically significant (Newman–Keuls test $q = 3.671$, $p < 0.05$).

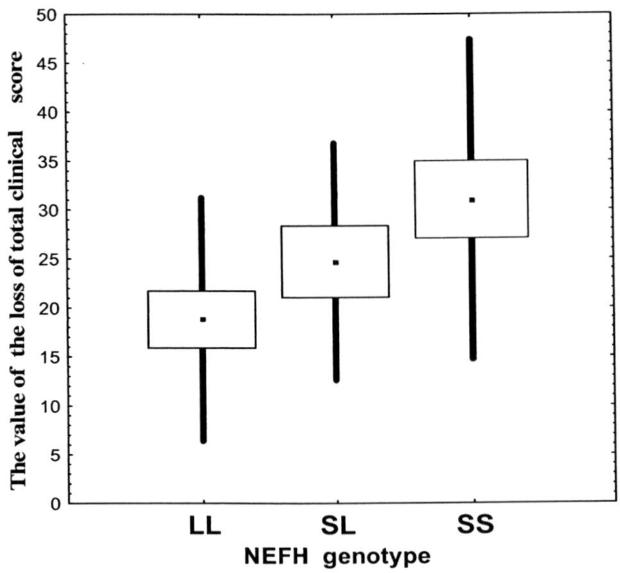

Figure 2. The first year loss of total clinical score (mean ± SD) according to the Norris Scale in MND patients with LL, LS and SS genotypes.

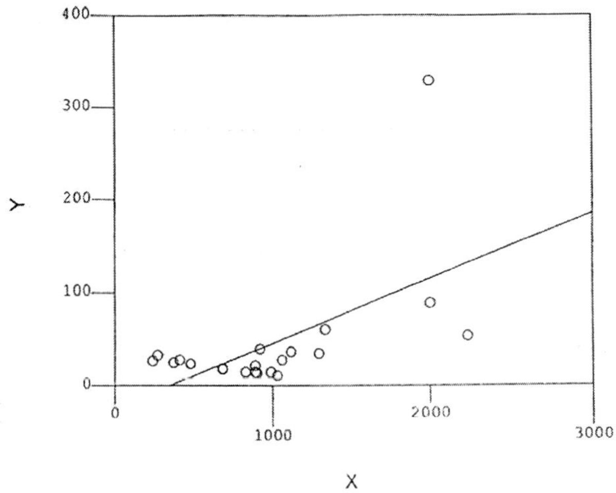

Figure 3. Positive correlation of total SOD activity in CSF and the duration of motor neuron disease. X-axis shows total SOD activity in CSF (U/g HB x 10^3), Y-axis shows duration of MND in months; $r= 0.57$; $p<0.01$.

Activity of SOD-1 in erythrocytes and total SOD activity in CSF in MND patients did not differ from those in the control group as well as from patients with spondylotic myelopathy ($p < 0.1$). SOD-1 activity in erythrocytes did not differ in patients with different rates of progression or sites or ages of MND onset (Table 7). However, total SOD activity in CSF in MND patients with slow progression was significantly higher than in controls as well as in patients with rapid and moderate progression rates ($p < 0.05$) (Table 7). The revealed conformity was confirmed by correlation analysis that showed significant positive correlation between total SOD activity in CSF and the duration of the disease ($r = 0.57$; $p < 0.01$) (Figure

3). Total SOD activity was also higher in patients with lumbar ALS than in controls, but no differences were revealed in relation to age of onset (Table 7).

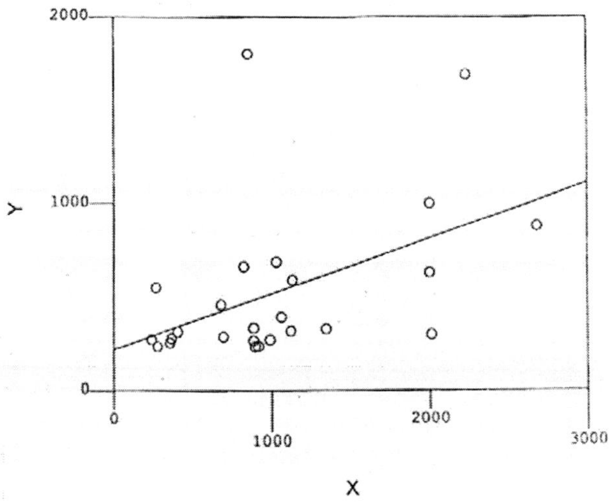

Figure 4. Positive correlation between total SOD activity and the level of TBARS in CSF. X-axis shows the level of TBARS in CSF (nmol/ml x 10^3), У-axis shows total SOD activity in CSF (U/g HB x 10^3); r=0.46; p<0.02.

Levels of TBARS in CSF and in blood serum of MND patients were significantly higher than in the control group ($p < 0.05$) and did not differ from those in patients with spondylotic myelopathy ($p > 0.1$) (Table 6). We found significant positive correlation between the level of TBARS in CSF and total duration of the disease ($r = 0.57$; $p < 0.02$), as well as total SOD activity in CSF ($r = 0.46$; $p < 0.02$) (Figure 4). We failed to find the same correlation for TBARS level in blood serum. The level of TBARS in CSF did not differ in patients with different progression rates, showing only a tendency to increase in patients with slow progression ($p < 0.1$). However, it prevailed in blood serum of patients with rapid and moderate progression rates over control values ($p < 0.05$) (Table 7). The level of TBARS in CSF prevailed in patients with cervical onset over those with PBP and controls ($p < 0.01$), and also in patients who became ill between 40 and 60 years of age vs controls ($p < 0.05$), while the level of TBARS in blood serum significantly predominated in patients who became ill after 60 years of age ($p < 0.05$) (Table 7).

We compared **level of TBARS in CSF and activity of SOD-1 in erythrocytes of MND patients with different variants of S/L-polymorphism of the NEFH gene.** Interestingly, the level of TBARS was higher in patients with SS genotype (^0.426 (0.347; 1.06)) vs control group (^0.307 (0.217; 0.36); $p < 0.02$) (Figure 5). The activity of SOD-1 in erythrocytes of MND patients with each of the NEFH S/L-polymorphic variants did not differ from that in control group; however, LL carrier SOD-1 activity (^677 (626; 704 U/gHb)) was lower than those of SL carriers (^726 (679; 745); $p < 0.05$) and, at a tendency level, of SS carriers (^735 (681.5; 758.5); $p < 0.1$).

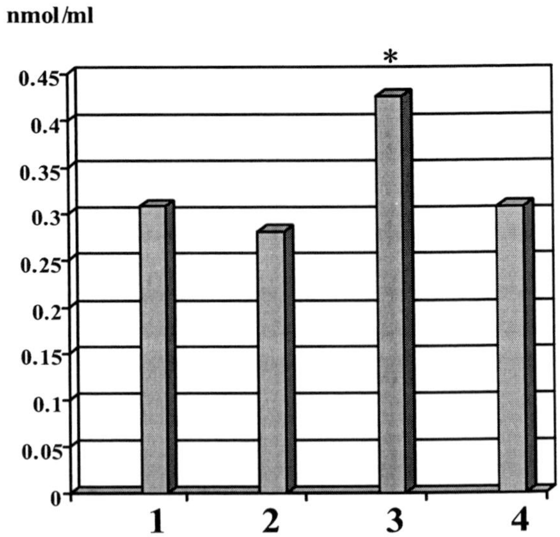

Figure 5. TBARS level in CSF in MND patients with different genotypes of S/L-polymorphism. 1 - MND patients with LL genotype; 2 - MND patients with SL genotype; 3 - MND patients with SS genotype; 4 - the control group. * $p<0.02$ vs the control group.

Discussion

The described homozygous D90A patient with very slowly progressive disease inherited ALS as a recessive trait. Patient V. was previously considered as a case of autosomal dominant D90A associated ALS with typical rapid progression in a low penetrance family taking her father's age into consideration. At first sight, there is a considerable interaction of endogenous and exogenous provocative factors in this patient. However, it is doubtful that such factors as connatal stress, old mechanical injury and short-term contact with lead do play any role here. The association of MND with lead exposure was noted by several authors only when the exposure was professional and lasted many years [29].

The presence of Scandinavian haplotype in our D90A heterozygous ALS patient allows us to reconsider the concept of inheritance pattern, as she occurs not to have dominant, but recessive D90A. However, P.M. Andersen [1] and A. Al-Chalabi et al. [5] analyzed many cases and have never seen any heterozygous relative of an ALS patient homozygous for D90A and Scandinavian haplotype who developed MND. The mechanism of "protection" against ALS in D90A homozygous patients still has to be elucidated. V's 96-year-old father is a heterozygous D90A carrier who has no MND probably due to Scandinavian haplotype and the genetically linked "protective" factor, which his daughter inherited from him. However, this factor obviously did not embody its properties in her. That does not deny the existence of the "protective" factor; however, to explain this strange and still only case worldwide is possible if it is suggested that V. had another independent ALS-causative factor, probably inherited from her mother, which was probably "stronger" than the putative "protective" factor.

Thus, we can suggest that individuals with heterozygous recessive D90A mutation are not guaranteed sparing from MND in that rare case when they carry another independent and stronger ALS-causative factor, which should be searched for in the relatives by maternal line in V's family.

MND associated with G12R SOD-1 mutation was first described in 2 Italian patients by S. Penco et al. in 1999 [30], and after that 3 additional cases appeared (SOD-1 Gene Mutation Database, www.alsod.org). All patients had slow progression, relatively early average age of onset (48.7 years) and average duration about 88 months. All patients had predominant UMN involvement with only flaccid paresis in heels within the site of onset. Patient C. differs from these cases in elder age of onset and rapid progression. SOD-1 activity in erythrocytes of the Italian patients was decreased to 20%, which is in agreement with our results and confirms the leading role of cytotoxic SOD-1 mutant properties rather than antioxidant failure in MND development. Such dissociation is characteristic for G93R, L38V, N96S, D76Y and I113T mutations. The first two of these are the most functionally significant, but disease duration may fluctuate from 2 to 15 years; as variable is also the age of onset [1]. Slight predominance of total SOD activity in CSF in patients with mutations vs those without them may reflect preservation of compensatory activation of extracellular SOD even in case of mild antioxidant deficit of SOD-1.

Monoclonal gammapathy is known to occur in 5–10% of MND cases [31]. We failed to find any data about its distribution among MND patients with SOD-1 mutations. In our opinion, its presence in an MND patient with known genetic causative defect as in V. speaks for its secondary character and argues against "autoimmune theory" of ALS. Monoclonal gammapathy may be a secondary autoimmune reaction to mutant SOD-1 protein or to toxic products from the extensive trophic ulcer.

The results of molecular genetic study suggest that A9V polymorphic variants of the SOD-2 gene are not associated wit MND development in the examined Russian population. These findings do correspond either to results of Tomblyn et al. that suggested association of the disease with VV genotype, nor with results of Van Landeghem et al. that suggested association of AA genotype with progressive bulbar palsy [12, 13]. This possibly reflects different significance of these polymorphism as a factor that plays a role in MND pathogenesis in various populations.

The potential importance of neurofilaments is underscored by the observation that abnormal accumulation of NF occurs in familial MND patients with various mutations in SOD-1 [32, 33]. Evidence of a primary role for abnormal NF in motor neurodegeneration also comes from animal models. Transgenic mice with point mutations of the light NF rod, overexpression of human heavy NF or overexpression of mouse light NF all develop motor neuron pathology. Moreover, transgenic mice carrying SOD-1 mutants develop NF accumulation [34, 35].

In this study, we investigated whether the L and S genotypes of the NEFH gene are associated with MND. We found a difference in SS genotype frequency between the control population and patients with sporadic MND. The SS genotype was significantly higher in these patients. These data suggest that the S genotype of the NEFH gene is involved in the pathogenesis of sporadic MND in the patients from Moscow. The observed divergences are not connected with the stratification of the compared cohorts, as we failed to reveal any differences in the spectra of the allelic variants of SOD-2 gene (which is probably involved in MND pathogenesis), ANG gene and ACE gene (genes of two proteins of the rennin–angiotensin system, that has not been reported to be involved in MND pathogenesis). In general, the distribution of S/L polymorphism of the NEFH gene in the random cohort from Moscow population and in the random cohort from Canadian population demonstrated quite a resemblance — thus the SS homozygotes in the Canadian population comprise 9% in frequency [36]. Moreover, patients with the SS genotypes had the highest values of loss of total clinical score. The findings about higher frequency of SS genotype and the highest loss of total clinical score in SS genotype carriers with MND in Moscow MND cohort have been reported in our previous publication [37].

However, Al-Chalabi et al. analyzed the L/S genotypes of the NEFH gene in ALS patients from Scandinavia and United Kingdom and found no association [16]. Thus, influence of the polymorphism on risk of MND development might be specific to ethnicity.

To summarize, we conclude that the NEFH gene is involved in the pathogenesis of sporadic MND and that the SS genotype could be a risk factor for the development and progression of sporadic MND in the Moscow population. Such an influence of heavy neurofilament subunit variants with different number of X-lysine-serine-proline-Y-lysine repeats may occur due to peculiarities of phosphorylation of the L and the S isoforms of neurofilaments. That may in turn lead to disruption of neurofilament transport due to increased pausing in neurofilament movement, which may contribute to motoneuron death [17].

The study confirmed that oxidative stress is present in sporadic MND patients. We found that it increases with the course of the disease coherently with elevation of total SOD activity in CSF. That may reflect compensatory mobilization of native antioxidant mechanisms. Along with that, there was no difference between the level of oxidative markers in MND and spondylotic myelopathy patients. This shows the nonspecific character of oxidative stress in the pathogenesis of sporadic MND. SOD-1 activity in erythrocytes and total SOD activity in CSF were compatible to those in the control group and patients with spondylotic myelopathy, which in consistent with the opinion of most authors [8, 38, 39] and argues specific deficiency of these antioxidant enzymes in sporadic MND, suggested by several others [7, 40]. The level of TBARS in CSF positively correlated with MND duration and did not differ in patients with different progression rates. Moreover, the lowest level was detected in PBP patients and no significant increase was registered in the oldest age group or patients with diffuse onset. However, it is known that MND progresses more rapidly in PBP, ALS with diffuse onset and in elderly [10]. These findings suggest that oxidative stress does not influence the disease prognosis. The level of TBARS in blood serum of MND patients was increased, but did not correlate with the duration of the disease. The same was shown by Bonnefont-Rousselot et al. [8], suggesting that oxidative markers in serum have no specific connection with the disease and may reflect disturbances in oxidation/reduction processes due to secondary MND complications such as muscle atrophy, immobilization, dysphagia, respiratory deficiency, or independent factors, such as old age and somatic pathology. The level of TBARS in our study was significantly increased in patients of the oldest age group and in those having rapid and moderate rates of progression, which may confirm the above opinion.

Along with negative results of therapeutic trials [11] and evidence of normal natural antioxidant status in MND [8], our findings argue the expediency of administering antioxidants in MND in order to alter the course of the disease. However, as far as the genetic basis of MND is not yet fully understood, it is possible that in some individuals with MND oxidative stress plays a more important pathogenic role than in others, and according to the above results, patients with the homozygosity for S allele of NEFH gene may be such a group. In the report by J. Crow et al. [41] that normal SOD-1 may produce nitration of light neurofilaments by peroxynitrite, so we can suggest that the same process may happen with "shorter" heavy neurofilaments, which leads to oxidative stress in homozygous carriers of SS genotype. It is unclear whether identical alterations in SOD-1 activity happen in motoneurons and erythrocytes in MND patients with different NEFH genotypes, but if they do the tendency towards the increase in SOD-1 activity in SS genotype carriers may reflect the inability of SOD-1 to compensate for oxidative stress, as it gains pro-oxidative function due to abnormal interaction with "shorter" heavy neurofilaments. Probably this genetically distinct group of MND patients can benefit from the differential administration of antioxidants.

Acknowledgements

This study was supported in part by a grant from the Russian Foundation for Basic Research (# 02-04-48999), the Russian Academy of Sciences programs "Physical and chemical biology", "From Basic Research to Medicine", and the Russian State programs "Genotherapy and genodiagnostics" and "Leading Scientific School".

References

[1] Andersen PM. Genetics of amyotrophic lateral sclerosis. *Zh Nevrol Psikhiatr im SS Korsakova*, 2001; 101 (3): 54-63 (in Russian).

[2] Miller RG, Bradley WG, Gelinas DF et al. Amyotrophic lateral sclerosis. Continuum, Lifelong Learning in Neurology, Aug 2002; 8 (4), pp. 227.

[3] Andersen PM, Sims KB, Xin WW et al. Sixteen novel mutations in Cu/Zn-superoxide dismutase gene in amyotrophic lateral sclerosis: a decade of discoveries, defects and disputes. *ALS and other motor neuron disorders*, 2003; 4: 62-73.

[4] Davidenkov SN. Genetics of amyotrophic lateral sclerosis. *Soviet neurology, psychiatry and psychohygiene*, 1933; 2 (8-9): 44-51.

[5] Al-Chalabi A, Andersen PM, Chioza B et al. Recessive amyotrophic lateral sclerosis with the D90A SOD1 mutation shares a common founder: evidence for a linked protective factor. *Hum Mol Genet* 1998; 13: 2045-2050.

[6] Skvortsova VI, Limborska SA, Slominsky PA, Levitskaya NI, Levitsky GN, Shadrina MI, Kondratyeva EA. Sporadic amyotrophic lateral sclerosis associated with the D90A CuZn-superoxide dismutase mutations in Russia. *Eur J Neurol*, 2001, vol. 8, pp. 167-172.

[7] Zakharova MN, Zavalishin IA, Boldyrev AA, Pavlova OA. The role of SOD in the pathogenesis of amyotrophic lateral sclerosis. *Bull Exp Biol Med* 1999; 127 (4): 460-462 (in Russian).

[8] Bonnefont-Rousselot D, Lacomblez L, Jaudon M et al. Blood oxidative stress in amyotrophic lateral sclerosis. *J Neurol Sci* 2000;178(1):57-62.

[9] Jansen GA, Wanders RJ, Jobsis GJ et al. Evidence against increased oxidative stress in fibroblasts from patients with non-superoxide-dismutase-1 mutant familial amyotrophic lateral sclerosis. *J Neurol Sci* 1996 Aug;139 Suppl:91-4.

[10] Andersen PM. Amyotrophic lateral sclerosis and superoxide dismutase. Doctoral dissertation. Umea: Umea University, 1997.

[11] Pioro E. Antioxidant therapy in ALS. Amyotrophic lateral sclerosis and other motor neuron disorders 2000 (Suppl 4), 5-15.

[12] Van Landeghem GF, Tabatabaie, Beckman L, Beckman G, Andersen PM. Mn-SOD Signal Sequence Polymorphism Associated with Sporadic Motor Neuron Disease. *Eur J Neurol* 1999; 6: 639-644.

[13] Tomblyn M, Kasarskis EJ, Xu Y, St Clair DK. Distribution of MnSOD polymorphisms in sporadic ALS patients. *J Mol Neurosci* 1998; 1: 65-66.

[14] Hirano A. Cytopathology of amyotrophic lateral sclerosis. *Adv Neurol.* 1991; 56: 91-101.

[15] Figlewicz DA, Rouleau GA, Krizus A, Julien JP. Polymorphism in the multi-phosphorylation domain of the human neurofilament heavy-subunit-encoding gene. *Gene* 1993; 132: 297-300.

[16] Al-Chalabi A, Andersen PM, Nilsson P et al. Deletions of the heavy neurofilament subunit tail in amyotrophic lateral sclerosis. *Hum Mol Genet* 1999; 8: 157-164.

[17] Al-Chalabi Am, Miller CCJ. Neurofilaments and neurological disease. *Bioessays* 2003; 24: 346-355.

[18] Brooks BR, Miller RG, Swash M, Munsat TL and Airlie House "Current Issues in ALS Therapeutic Trials" Workshop Contributors (1998). El Escorial Revised: Revised Criteria for the Diagnosis of Amyotrophic Lateral Sclerosis. http://www.wfnals.org/Articles/elescorial1998.html (The WFN/ALS Website).

[19] Norris FH. Onset, natural history and prognosis of adult motor neuron disease. *J Neurol Sci* 1993, 118: 48-55.

[20] Norris FH, Callachini PR, Fallat RJ et al. Administration of guanidine in amyotrophic lateral sclerosis. *Neurology* 1974; 24:721-728.

[21] Miller SA, Dykes DD, Polesky HF. A sample salting out procedure for extracting DNA from human nucleated cells. *Nucleic Acid Res* 1988; 16: 1215.

[22] Figlewicz DA, Krizus A, Martinoli MG et al. Variants of the heavy neurofilament subunit are association with the development of amyotrophic lateral sclerosis. *Hum Mol Genet* 1994; 3: 1757-1761.

[23] Grasbon-Frodl EM, Kosel S, Reiss O et al. Analysis of mitochondrial targeting sequence and coding region polymorphisms of the manganese superoxide dismutase gene in German Parkinson disease patients. *Biochem Biophys Res Commun* 1999; 255: 749-752.

[24] Hingorany AD, Sharma P, Jia H et al. Blood pressure and the M235T polymorphism of the angiotensinogen gene. *Hypertension* 1996;28: 907-911.

[25] Rigat B, Hubert C, Corvol P et al. FPCR detection of the insertion/deletion polymorphism of the human angiotensin converting enzyme gene (DCP1)(dipeptidyl carboxypeptidase 1). *Nucl Acids Res* 1992; 20: 1433.

[26] Cohen G., Heikkila R. E. The generation of hydrogen peroxide, superoxide radical and hydroxyradical by 6-hydroxydopamine. *J. Biol. Chem.* 1974, 249(8), 2447-2453.

[27] Beauchamp C, Fridovich I. Superoxide dismutase: improved assays and an assay applicable in acrylamide gels. *Anal Biochem* 1971; 44: 276-287.

[28] Ohkawa H., Ohishi N., Yagi K. Assay for lipid peroxides in animal tissues by thiobarbituric acid reaction. *Anal. Biochem.*, 1979, 95 (10), 351-358.

[29] Armon C, Kurland LT, Daube J et al. Epidemiological correlates of sporadic amyotrophic lateral sclerosis. *Neurology*, 1991; 41: 1077-1084.

[30] Penco S, Schenone A, Bordo D et al. A SOD1 gene mutation in a patient with slowly progressing familial ALS. Neurology 1999 Jul 22; 53(2): 404-6.

[31] Shy ME, Rowland LP, Smith T et al. Motor neuron disease and plasma cell dyscrasia. *Neurology* 1986; 36: 1429-1436.

[32] Hirano A, Donnefeld H, Sasaki S, Nakano I. Fine structural observation of neurofilamentous changes in amyotrophic lateral sclerosis. *J Neuropathol Exp Neurol* 1984; 43: 471-480.

[33] Shaw CE, Enayat ZE, Powell JF, et al. Familial amyotrophic lateral sclerosis. Molecular pathology of patient with a SOD1 mutation. *Neurology* 1997; 49: 1612-1616.

[34] Julien JP, Cote F, Collard JF. Mice overexpressing the human neurofilament heavy gene as model of ALS. *Neurobiol Aging* 1995; 16: 487-490.

[35] Xu Z, Cork LS, Griffing FW, Cleveland DW. Increased expression of neurofilament subunit NF-L produces morphological alterations that resemble the pathology of human motor neuron disease. *Cell* 1993; 73: 23-33.

[36] Figlewicz DA, Rouleau GA, Krizus A, Julien J-P. Polymorphism in the multiphosphorylation of the human neurofilament heavy-subunit-encoding gene. *Gene* 1993; 132:297-300.

[37] Skvortsova VI, Shadrina MI, Slominsky PA, Levitsky GN, Kondratieva EA, Zherebtsova AL, Levitskaya NI, Alekhin AV, Serdyuk AV, Limborska SA. Analysis of heavy neurofilament subunit gene polymorphism in Russian patients with sporadic motor neuron disease (MND). *European Journal of Human Genetics advance online publication* 14 January 2004; doi:10.1038/sj.ejhg.5201144.

[38] Fujita K, Yamauchi M, Shibayama K et al. Decreased cytochrome c oxidase activity but unchanged superoxide dismutase and glutathione peroxidase activities in the spinal cords of patients with amyotrophic lateral sclerosis. *J Neurosci Res.* 1996; 1; 45(3): 276-81.

[39] Oteiza PI, Uchitel OD, Carrasquedo F et al. Evaluation of antioxidants, protein, and lipid oxidation products in blood from sporadic amyotrophic lateral sclerosis patients. *Neurochem Res* 1997 Apr; 22(4):535-9.

[40] Iwasaki Y, Ikeda K, Kinoshita M. Decreased cerebrospinal fluid superoxide dismutase in amyotrophic lateral sclerosis. *Lancet* 1993; 342: 1118.

[41] Crow JP, Ye YZ, Strong M, Kirk M, Barnes S, Beckman JS Superoxide dismutase catalyzes nitration of tyrosines by peroxynitrite in the rod and head domains of neurofilament-L. *J Neurochem.* 1997a; 69(5): 1945-53.

Index

A

B

C

D

E

F

G

H

I

J

K

L

M

N

Q

R